Persisting Speech Difficulties in Children

Children's Speech and Literacy Difficulties: Book 3

Persisting Speech Difficulties in Children

Children's Speech and Literacy Difficulties: Book 3

Michelle Pascoe, PhD
Joy Stackhouse, PhD
and
Bill Wells, DPhil

Department of Human Communication Sciences
University of Sheffield

Consulting Editor: Professor Margaret Snowling
University of York

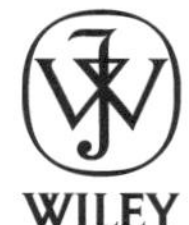

Whurr Publishers Limited (a subsidiary of John Wiley & Sons Ltd)
The Atrium, Southern Gate, Chichester,
West Sussex PO19 8SQ, England
Telephone (+44) 1243 779777

Email (for orders and customer service enquiries): cs-books@wiley.co.uk
Visit our Home Page on www.wiley.com

Other Wiley Editorial Offices

John Wiley & Sons Inc., 111 River Street, Hoboken, NJ 07030, USA

Jossey-Bass, 989 Market Street, San Francisco, CA 94103-1741, USA

Wiley-VCH Verlag GmbH, Boschstr. 12, D-69469 Weinheim, Germany

John Wiley & Sons Australia Ltd, 42 McDougall Street, Milton, Queensland 4064, Australia

John Wiley & Sons (Asia) Pte Ltd, 2 Clementi Loop #02-01, Jin Xing Distripark, Singapore 129809

John Wiley & Sons Canada Ltd, 22 Worcester Road, Etobicoke, Ontario, Canada M9W 1L1

Wiley also publishes its books in a variety of electronic formats. Some content that appears in print may not be available in electronic books.

Library of Congress Cataloging-in-Publication Data
Pascoe, Michelle.
Persisting speech difficulties in children : children's speech and literacy difficulties 3 / Michelle Pascoe, Joy Stackhouse, and Bill Wells.
p. cm.
Includes bibliographical references and index.
ISBN 0-470-02744-4 (pbk.)
1. Language disorders in children. 2. Speech disorders in children. I. Stackhouse, Joy. II. Wells, Bill, D.Phil. III. Title.

RJ496.L35P37 2006
618.92'855 - dc22

2006007374

A catalogue record for this book is available from the British Library

ISBN-13 978-0-470-02744-8
ISBN-10 0-470-02744-4

Typeset in 10.5/12.5 Garamond by SNP Best-set Typesetter Ltd., Hong Kong
Printed and bound in Great Britain by TJ International Ltd, Padstow, Cornwall

This book is printed on acid-free paper responsibly manufactured from sustainable forestry in which at least two trees are planted for each one used for paper production.

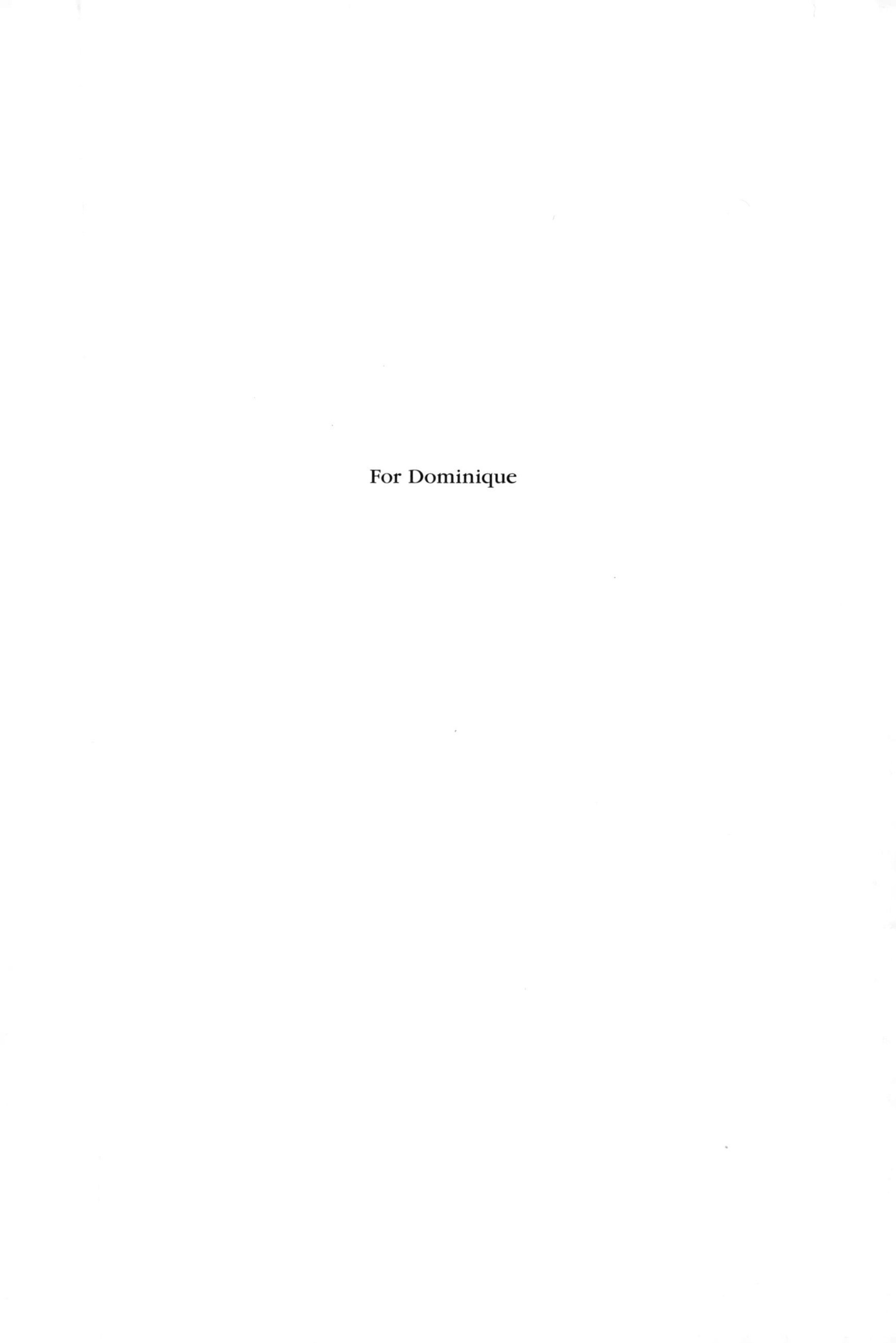

For Dominique

Contents

Foreword

Many therapists and teachers feel despondent when faced with a school-age child with a persisting and significant speech and language problem. It is clear that there are many learning, psychological and emotional difficulties that need to be considered. However, all those involved will be aware that these children have frequently run the gamut of assessments and interventions, and these have had limited impact. This group has often been associated with the phrase 'heart sink'. Thus it is most heartening to have, captured in this book, a positive framework which can assist speech and language therapists, teachers and students to be refreshed in their approach and encouraged with regard to what can be achieved.

This book follows on from the previous books by Joy Stackhouse and Bill Wells in the Children's Speech and Literacy Difficulties series. The first book introduced a psycholinguistic framework and the second focused on identification and intervention for children with speech and literacy difficulties. This book, although incorporating the psycholinguistic approach, also includes different drivers leading to an eclectic and dynamic approach to management of school-age children with persisting speech difficulties. It helps by clearly defining the difficulties of these children, clarifying methods of investigation and carrying out intervention. Because of the entrenched nature of these children's difficulties, they are considered (quite appropriately) 'hard to treat' and this text specifically focuses on this client group in a structured, principled and positive manner.

Many practical handbooks for teachers and therapists divorce themselves from the underpinning theory and research. This book does not do so. While being accessible and providing clear guidance for implementation, it still is based on the evidence and assists the reader in accessing more academic literature. With this client group it is often necessary to try different approaches to see which ones suit particular children and are likely to lead to better outcomes. The book, which incorporates detailed case studies, helps the reader to structure therapy trials in order that the most salient approach is identified.

As a therapist and researcher, I particularly appreciated this meshing of the worlds that help teachers and therapists to benefit from, implement and contribute to research; researchers will benefit from the clarity of the pragmatic exposition and structured approach to intervention. But those who will benefit the most are children with longstanding speech and language difficulties.

Pam Enderby
School of Health and Related Research (ScHARR)
University of Sheffield
Sheffield, UK

Preface

'Don't worry he'll grow out of it'

How many times have you heard this applied to children with speech difficulties by well meaning professionals and friends? Of course, many children do grow out of their speech difficulties, but others do not and can have associated literacy and behaviour problems. There is now more information about which children will go on to have **Persisting Speech Difficulties** - or PSDs for short - and what best practice might be. As these children are often considered 'hard to treat' and may not always be receiving the intervention they require, particularly as they get older, we felt there was a need for a text that specifically focuses on such a client group in a principled way.

This third book in the series *Children's Speech and Literacy Difficulties* is written mainly for speech and language therapists/pathologists (practitioners, researchers and students) and others who have a knowledge of the psycholinguistic framework presented in Books 1 and 2. It also assumes the reader has a basic knowledge of phonetics and speech difficulties in children. Book 1 introduced a psycholinguistic framework for research and practice, while Book 2 focused on using this framework for identification and intervention for children with speech and literacy difficulties. Book 3 uses this framework in combination with other approaches to examine in more detail intervention approaches with school-age children with specific speech difficulties.

The main themes running through this book are as follows.

- A range of perspectives is needed in order to treat school-age children with PSDs effectively, e.g. educational, psycholinguistic, linguistic, psychosocial and medical.
- Combining psycholinguistic and linguistic (specifically phonological) knowledge and skills is essential for planning appropriate therapy for individual children with PSDs.
- Theory and therapy are inseparable. Theory can be used to drive therapy but, in turn, experience of therapy helps to reshape the theory.

- In order to build the evidence base we need to carefully evaluate therapy outcomes using wide-ranging outcomes measures that can evaluate change at a variety of levels.

The aims of the book are to:

- summarize findings about research and practice;
- explain further the psycholinguistic approach; how to implement it and integrate it with other approaches;
- share how intervention has been carried out with specific children with PSDs in order to stimulate further thought and discussion about therapy;
- stimulate readers to pursue appropriate research designs for evidence based practice;
- highlight the importance of detail when carrying out and evaluating practice, e.g. stimuli selection, and scoring procedures;
- motivate for changes to service delivery for children with persisting speech difficulties as needed;
- engage the reader in actively thinking about issues presented through a range of Activities with keys for further discussion;
- provide a practical handbook through the inclusion of: bulleted summaries of main findings at the end of each chapter, stimuli lists, therapy tips, and sheets for photocopying;
- facilitate shared terminology through the provision of a glossary; particularly for students embarking on the study of PSDs.

Chapter 1 starts from the point of what the reader might know already about PSDs and then goes on to define the term, present the nature of the associated problems and review what is known about intervention for children with speech difficulties. Chapter 2 summarizes the three components of the psycholinguistic framework (the speech processing profile, box model, and developmental phase model) and provides an overview of research methods used in intervention studies. Combining the psycholinguistic approach with a linguistic one in order to ensure that appropriate stimuli are selected as targets in intervention is the main theme of Chapter 3, with Chapter 4 showing how to put this into practice through a case study of a child who was receiving therapy targeting segments in single words. Similarly, Chapter 5 focuses on stimuli design for working on clusters and Chapter 6 illustrates this through an intervention case study. Chapter 7 moves on to the connected speech level and Chapter 8 illustrates the principles involved through another intervention case study. Chapter 9 considers the important phenomenon of generalization in intervention, reviews what is known about it and considers ways in which it might be maximized. Chapter 10 discusses the link between speech and literacy and the role of the speech and language therapist in this domain;

again a case study is included. Chapter 11 tries to unpick what is meant by 'intelligibility' and how to use it as an outcome measure. This is developed in Chapter 12, which considers a range of intervention outcomes and how they might be selected and measured. Practical issues about service delivery are at the heart of Chapter 13. This discusses some of the daily challenges facing practitioners and managers in trying to deliver an effective service for school-age children with PSDs and examines what might be time- and cost-effective. Finally, Chapter 14 pulls together the main themes of the book and sets us all the challenge of putting the 'speech back into speech therapy'.

In this book we have emphasized the reciprocal relationship between theory and therapy and the importance of 'thinking like a researcher' in everyday practice. Building the evidence base is vital if the support and services offered to children with PSDs are to be developed. The case studies in particular can inform our knowledge of how children develop their speech processing system and the difficulties that arise if this system is not intact. The cases presented are real. They were not selected specifically for research but are typical of children in mainstream schools. Their names and identifying details have been changed and parental permission has been obtained to publish their therapy stories. These case studies are not to show how intervention *should* be done but rather to *share* how therapy *might be* done. They are used to reflect on practice and to make comparisons with other approaches. We are not claiming to know how best to manage children with PSDs – that is a long journey of discovery for all of us and one that is ongoing given the individual nature of the children involved and their circumstances.

Michelle Pascoe, Joy Stackhouse and Bill Wells
November 2005

Acknowledgements

We would like to thank all our colleagues who read and commented on draft chapters of this book: Beth Busani; Pam Enderby; Ruth Herbert; Maria Isernhinke; Jenny Leyden; Dariel Merrills; Blanca Schaefer; Jane Speake; Jennifer Teal; Wendy Wellington.

Thank you also to all the children - and their parents and schools - who appear in these pages. Without you there would be no book - and life would be a lot less interesting.

Michelle Pascoe was funded by an ESRC/MRC Interdisciplinary Post-doctoral Fellowship while working on this book, and also received funding from the University of Sheffield (UK), University of Cape Town (South Africa) and an Overseas Research Students (ORS) Award while carrying out the case studies included in this book as part of her PhD.

Conventions

TIE	spoken real word stimulus, as in real word repetition test, rhyme production test, spelling to dictation of real words; also used for picture target/stimulus, as in naming test, or silent rhyme detection.
[strai]	spoken non-word stimulus as in non-word repetition or discrimination test; spelling non-words to dictation; also used for real word target when phonological information is required.
<tie>	written stimulus or response, as in a test of single word reading (real or non-word).
[taɪ]	spoken response where phonetic information is required.
‘tie’	spoken response where phonetic information is not required.
[b]~[p]	[b] contrasted with [p].
SKY → [taɪ]	target SKY is produced as [taɪ].

CVC word structure where C = consonant; V = vowel.

Children’s chronological ages (CA) are given using the convention of years; months, e.g. 5;6 = 5 years and 6 months.

Chapter 1
Persisting Speech Difficulties

Many young children with early speech difficulties receive intervention that brings about rapid and long-lasting normalization of their speech. For this group of children, intervention is a brief and usually positive episode in their young lives, easily forgotten as they move forward with normal language, speech and literacy attainments. Speech and language therapists often find working with these children a rewarding experience as they are quickly able to see positive evidence of their input.

However, not all children with speech difficulties will fall into this group. Ruscello (1995) described children who do not respond to intervention and whose speech difficulties persist through the school years and often into adulthood. Wood and Scobbie (2003) refer to children who receive many years of therapy and are either very slow to resolve or are eventually discharged with residual errors. Woodyatt and Dodd (1995, p. 199) note:

> Whereas children with articulation difficulties and delayed acquisition of phonology are often referred to community speech pathology clinics, they would not be considered difficult cases for treatment by most experienced practitioners. The literature, then, rarely addresses the treatment of children whose speech disorder appears severe and resistant to therapy.

This volume aims to redress this imbalance by focusing on children whose speech difficulties are severe and resistant to intervention. There are a large number of children with speech difficulties that have persisted. Estimates suggest that approximately 5% of primary school children have speech difficulties (Weiss, Gordon and Lillywhite, 1987) and that 48 000 children per year in the UK present with primary speech difficulties (Broomfield and Dodd, 2004). We aim to explore and discuss ways of maximizing the effectiveness of intervention with children with persisting speech difficulties (PSDs). Let us start by considering what is meant by the term persisting speech difficulties in Activity 1.1.

ACTIVITY 1.1

Consider what you understand by the term persisting speech difficulties. List any features of persisting speech difficulties or PSDs you can think of. How would you know if a child of school-age has a speech difficulty?

See Key to Activity 1.1 at the end of this chapter for some of the words you may have written down, then read the following account of how we see persisting speech difficulties.

What are Persisting Speech Difficulties (PSDs)?

Persisting speech difficulties are exactly that. They are difficulties in the normal development of speech that do not resolve as the child matures or even after they receive specific help for these problems. There are similar terms used to describe the same sort of difficulties. Shriberg, Gruber and Kwiatkowski (1994) refer to children with 'residual phonological errors'. Wood and Scobbie refer to 'intractable speech disorders,' and define these as:

> systematic speech production errors that are judged not to have responded to conventional clinical intervention, or those in children who are 10 years or older but who have not been referred to speech therapy until very late.
>
> (Wood and Scobbie, 2003, p. 1)

We favour the term persisting speech difficulties since it covers a broad range of speech problems and causal factors. As we use it, the term may include both articulation and phonological difficulties as well as fluency difficulties. It does not imply that the child has a specific medical diagnosis, although in some cases they may have been given a diagnostic label such as childhood apraxia of speech, dyspraxia or dysarthria. As for the previous books in this series, in this volume the term 'speech difficulty' is used to refer to children who have difficulties with producing speech segments in isolation, single words or in connected speech regardless of origin of difficulty. Whatever term we choose to refer to these speech difficulties, those who have investigated them are broadly agreed on the basic characteristics of this client group. PSDs are usually identifiable through the

- child's age;
- primary nature of the speech difficulties;
- associated problems.

Each of these points is discussed in greater detail below.

Child's Age

By definition, PSDs are found in older children in their school years, typically age 5 or 6 years and beyond. These hard-to-treat children make slow progress so that their difficulties will typically not have resolved by the time they enter formal education. Bishop and Adams' (1990) critical age hypothesis suggests that 5;6 years, i.e. the age around which most children are receiving formal schooling in the UK, is the critical point at which a child's risk increases for other associated problems, e.g. literacy, if their speech difficulties have not yet resolved. Clearly this exact age will vary in other parts of the world. Shriberg, Austin, Lewis, *et al.* (1997) use the term 'residual speech difficulties' to refer to children whose difficulties remain beyond the age of 9. Between 6 and 8;11 years they prefer the term 'questionable residual difficulties'.

Research has attempted to distinguish between children who do and do not resolve their speech difficulties by the time they start school. When a young child is referred for a speech assessment for the first time, the practitioner may wonder whether therapy will prove a relatively straightforward and short-term exercise, or whether the child's difficulties will persist with more long-term sequelae and require ongoing intervention and support. Until fairly recently, the only way of answering this question was to carry out intervention and evaluate the progress made by the child. However, longitudinal studies have indicated some early predictors which might distinguish between the two groups. Nathan, Stackhouse, Goulandris and Snowling (2004a) investigated 47 children aged 4–7 years who had primary speech difficulties. They examined possible clinical markers for identifying children at risk for PSDs and associated literacy problems. Approximately 25% of the children with speech difficulties in their study resolved their speech difficulties by the end of the study when the children were aged approximately 7 years. Those children who had PSDs generally had more severe speech difficulties; speech input processing problems (auditory discrimination difficulties) and delayed language skills. The persisting speech difficulties were associated with poorer literacy development.

Primary Nature of the Speech Difficulties

Some children with PSDs may have an identifiable aetiology, e.g. cleft lip/palate or hearing impairment. Many others have speech difficulties with no known cause. Irrespective of whether aetiology has been identified or a diagnosis made, the nature and severity of PSDs varies widely and it is generally held that children with speech difficulties are a heterogeneous group (e.g. Dodd, 1995, 2005; Stackhouse, 1996). For all children with PSDs, speech problems can result from difficulties with the following:

- input processing, e.g. auditory discrimination of sounds;
- lexical representations, e.g. imprecise knowledge is stored about the sounds comprising a word;
- speech output, e.g. assembly of sounds needed for speech.

Stackhouse and Wells (1997) conceptualize these three aspects of potential difficulty in a simple speech processing model shown in Figure 1.1. The basic tenets of a psycholinguistic approach to understanding children's speech difficulties are encapsulated in this figure; difficulties in speech processing occur as a result of breakdown at some point or points along this processing path.

In Book 1 of this series, Stackhouse and Wells (1997, p. 3) reviewed different approaches to classifying speech problems in children. They outlined medical approaches that use diagnostic labels to group children; linguistic approaches which use linguistic terminology to describe children's difficulties; and psycholinguistic approaches which attempt to understand children's speech difficulties in terms of individual profiles of strengths and weaknesses and in terms of underlying points of breakdown in a speech processing chain or model. Using the medical approach, we might describe a child as having childhood apraxia of speech should they meet the cluster of symptoms typically linked to this label, e.g. see Ozanne, 2005. That same child's speech difficulty might be described in linguistic terms of a series of phonological processing rules, e.g. they exhibit cluster reduction word initially and finally, as well as metathesis in multi-syllabic words.

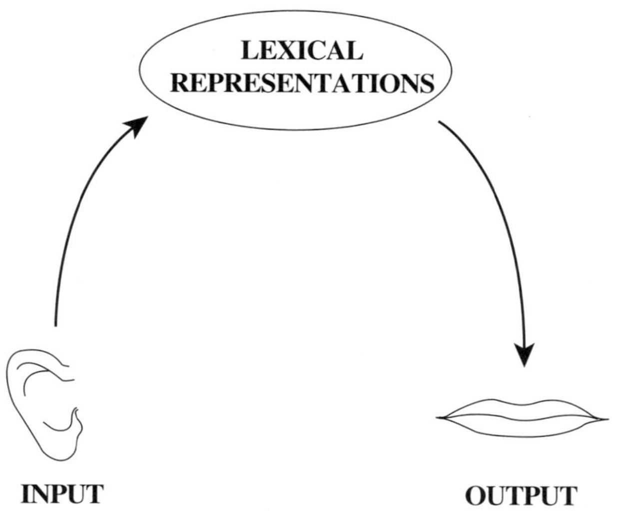

Figure 1.1: The speech processing chain: A simple speech processing model (reproduced by kind permission of Whurr Publishers from Stackhouse and Wells, 1997, p. 9).

Shriberg, Austin, Lewis *et al.* (1997) devised an aetiological classification system for children's phonological difficulties. This classification system relies on causal sub-groups among developmental phonological disorders and includes (1) unknown origin, possibly genetic, (2) otitis media with effusion (OME), (3) developmental verbal apraxia, (4) developmental psychosocial involvement, and (5) special populations such as those with craniofacial and sensory motor involvements. However, in many cases a detectable aetiology is not always present, and some children fall into more than one of Shriberg's classifications. Fox, Dodd and Howard (2002) attempted to classify 66 children according to Shriberg's system and found that around half could not be readily classified.

There are many different ways of describing children's speech difficulties. We are likely to select these and use these in ways which reflect our own background and training. Our choice of labels or descriptors is likely to vary depending on the settings in which we work and the practical demands of the situations in which we find ourselves. Diagnostic medical labels can be useful in obtaining support for children with severe speech difficulties, e.g. through the statementing process in the UK whereby the needs of children with specific educational difficulties are legally acknowledged. However, labels such as childhood apraxia of speech, dysarthria and hearing impairment may convey a set of assumptions about where the breakdown is occurring in the speech processing system that may not represent the whole picture. For example, Ebbels (2000) investigated the speech and language processing skills of a 10-year-old child with a hearing impairment. Specific points of breakdown for individual phonological contrasts were identified, with detailed input and output phonological analyses interpreted within a broader psycholinguistic framework. The results of the investigation showed that for this child there was not merely one level of breakdown with hearing, but rather there were multiple levels of difficulty with specific phonological contrasts implicated at particular levels.

A child with PSDs will have areas of weakness in his/her speech processing chain. To compliment this psycholinguistic perspective, we can use linguistic descriptive terms to describe the difficulties observed in speech output. The paper by Susan Ebbels effectively shows how the psycholinguistic and linguistic (in this case phonological) perspective can be combined. For some children with PSDs individual speech sounds may be affected. Shriberg, Gruber and Kwiatkowski (1994) suggest that in English the fricative and liquid sound classes are most vulnerable. In school-age children the most common and persisting speech sound difficulties are:

- /θ/ produced as /f/, e.g. THIN → [fɪn]
- /ð/ produced as /v/, e.g. THEN → [vɛn]
- /r/ produced as /w/, e.g. RUN → [wʌn]

In some local accents these sound substitutions are the norm, and if this is the case then they should clearly not be labelled as speech errors. Nevertheless, Stackhouse cautions, 'The child's production should be compared with the peer group at school as well as with other members of the family' (1996, p. 27). While we know that PSDs can be manifested in problems with individual sound production, this is not always the most striking characteristic. For some children, connected speech – the production of longer strings of sounds beyond the single word – poses real challenges. Children's speech may be unintelligible to unfamiliar listeners because of difficulties not only at a segmental level but also with prosody, timing and the 'glue' that joins words together. Shriberg, Austin, Lewis *et al.* (1997) refer to 'imprecise speech'. By the time a child starts school he or she should be using a full range of sounds and should be intelligible for most of the time. By 7 years of age, the child should not have noticeable speech problems. Sadly, this is not the case for children with PSDs. Moving beyond the production of individual sounds means that it can sometimes be difficult to pinpoint the reasons for a child's low intelligibility. Single word assessments may suggest that the child has no difficulties. Wood and Scobbie (2003) describe a 10-year-old girl with a repaired cleft of the soft palate. This child had received 6 years of regular speech therapy targeting the production of a range of speech sounds. At 10 years of age she was now able to articulate velars at word level but was unable to transfer this to other levels. The authors used the instrumental technique of electropalatography (EPG) to arrive at this conclusion.

Associated Problems

Persisting speech difficulties place children at increased risk for experiencing other associated problems. The impact of PSDs on other aspects of the children's development should not be underestimated. Research has shown that these children are at increased risk of having difficulties in the normal acquisition of literacy, and that their psychosocial development may also be affected, e.g. having low self-esteem and being at increased risk of bullying. We explore these two associated problems in the following sections.

Literacy Acquisition

It is known that children with PSDs can face an increased risk of experiencing problems in the acquisition of literacy. However, the relationship between speech and literacy is not a straightforward one. It is important to consider the nature of the speech difficulties when making predictions about literacy and long-term outcomes. There are shared phonological underpinnings for speech processing and literacy. If a child's speech difficulty reflects problems with phonological processing then it is likely that the foundation for developing literacy will not be a firm one. Children with PSDs may be at risk for later spelling difficulties due to poor phonological awareness and difficulties in phonological coding in verbal memory. Volume 1 of this series emphasized the links between speech and literacy (Stackhouse and Wells, 1997, p. 3) and the need for children to have an intact speech processing system in order to acquire literacy in the normal way.

Speech difficulties assume greater importance for literacy outcomes when they co-occur with language difficulties. Bishop and Clarkson (2003) reported that their group of children with both speech and language disorders were the poorest performers in their study, and the results from a longitudinal study by Nathan, Stackhouse, Goulandris and Snowling (2004a) confirmed this finding. Bishop and Adams (1990) contrasted literacy outcomes for two groups of 8-year-old children: a group whose speech difficulties had resolved, and a group whose speech difficulties remained. They found that a significant number of the children with persisting speech problems had literacy difficulties, while their resolved counterparts did not. Their critical age hypothesis suggests that children whose speech difficulties have not resolved by 5;6 face an increased risk of experiencing difficulties with literacy as they get older.

Children with PSDs are at particular risk of being poor spellers due to the shared phonological underpinnings for speech and spelling (Lewis, Freebairn and Taylor, 2002). A study by Clarke-Klein and Hodson (1995) revealed that children with histories of speech difficulties made more phonologically deviant misspellings than their normally developing peers. Speech sound errors do not necessarily map directly onto spelling errors (McCormack, 1995), but rather difficulty with speech may result in imprecise phonological representations of words in the lexicon (Treiman, 1985; Stackhouse, 2006), resulting in inconsistent erroneous spellings. Bishop and Clarkson (2003) observe that spelling skills are frequently overlooked when evaluating children with speech and language difficulties. These authors note that literacy research has tended to focus more on reading than spelling, and that it is often argued that spelling performance can be deduced from reading performance since the two are typically highly correlated. They argue that spelling offers an important window into the developing speech and language system since it is a late-acquired and complex skill. Children with speech difficulties, indicative of underlying speech processing problems, are not likely to be able to progress in their literacy development with the ease of their normally developing classmates.

However, it is also important to note that a child whose speech difficulty comprises an isolated articulatory difficulty arising from a physical abnormality may be no more likely to develop literacy difficulties than a child with normally developing speech (Stackhouse, 1982). Studies of children with motor speech difficulties, e.g. dysarthria, have found that such speech difficulties are not linked to spelling problems (Bishop and

Robson, 1989). Similarly, children with articulation difficulties are not at an increased risk of having literacy problems provided that they have good language skills and the articulation difficulties are not severe (Bishop and Clarkson, 2003). Literacy difficulties in children with PSDs are discussed in greater detail in Chapter 10.

Psychosocial Development

Given the importance of speech in everyday communication, it is not hard to imagine the psychosocial impact of having PSDs. Rebecca, a girl aged 11;3 with PSDs emphasizes the social importance of communication:

> talking is important because . . . if you couldn't use another way, would be no other way people could connect . . . you wouldn't make friends, then wouldn't get married and wouldn't be any kids

Children with PSDs are at increased risk of experiencing psychosocial difficulties, and a fairly large body of research attests to this fact. Hadley and Rice (1991) found that children with communication difficulties were more likely to be ignored by peers and not invited to join in with social interactions, and it is known that even minor speech errors may be negatively perceived by peers (Crowe Hall, 1991). The psychosocial impact of PSDs varies from minor to severe, and is not necessarily correlated with the severity of the speech problem. For some children, minor speech difficulties assume great psychosocial significance, while other children seem better able to cope with the impact of more severe speech difficulties. Psychosocial difficulties - whether resulting from mild or severe speech difficulties - need to be addressed.

A study carried out by Knox and Conti-Ramsden (2003) investigated 100 children diagnosed with specific language impairment (SLI) who were attending school in a variety of settings, e.g. mainstream schools and special schools. They found that these children faced significantly higher risks than the general population for being bullied, and that educational placement had no significant impact on this risk, i.e. it did not matter if the children were in a mainstream or special school as the risk of being bullied remains the same. Conti-Ramsden and Botting (2000) found that children with severe communication difficulties may also be at risk for behaviour problems and higher incidence of attention deficit hyperactivity disorder (ADHD). These authors along with others such as Nash, Stengelhofen, Toombs, et al. (2001) and Nash (2006) describe a cycle of disadvantage in which poor communication skills reduce peer interaction, which results in fewer friends, increased risk of victimization and low self-esteem.

Lindsay, Dockrell, Letchford and Mackie (2002) investigated the self-esteem of 69 children with specific speech and language difficulties in Years 6 and 7, i.e. aged approximately 10–11 years. Results revealed that these children not only had educational difficulties, but that they also had lower estimates of their own academic ability and their competence in peer relationships. Bryan (2004) carried out speech and language screening of young offenders in a British prison. Forty-seven per cent of the offenders were rated as having moderate speech difficulty with over half of this group reporting that they had a stammer or that they had been told they stammered. While this does not mean there is a causal link between crime and PSDs, the data speak to the psychosocial difficulties that some individuals with PSDs may face. The studies presented in this section are sobering for anyone involved with children with PSDs.

ACTIVITY 1.2

By now you should have a clearer idea of what is meant by PSDs. In this activity, consider the reasons why some children's speech difficulties persist. List any reasons you can think of.

See Key to Activity 1.2 at the end of this chapter for some of the reasons you may have written down, then read the following account of how we would answer this question.

Why Do Some Children's Speech Difficulties Persist?

There are different ways in which this question might be considered. On the one hand, responses may focus on 'nature' looking to the medical literature on speech disorders and transmission of genes. On the other hand, one might suggest that 'nurture' is the key factor with the nature of intervention and social circumstances giving rise to the difficulties. The answer most likely varies from child to child with both nature and nurture contributing in different measures. We outline some of the factors which may contribute to the persisting nature of speech difficulties.

Medical Diagnoses and Genetics

Experience and research with some client groups has suggested that the prognosis for developing normal speech is limited. Some children with conditions such as cerebral palsy, hearing impairment, Down and other syndromes may never acquire intelligible speech. These children may be severely limited by their cognitive skills, motoric skills or sensory–perceptual skills. However, for most medical conditions there is a range of outcomes. Many children with Down syndrome cope in mainstream classrooms and go on to achieve speech that is intelligible. For some children with hearing impairment, speech outcome assumes less significance as the child develops successful communication through signing and written communication. Pascoe, Stackhouse and Wells (2005) described the speech processing profile of a 6-year-old girl, called Katy, diagnosed with ataxic cerebral palsy. Contrary to initial assumptions based on her diagnosis, her difficulties were not limited to peripheral articulatory difficulties but included both output and input levels of the speech processing profile. The progress she made as a result of the intervention was perhaps greater than many would think given the prognosis typically associated with that condition. Katy is discussed in greater detail in Chapters 7 and 8 of this volume.

Childhood apraxia of speech (CAS) (also sometimes called developmental verbal dyspraxia) is a controversial diagnosis but usually one that is given to children who are unable to perform the coordinated movements required for speech. Diagnoses of CAS do not necessarily inform intervention planning: in many cases, only when children fail to respond to traditional phonological intervention, are they labelled as 'apraxic', thus intervention can give rise to the diagnosis, rather than vice versa. It is well documented however that such children typically respond extremely slowly to intervention (Shriberg, Aram and Kwiatkowski, 1997a, b).

There is further information about the nature of childhood apraxia of speech/developmental verbal dyspraxia from gene studies. PSDs are sometimes observed to run in families. Vargha-Khadem and her co-authors (e.g. Vargha-Khadem, Gadian, Copp and Mishkin, 2005) describe the discovery of a mutation in a gene known as FOXP2, which is thought to give rise to apraxia in those with the affected gene. Investigations of the speech and language skills of the so-called KE family, half of whose members have CAS, have suggested that this mutated gene gives rise to the cluster of deficits associated with apraxia. This type of study is extremely useful in shedding light on the neural mechanisms involved in speech. While it informs our knowledge about why some children have conditions such as apraxia, it does not tell us why these difficulties persist or how they might be addressed. There is a great deal of further work to be done in considering how genes and environment interact.

A Psycholinguistic Perspective

Using a psycholinguistic approach can help explain why some children have PSDs. Psycholinguistic approaches consider that speech processing involves successive levels of input processing, stored representations and output. Such models can be simplistically represented as in Figure 1.1. Children with persisting difficulties are thought to have multiple, and often severe, levels of breakdown throughout the system. Difficulties in one part of the system can affect processing in other parts, and it is a challenge for intervention to tap into the appropriate level and at the same time to take account of how the different levels affect each other. Psycholinguistic models are useful in helping us understand the nature and extent of a child's underlying speech processing difficulties. Once this is understood more fully, beyond surface speech errors or diagnostic labels, it may not be entirely surprising that a child is only capable of making slow progress with their speech processing.

Returning to childhood apraxia of speech, Ozanne (1995, 2005) and Stackhouse and Wells (1997, 2001) suggest that children diagnosed with CAS have a multi-deficit disorder: they are likely to have difficulties in devising new motor programs (i.e. templates or blueprints of how to produce a word), but they may well also experience difficulties with other aspects of speech processing such as motor planning (i.e. the actual realization of the template in connected speech) and auditory discrimination. These levels of processing are discussed in Chapter 2. Such multi-deficit conceptualizations can account for the fact that children with CAS often present with severe difficulties, and also the fact that intervention typically yields slow results, since intervention is unlikely to tap into all deficit areas at one time in what Ozanne (1995, p. 109) terms a 'sabotaging effect'.

Social Circumstances

Communication takes place in social settings, and it is clear that for some children environmental circumstances have a role to play in the outcome of speech difficulties. Locke, Ginsborg and Peers (2002) investigated the spoken language skills of pre-school children being raised in poverty. They found that more than 50% of the 240 children participating in the study had spoken language skills significantly delayed for their age. They discuss the implications of this in terms of the critical age hypothesis and the likely outcome on the children's literacy achievement.

Broomfield and Dodd (2004) investigated the socio-economic status of pre-school children referred to their local paediatric clinic. They found that the distribution of speech disability across socio-economic status was similar to that of the local population. There were, however, slightly more children from affluent backgrounds referred with articulation difficulties and phonological delay. Affluent parents may find it easier to bring children to the clinic and access the referral system. Some children with PSDs have not been able to access the support and intervention needed to address their difficulties.

Intervention Itself

Thus far the question of 'Why do some children's speech difficulties persist?' has been answered mainly in terms of the children themselves, and the characteristics that seem to distinguish them from their normally developing or readily-resolving peers. However, phonological intervention is a complex process and there are a great many factors that can affect outcome. These include:

- the child: the nature and severity of the difficulties; personality; learning style, motivation and previous experience of intervention;
- the assessment;
- the intervention procedure and process;
- the child's communication partners and opportunities for communicating.

It is clear that intervention has an important part to play in outcome, although there are a great many questions unanswered about its contributions. For example, it might be asked whether the difference between the resolved and unresolved groups of children is due to the nature and type of intervention that they receive. Do the children with resolved difficulties receive more or better intervention than their unresolved peers? Research suggests that this is not the case, although few studies have used methodologies that would be appropriate for investigating this question. Nathan *et al.* (2004a) included detailed questionnaires for speech and language therapists in their longitudinal study of children with PSDs, asking about the frequency and type of intervention that each child was given. They found that the children who went on to have the PSDs, had on average received more intervention than the other children. This suggests that intervention is given where it is most needed but despite getting larger intervention dosages than their resolving peers, these children's intractable difficulties remain. Their limited progress and persisting problems suggest to practitioners that further intervention is warranted. Nathan *et al.* (2004a) found no substantial difference in the type of therapy that was delivered to the children who did or did not resolve their difficulties.

Bernhardt (2004) describes studies in the United States that she and her colleagues carried out to evaluate the effectiveness of phonological therapy with 22 pre-school children. At the end of the study the participating speech and language therapists completed questionnaires about their own education, confidence in the therapy approaches, and treatment style. The only factor linked to outcomes was whether the therapist had specific and advanced training in linguistics in addition to their Speech–Language Pathology qualification. Children who were treated by therapists who had linguistics degrees in addition to their Speech–Language Pathology qualification made more rapid gains in word structure development (CV, CVC, CCVC) and acquired more segments accurately. Bernhardt concluded:

> There is much yet to learn about practitioner training and intervention outcomes, . . . [and] the effects of the interactions between participants

> in the intervention process, for example, between practitioners and child, between the teacher and the speech and language therapist.
>
> (Bernhardt, 2004, p. 197)

We have outlined some of the ways in which children's persisting speech difficulties might be explained and accounted for. For most children the answer to the question, 'Why do speech difficulties persist?' will be answered by drawing on a combination of the factors suggested above. A combination of medical, genetic, psycholinguistic or social reasons may help us answer that question for any individual child. We should also remember that children with PSDs are a diverse group and no two children will present with the same difficulties or the same background history. There are always children who do not fit in with the general pattern. Some children are resilient. Despite difficult social circumstances they seem to cope better with their persisting speech difficulties, and their PSDs do not seem to affect their literacy or social success, or do so only in very limited ways. The concept of resilience is an interesting one that has been little researched in relation to speech and language. Some authors (e.g. Werner and Smith, 1982) have attempted to profile resilient children, looking at factors which seem to predispose at-risk children to cope with their particular environment and difficulties in a positive way. Although the focus of this research is not specifically on speech and language, findings have suggested that autonomous children with good social skills are ones who are likely to cope best with difficulties faced.

What Do We Know about Intervention for Children with Speech Problems?

A Historical Perspective

In the 1960s speech therapy was heavily influenced by behaviourism with speech regarded as a specialized behaviour that could be modified by altering the environment and its associated precedents and consequences (e.g. Gray and Fygetakis, 1968; Sloane and MacAulay, 1968). In the 1970s the influence of linguistics became more strongly felt. A shift was seen from articulatory approaches concerned with individual segments (e.g. Van Riper, 1963) to phonological therapy (e.g. Ingram, 1974, 1976), which focused on targeting phonological processes as a more effective way of carrying out therapy. Phonological approaches - like their articulatory predecessors - have the ultimate goal of improving a child's speech production and of helping a child to become more intelligible. In addition, phonological intervention has the goal of 'facilitating cognitive reorganisation of the child's phonological system and his [or her] phonologically-oriented processing strategies' (Grunwell, 1985, p. 99). There are many different approaches to phonological intervention based on these broad principles. These include:

- Minimal pair contrast therapy or 'meaningful minimal pairs'. Children's attention is drawn to the distinct meanings associated with words that differ by only one feature such as the voicing contrast in GATE and KATE. The particular contrasts are selected based on the child's specific difficulties. See Weiner, 1981; Dodd and Bradford, 2000.
- Maximal pair contrast therapy or maximal opposition approach. Children's attention is drawn to the distinct meanings associated with words that differ on several features, e.g. PIN and GIN differ in the word initial consonants in terms of place, manner and voicing. The particular contrasts are selected based on the child's specific difficulties. See Gierut, 1991, 1992.
- Multiple opposition contrasts. Children's attention is drawn to a set of words and the focus is on developing contrasts between all words in the set. The particular contrasts are selected based on the child's specific difficulties, e.g. the set of words addressed in intervention might include TWO, SHOE, CHEW, SUE for a child who produced /tu/ for targets TWO, SHOE, CHEW, SUE. See Williams, 2000a, b.
- Metaphon and other metaphonological approaches. The child is made explicitly aware of the sound properties that need to be contrasted in order to improve their speech, e.g. if a child has difficulty with the voicing contrast then intervention would focus attention on the concepts of 'noisy' (voiced) and 'quiet' (voiceless). See Howell and Dean, 1994.

Baker and McLeod (2004) review a range of phonological intervention approaches. They emphasize that evidence-based practice is about selecting and applying the right approach with the right type of child. Each of the approaches above would be most appropriate with particular types of children. For example, for the metaphonological approach to be effective the child needs to have the cognitive skills to understand the concepts being taught (e.g. noisy and quiet) and be able to apply these concepts to their own speech. The multiple oppositions approach is best for children with severe phonological difficulties, and those who have sufficient semantic knowledge to keep track of the entire word set, e.g. TWO, SHOE, CHEW, SUE. Joffe and Serry (2004) provide a useful longitudinal perspective of speech and language therapy in the phonological domain. These authors, in describing the shift from articulation to phonology therapy in the 1970s, suggest that discarding articulation frameworks 'had the unfortunate consequence of throwing the baby out with the bath water' (p. 259).

There may of course be children for whom an articulatory approach is required. The *Diagnostic Evaluation of Articulation and Phonology*

(*DEAP*) (Dodd, Hua, Crosbie, *et al.*, 2002) specifically distinguishes between phonological and articulation difficulties. This assessment is based on Dodd's (1995, 2005) work in which children are grouped into categories based on the nature and underlying cause of their speech problems. The sub-groups outlined by Dodd include:

- Articulation. Children who are not able to produce acceptable versions of particular phones. The difficulties are at the level of the mouth (see Figure 1.1)
- Phonological delay. Children whose phonology resembles that of a younger child. They show normal speech processes exhibited by younger children. The entire speech system (shown in Figure 1.1) is slow in developing.
- Consistent deviant phonology. Children who show non-developmental errors and unusual processes, and are consistent in their application of these rules. These children have difficulties with their phonological knowledge, the lexical representation shown in Figure 1.1.
- Inconsistent deviant phonology. These children may show delayed and non-developmental errors, but in addition they show significant variability in their speech production which does not reflect a maturing system.

Undoubtedly, however, the contribution of linguistics to speech and language therapy has been considerable, and has enabled therapists to develop a more comprehensive understanding of the complexities of communication beyond that of articulation. Linguistic contributions are not limited to phonology. Gallagher (1998) observes the wide-ranging influence of pragmatics and metalinguistic knowledge in the 80s and 90s, and the increased attention given to functional and psychosocial aspects of communication. These are aspects that have influenced the way in which all speech and language interventions are carried out, including phonological therapy. In terms of service delivery there have also been considerable changes since the early years of the profession. Bowen and Cupples (1998) comment on the increasing role of parents - and other involved parties - in the therapeutic process. The effectiveness of different types of phonological therapy and its delivery has been evaluated to varying degrees, and this is discussed in subsequent sections.

An Eclectic Approach for Children with Persisting Speech Difficulties

Faced with children with PSDs, we need to 'pull out all the stops' to maximize the success of intervention. Using an eclectic approach may offer the best chance of success with these hard-to-treat children. A psycholinguistic approach is a useful starting point in that it may:

> . . . provide a framework for explaining the descriptive or symptomatic information about impaired phonological systems derived from linguistic-based assessments by attempting to identify the level at which speech processing is disrupted.
>
> (Baker, Croot, McLeod and Paul, 2001, p. 686)

However, psycholinguistic models have inherent limitations, and even if further refined, it is doubtful if they could ever shape the therapy process in isolation. Psycholinguistic approaches need to be integrated with linguistic and other knowledge in order to be effective. The psycholinguistic approach is useful in answering the question: 'How?' – How is intervention going to work, i.e. how is change to be brought about in the individual's speech processing system? Knowledge from linguistics, in this case phonology, enables us to answer the more specific 'what?' question, i.e. what is the content of intervention?, e.g. what are the stimuli that will be used in the activities? We also need to consider social and psychosocial aspects since all children will bring their own personality, likes and dislikes, and network of support to intervention.

Many single case studies have relied mainly on linguistic theory and phonological analyses (e.g. Weiner, 1981; Monahan, 1986; Saben and Ingham, 1991; Bernhardt, 1992; Barlow, 2001) in planning and evaluating interventions, and this body of knowledge should be brought to bear alongside a psycholinguistically-oriented approach. Edwards, Fourakis, Beckman and Fox (1999) outline the evolution of representation-based approaches to understanding children's phonology, and suggest that characterizing children's phonological competence in terms of representations and the constraints acting on them allows for a richer conceptualization of phonological development than traditional derivational and normalizing approaches. A further reason for careful investigation of underlying phonological representations and phonological processing ability is because of the close relationship between these skills and reading and spelling abilities. The association between phonological processing difficulties and reading and spelling problems has been shown in a number of single case studies (e.g. Campbell and Butterworth, 1985; Snowling, Stackhouse and Rack, 1986) and experimental investigations comparing children with dyslexia with normally-developing readers (e.g. Wagner and Torgeson, 1987). For school-age children with persisting speech difficulties, understanding of the child's underlying difficulties can have important implications for speech, language and literacy support. This is discussed further in Chapter 10. Again, we need to be careful not to wholly discard the more traditional linguistic approach.

Waters, Hawkes and Burnett (1998) combined psycholinguistic and phonological factors, as well as consideration of the 'child as learner' in their intervention with a child called Alan aged 5 years, with unintelligible speech. They suggested that while phonological analysis and psycholinguistic assessment are essential for a principled approach to intervention, they may not always be sufficient: children's attitudes, behaviours and preferred learning styles also need to be taken into account (see also Waters, 2001).

There are other model-based intervention case studies that have attempted to couch phonological intervention within an explicit psycholinguistic framework. Bryan and Howard (1992) described intervention for a five-year-old child with severe phonological difficulties. The child's speech processing difficulties were investigated through a series of psycholinguistically-motivated tasks and interpreted in the light of current models of speech and language processing. In addition a phonological analysis of the child's surface speech errors took place, with both sets of data used to inform intervention planning. This paper emphasises many of the key aspects emphasized in this book, e.g. the need for levels of analysis which vary in terms of sensitivity, and the importance of understanding the difficulties underlying surface speech errors. Although this volume emphasizes the application of phonological intervention in a psycholinguistic framework, it is acknowledged that psychosocial and emotional interventions have an important role to play in the overall management of children with PSDs.

Medical and educational approaches are also part of the eclectic perspective used with children with PSDs. A medical approach can suggest long-term prognosis. Children with cleft lip and palate, and physical conditions such as cerebral palsy may continue to receive medical and surgical monitoring or intervention related to their condition. As they develop and grow, different interventions may become more or less appropriate. We have noted previously that children with PSDs are by definition of school-age, and will spend a great deal of time in school. Therapists working with this client group will typically be seeing the child in school and working together with school staff to meet the needs of children with PSDs and support them in accessing the school curriculum.

Outcomes Research

Speech and language therapy for children is generally held to have positive outcomes (Nye, Foster and Seaman, 1987; Gierut, 1998b; Law, Boyle, Harris, *et al.*, 1998; Goldstein and Gierut, 1998; Law and Garret, 2003). It is in the area of speech difficulties that much of the outcomes research in speech and language therapy has focused, and shown generally positive results (e.g. see Shriberg and Kwiatkowski, 1994; Law and Garret, 2003).

There are a great many challenges associated with intervention research with children. Enderby and Emerson note 'there is no other client group . . . that demonstrates so many challenges to the researcher' (1995, p. 35).

ACTIVITY 1.3

Consider the quote from Enderby and Emerson above. Make a list of reasons why children, in general, pose enormous challenges to researchers. Consider the population of children with PSDs specifically, and the challenges they pose for intervention researchers. See Key to Activity 1.3 page 24 for some of the reasons you may have written down, then read our account of these challenges below.

Intervention research with children with PSDs is a challenge for the following reasons:

- Children with PSDs are a heterogeneous group. A range of different diagnostic and classification systems are used and can make comparisons between outcomes studies difficult.
- A range of different outcomes measures are used to evaluate the effectiveness of intervention, again making comparisons between studies a challenge.
- Intervention outcomes depend on wide-ranging factors such as the child, practitioner, intervention.
- Children's development is dynamic. They are constantly changing and developing anyway.

Despite these challenges, intervention research is important for a number of reasons. There is the obvious need to serve individual clients in ways that are effective and efficient. Children with PSDs face an increased risk of social, literacy and academic difficulties and it is imperative to address their difficulties as soon as possible to prevent any more widespread negative academic and social consequences. In addition, there is a need to demonstrate the value of speech and language therapy services within a broader setting. If the profession aims to develop and grow, it needs to be able to show its benefit in demonstrable, scientific ways. Current professional concerns in healthcare and education have continued to necessitate more evidence of knowledge-based practice to underpin service delivery and development (Byng, Van der Gaag and Parr, 1998; Baker and McLeod, 2004). The rationale for evaluating effectiveness of therapy lies not only in accountability, but is also important to direct in therapy planning, and to enhance work satisfaction (Dodd, 1995).

Evidence-based Practice: Theory and Therapy Together

Intervention planning can be a complex process. When therapists are faced with children with a range of surface speech errors and underlying processing deficits, it may be difficult to know where to begin and how to structure intervention. The psycholinguistic framework, combined

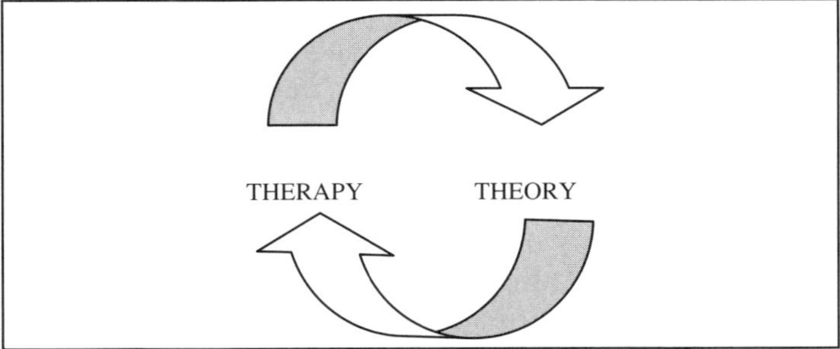

Figure 1.2: The cyclical and symbiotic relationship between theory and therapy (based on Reilly, 2004, p. 12).

with knowledge of linguistic theory, can help to make the process more transparent and explicit. If intervention is carefully targeted at an individual's specific point of breakdown, and carried out with an awareness of the strengths and weaknesses that underlie the individual's speech processing system, then it seems more likely that (a) intervention will be successful in bringing about change in the speech processing system, and (b) if intervention is *not* successful then it is possible to isolate the level of the speech processing system that therapy tasks were tapping, and make appropriate revisions. For some children, generalization is minimal and progress is limited to specific targeted segments. Monitoring the extent of generalization and patterns that occur, informs decision-making as well as our knowledge of how the speech processing system works.

Reilly describes the theory–practice gap: 'Often, tensions exist between practitioners who fear that research will become the sole driver of clinical practice and academics who value basic science over clinically relevant research' (2004, p. 12). One of the aims of this volume is to show that both views are vital and can be knitted together. Figure 1.2 outlines the cyclic, symbiotic relationship between theory and therapy (based on Reilly, 2004). Aspects of the intervention process such as generalization are shown in each chapter to be key to evaluations of efficiency as well as for the way in which they inform our theoretical knowledge.

Towards a Theory of Therapy

Sometimes therapists are reticent to discuss the content of their therapy. A likely reason for this is the perceived mismatch between theory and practice: theoretically-motivated work from a variety of viewpoints has provided detailed analyses of the deficits underlying some difficulties. Compared with these sophisticated analyses, many therapists' treatment techniques used in day-to-day practice appear very simple; therapists may not feel that they do justice to the complexity of the problem. Howard and Hatfield (1987) relate this to the fact that there is no 'metatheory' available which explicitly relates a deficit analysis to the process of treatment. What is a metatheory? What should it contain? And how close are we to devising one?

A metatheory or 'theory of therapy' is an account of intervention that involves systematically relating an analysis of the client's strengths and weaknesses to the process of treatment. The development of a metatheory is a prerequisite for the development of specific and motivated therapy methods with decisions taken at each step being conscious and explicit. Only if we know exactly how a particular treatment task is meant to affect what ability and why it does so, can therapy progress. The results of intervention can support or refute hypothetical answers to these questions; but until these hypotheses are put to empirical test, we will have no means to improve our treatments. Stackhouse and Wells' (1997, 2001) psycholinguistic framework goes some way towards providing a theory of therapy. Therapists adopting this approach may be carrying out games and activities that seem simple on the surface. Yet, if they are carried out with an awareness of the parts of the child's speech processing system that are being tapped, and why this is important in terms of their overall profile, then there is no mismatch between theory and therapy. Nevertheless there is further work to be done in developing a theory of therapy using this approach, e.g. what are the mechanisms for bringing about change, and how does the interaction between therapist and child affect therapy outcomes? Horton and Byng's (2000) ATICS is a system used to examine interactional aspects in adult treatment which might have application to children.

Bunning (2004) attempts to elucidate intervention by applying theoretical frameworks drawn from sociological, medical and psychological literature to speech and language interventions. One of Bunning's aims is to draw together the range of specialisms within the speech and language therapy field, and highlight commonalties they share in terms of intervention. This is philosophically interesting, but ultimately the frameworks may be too broad to account for the complex, highly-specific difficulties encountered by different client groups, e.g. children with PSDs. Bunning's frameworks may be helpful in carrying out a retrospective analysis of what occurred in an intervention episode, but would not be able to effectively inform intervention planning, for example, for the children presented in this book.

Evidence-based practice offers guidelines for decision-making. Reilly (2004) emphasizes the disparity that exists between clinical practice and research evidence, suggesting that in some cases although evidence exists it is not applied in clinical situations. She cites the example of Rousseau, Onslow, Packman and Robinson (2001) who investigated the Lidcombe programme for addressing stammering in young children. Only about 50% of practitioners were using the programme in the recommended way with most making compromises in terms of dosage to suit service delivery constraints, and selecting parts of the programme that they felt were relevant. This was despite published evidence from Onslow, Packman and Harrison (2001) that the programme is most effective when employed in a particular way. Rousseau *et al.* (2001) concluded that those therapists not using the prescribed programme were almost certainly carrying out interventions for which there is as yet no evidence of effectiveness. This finding, surely not specific to the area of dysfluency, raises some important issues.

1. Speech and language therapy is a relatively young profession. Thus it is not surprising that the academic underpinning of the work is limited.
2. Demands for services and clinical priorities mean that academic underpinnings are often seen as added extras for the workforce rather than fundamental. Clearly, there is a need for theoretical underpinnings and this is something which needs to be strongly emphasized in undergraduate training courses and throughout professional development. Howell and Dean have suggested that speech and language therapists are in a unique position to synthesize knowledge from a variety of fields including that of clinical practice to 'create a viable theoretical underpinning for rehabilitation' (1994, p. 2).
3. Evidence-based practice guidelines do not necessarily define best practice since the evidence may be weak or insufficient to make that determination. The evidence-base needs to be critically judged and continually re-evaluated in the light of new evidence.

What Can We Do?

This volume aims to discuss the challenges of intervention for practitioners working with school-age children with persisting speech difficulties: It includes how to select appropriate stimuli for intervention and in what ways to target these; how to obtain maximum generalization; how to measure and understand intelligibility; how to make links with literacy; and how to evaluate intervention in clinical and research settings. We are not able to supply definitive answers for all these questions. We aim to share the intervention we have carried out with some children with PSDs, and discuss the outcome of this and how the process might have been handled differently. The book has three key themes.

1. Using an eclectic approach will maximize our chances of successfully understanding and treating children with intractable speech difficulties. In the case studies we present of children with PSDs,

we typically use a psycholinguistic approach as a starting point in investigating the child's difficulties and then combine this with other perspectives.

2. Practitioners should carry out their intervention with strong and explicit theoretical underpinnings. Theory should drive our therapy, but in turn the results of the intervention should be used to inform our theory.
3. Evaluation of outcomes is essential and can be achieved in routine practice with minimal extra effort. Intelligibility and connected speech are key outcomes measures for children with PSDs.

There is a great need for intervention case studies, especially those that have school-age children with speech and literacy problems as their focus. Dorothy Bishop suggests:

> It is time for researchers to recognize that intervention studies are not just an optional, applied adjunct to experimental work, but that they provide the best method available for evaluating hypotheses and unconfounding correlated factors . . . Intervention studies . . . generate excitement.
>
> (Bishop, 1997a, p. 240)

There is a great deal to be gained from outcomes measurements for the individual client and therapist, and also for the profession and its knowledge base more generally.

In this book you will meet several children. The book was inspired by intervention that took place with school-age children with PSDs. The children and their difficulties, interventions and outcomes are referred to throughout this book. The children's names and identifying details have been changed, and parental permission has been obtained to publish their therapy stories.

Summary

This chapter has described the population of children that form the focus of the book: school-age children with persisting speech difficulties. The key points are as follows.

- PSDs are characteristic of children in their school years whose speech difficulties have not resolved.
- Core speech difficulties include difficulties with individual speech sounds and/or connected speech.
- Difficulties with literacy and psychosocial issues are common associated factors for these children.

- Children with persisting speech difficulties form a heterogeneous group.
- The group of children with PSDs may include children who have been given a diagnosis such as childhood apraxia of speech, or have a cleft-lip and palate, or whose speech difficulties are not linked to any identifiable condition or cause.
- Children with PSDs pose a challenge for practitioners and require long-term management.
- In order to maximize our chances of successful intervention, an eclectic approach to intervention may be the most helpful.
- A psycholinguistic approach can suggest what aspects of speech processing should be treated, while the linguistic (phonological) approach suggests how this should be done, i.e. what specific stimuli should be used.
- The management of psychosocial factors such as self-esteem is vitally important for these children.
- Medical and educational perspectives are also key aspects of the eclectic management approach.
- Intervention studies with children with PSDs are challenging, but important in adding to the evidence base.
- Evaluations of intervention should be done not only in research settings, but also in routine therapy situations where it can have important impacts on clients, therapist and the profession more generally.
- Access to effective intervention can contribute to positive long-term outcomes for children with PSDs.

KEY TO ACTIVITY 1.1

You may have written down some of the following words to describe persisting speech difficulties:

ongoing problems;
don't respond to intervention;
don't spontaneously resolve as child matures;
speech problems that occur regularly, i.e. not 'one-off' errors;
errors may be systematic rather than random;
help is needed to address the speech difficulties;
individuals cannot correct their own speech errors;
stuttering/stammering;
problems with specific speech sounds or words;
'mumbley' speech;
slurred speech.

You may have written down some of these points about identifying school-age children with PSDs:

avoidance behaviours/child is hesitant to speak in front of class;
child cannot correct his or her own speech errors;
child is shy and withdrawn;
child is reluctant to participate in group activities;
child's speech problems affect reading and spelling;
child's speech differs markedly from others in classroom;
other children draw attention to the child's speech.

KEY TO ACTIVITY 1.2

You may have written down some of the following as reasons for persisting speech difficulties:

The child hasn't had intervention (or cannot access intervention).
Parents or school staff do not recognize the problem or know what to do about it.
The child has:

- a hearing impairment
- cleft lip or palate
- learning difficulties
- emotional/psychiatric problems.

KEY TO ACTIVITY 1.3

You may have written down some of the following reasons that children are challenging for intervention researchers:

lack of cooperation especially in younger children;
if children have input problems they may not understand the task;
children change and grow all the time;
may lack motivation, especially if older child who has had a lot of therapy;
older children may be withdrawn or embarrassed;
intervention is complex. It's hard to pick apart what is bringing about change;
hard to know if children would have matured and got better anyway, without intervention.

Chapter 2
Theory, Therapy and Methodology

Working with children with persisting speech difficulties is a privilege, and also a great challenge. In order to maximize the success of our interventions with children with PSDs, we need to approach therapy in a logical way with a clearly thought-out and justifiable rationale for what we are doing. Schuell, Jenkins and Jimenez-Pabon (1964) note of speech and language therapy, 'A good therapist should never be taken unawares by the question: "Why are you doing this?"' (p. 333).

Although therapy might not always work as well as we hope, if we have a clear answer to the question 'Why are you doing this?' then we will be in a better position to revise our intervention and reconsider why the outcome may have been less than what was envisaged. For example, carrying out listening activities with a child with PSDs may seem strange to parents or teachers if the child has no known difficulties with hearing. A speech and language therapist might respond to the question 'Why are you doing this?' by suggesting that the child's speech problems are because he or she has stored inaccurate or fuzzy representations of words. Therapy aims to improve the accuracy of stored word knowledge as doing so may result in improved speech production. If the therapy results in improved speech production then the original hypothesis is confirmed. If therapy does not bring about the desired changes, then the hypothesis may need to be reconsidered. Working within an explicit theoretical framework helps us to answer the question 'Why are you doing this?' and to continually revise and reformulate hypotheses about a child's difficulties.

A psycholinguistic approach is one theoretical approach that we have found useful when working with children with PSDs. In Book 1, Stackhouse and Wells described the psycholinguistic approach as follows:

> [it] involves the use of a theoretical model of speech processing from which hypotheses are generated about the level of breakdown that

gives rise to disordered speech output. These hypotheses are then tested systematically . . .

(Stackhouse and Wells, 1997, p. 7)

The psycholinguistic approach needs to be combined with other approaches, such as linguistic, educational and psychosocial approaches, when working with children with PSDs. However, it is a useful starting point when working with these children. In this chapter we start by reviewing the psycholinguistic approach in order to give a framework by which to structure intervention. Every child is unique, and all children with PSDs have their own strengths and weaknesses. Intervention needs to be tailor-made to meet these needs. The psycholinguistic approach is not a programme or a package, but rather a way of thinking that a therapist can use to guide assessment and intervention.

While it is helpful to have access to an explicit theoretical framework and to actively use a hypothesis-forming and testing approach, practitioners working with children with PSDs do not need to reinvent the wheel each time. Evidence-based practice (EBP) is about looking at what others have done before and using information from such studies to guide our own decision making. This means considering how a particular intervention reported in the literature might be applied or adapted for use with an individual child. Consideration of the individual is central to EBP (Baker and McLeod, 2004). This book describes the interventions we carried out with children with PSDs. The aim is to share what was done with these children. Making sense of intervention studies is, however, not always easy. The second part of this chapter therefore introduces some methodological issues related to single-case studies. Terminology commonly used in intervention studies is introduced, and some intervention studies carried out with children with PSDs are presented. But first, let us explain the psycholinguistic framework further.

The Psycholinguistic Framework: A Review

Psycholinguistic approaches view children's speech and language problems as being derived from a breakdown at one or more levels of input, stored knowledge or linguistic output. In Figure 1.1 in Chapter 1 (page 4) we presented a simple speech processing chain showing these three key stages: input, stored lexical representations and output. Psycholinguistic models allow us to move away from mere observation and description of symptoms (e.g. a child produces /t/ for /k/) towards explanation in terms of underlying processing representations and mechanisms (e.g. a child produces /t/ for /k/ because he or she is not able to discriminate between the two sounds). The psycholinguistic approach uses assessment findings to provide explanatory accounts of different underlying strengths and weaknesses in children whose speech and language difficulties may appear superficially similar, thus dealing with the diversity of the population. Therapy that is designed to specifically target children's needs, taking into account their speech processing strengths and weaknesses, is more likely to be effective. In cases where it is minimally effective it will at least be possible to identify why, e.g. isolate the level of the speech processing system that intervention tasks were tapping, and make appropriate revisions.

Stackhouse and Wells introduced a psycholinguistic framework in Book 1 (1997) and Book 2 (2001) of this series. The framework comprises three parts:

- A speech processing profile
- A speech processing box-and-arrow model
- A developmental phase model

In the following sections we review each of these components.

The Speech Processing Profile

The speech processing profile is a practical tool for organizing data from an individual child's assessment. It is shown in Figure 2.1. We have included the simple model of the speech processing chain (from Figure 1.1) together with the profile to remind readers that the profile is based around this simple concept. A blank profile is presented in Appendix 1 for photocopying purposes. If you are not familiar with the speech processing profile at all, you should read Chapter 4 in Book 1 (Stackhouse and Wells, 1997).

The speech processing profile poses a series of questions, which allows data from assessments to be systematically organized into a summary profile of the child's strengths and weaknesses. The profile is organized around the simple speech processing chain presented in Figure 1.1, with questions related to input processing on the left (e.g. 'Can the child discriminate between real words?') and questions about output on the right-hand side of the profile (e.g. 'Can the child articulate real words accurately?'). More specifically, the levels of the profile ask the following questions.

Input Processing

Level A: Does the child have adequate auditory perception?

This level of the speech processing profile focuses on a child's hearing acuity or the ability to carry out non-speech discrimination tasks.

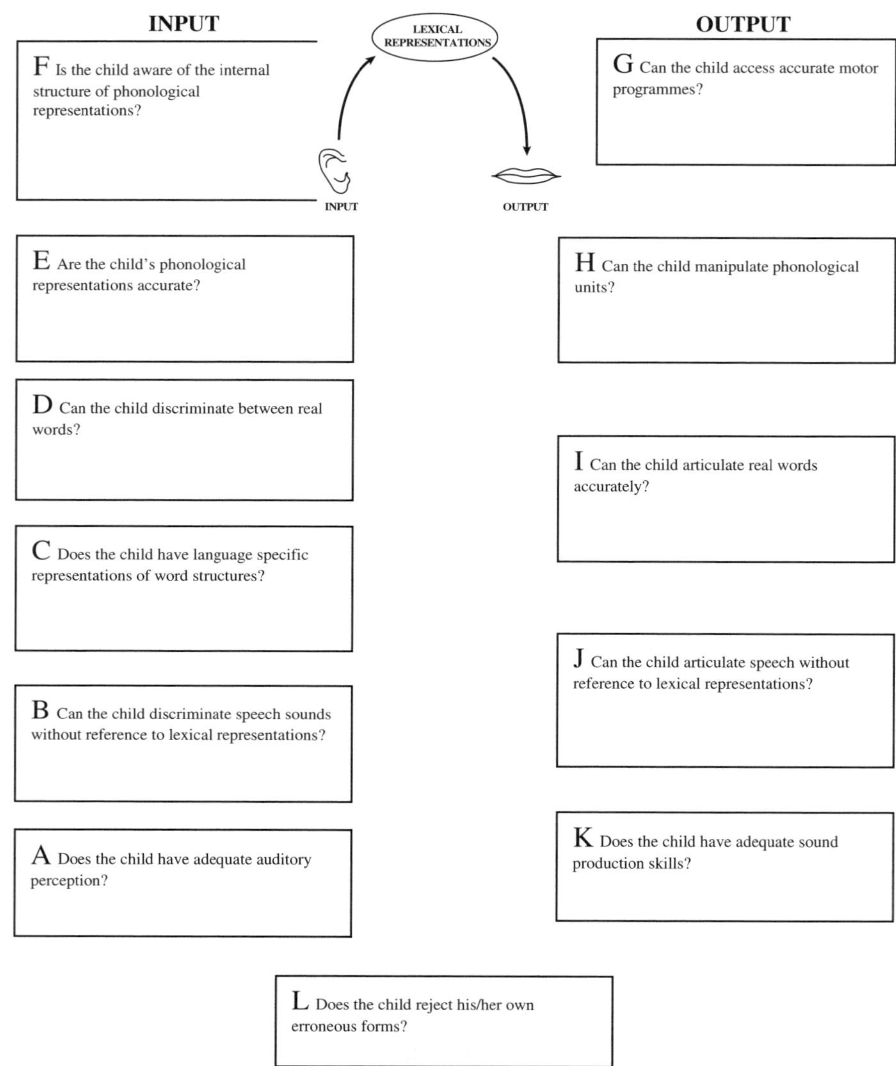
INPUT
LEXICAL REPRESENTATIONS
OUTPUT
F Is the child aware of the internal structure of phonological representations?
G Can the child access accurate motor programmes?
INPUT
OUTPUT
E Are the child's phonological representations accurate?
H Can the child manipulate phonological units?
D Can the child discriminate between real words?
I Can the child articulate real words accurately?
C Does the child have language specific representations of word structures?
J Can the child articulate speech without reference to lexical representations?
B Can the child discriminate speech sounds without reference to lexical representations?
K Does the child have adequate sound production skills?
A Does the child have adequate auditory perception?
L Does the child reject his/her own erroneous forms?

Figure 2.1: Speech processing profile (adapted from Stackhouse and Wells, 1997).

Level B: Can the child discriminate speech sounds without reference to lexical representations?

This level of the speech processing profile focuses on a child's ability to discriminate between non-words, e.g. a child might be asked to say whether there is a difference between pairs of words such as VOS and VOT. Unlike level A it does involve linguistic stimuli, although these are not familiar to the child.

Level C: Does the child have language specific representations of word structures?

This level of the speech processing profile is not routinely used with monolingual children. However, for bi- or multi-lingual children, the level would be used to determine whether the child is able to determine which words are legal or acceptable in a given language, e.g. a child might be asked to determine if words like BLICK and BNICK are legal words that one might find in English.

Level D: Can the child discriminate between real words?

This level of the speech processing profile focuses on a child's ability to discriminate between real words, e.g. a child might be asked to say whether there is a difference between pairs of words such as RATE and RACE. It involves linguistic stimuli that are familiar to the child.

Level E: Are the child's phonological representations accurate?

This level of the speech processing profile aims to determine whether the child has stored an accurate internal representation of a word. Tests at this level all involve a stimulus word spoken by the tester which is then matched to a picture. The child is asked to say whether the tester has said the word properly.

Level F: Is the child aware of the internal structure of phonological representations?

This level of speech processing is concerned with children's knowledge about their own stored phonological representations. All tests at this level do not involve the tester naming the items. The tests all involve pictures which will trigger the child's own phonological representation. Children might typically be asked to point to the 'odd-man out', i.e. a picture which does not rhyme with the others or starts with a different sound.

Output Processing

Level G: Can the child access accurate motor programs?

This level of the speech processing profile investigates whether the child has stored accurate motor programs for particular words. Picture naming tasks are often used at this level.

Level H: Can the child manipulate phonological units?

This level of the speech processing profile taps a child's ability to take a motor program and do something with it, i.e. manipulate it in a phonological awareness task. Tasks at this level will typically involve the tester giving the child the stimulus item (unlike Level G) and requiring, for example, the child to generate further words that rhyme with it.

Level I: Can the child articulate real words accurately?

This level of the speech processing profile investigates a child's ability to produce real words, without necessarily having to access their own stored representation of the words. This is most often done using a repetition format so that, unlike Level G, children can carry out this task without knowing what the words mean.

Level J: Can the child articulate speech without reference to lexical representations?

This level of the speech processing profile investigates a child's ability to repeat non-words, i.e. words that the child will not have produced before and cannot have any stored knowledge about.

Level K: Does the child have adequate sound production skills?

This level of the speech processing profile is concerned with a child's physical and functional motor execution abilities. It focuses on the child's physical capability to perform non-linguistic tasks, e.g. syllable repetition and oral–motor exercises.

Level L: Does the child reject his or her own erroneous forms?

This level of the speech processing profile taps children's own self-monitoring ability. It is not possible to formally test this level, but observations of children's responses to their own errors yield useful information about the 'feedback loop' we all have linking output and input processing.

It is important to note that the organization of the profile does not reflect hierarchical levels of difficulties, i.e. a level near the top of the profile (e.g. Level F) is not intrinsically harder than a lower level (e.g. Level B). Within each level, different tasks can be designed to tap into different levels of skills, i.e. discrimination of CVC words would be a fairly simple assessment task at Level D, whereas discrimination of multi-syllabic words would be more challenging within the same level. Many of the cases presented in this volume involved the collation of assessment data onto a speech processing profile, and this was then used in intervention planning and in some cases for evaluating intervention outcomes.

The speech processing profile can be used in a number of different ways. Typically, ticks (√) or crosses (x) are placed at appropriate levels of the profile. Ticks (√) are used to indicate that a child has performed in an age-appropriate way on a particular task. Crosses indicate that they have scored below the expected norm for their age, usually with one cross (X) indicating a score that is one or more standard deviations below the mean (average) for their age; two crosses (XX) indicating that the child performed more than two standard deviations below the mean for their age, and three crosses (XXX) indicating that the child scored more than three standard deviations below the mean for their age. Mean and standard deviation data are usually provided in the test manuals of published assessments. However, for some tests this information is not given and in that case a qualitative comment can be written in the appropriate box and used to yield a picture of the child's own relative strengths and weaknesses. In Book 1 of the series, appendices were presented listing assessments (both published and unpublished procedures) that tapped into the different levels of the profile. This list has been revised and updated for the current volume (see Appendix 2).

ACTIVITY 2.1

Aim: To revise the speech processing profile introduced in Stackhouse and Wells (1997) by interpreting a child's speech processing profile.

Nicholas is 7;4 and has PSDs. Look at Nicholas's speech processing profile presented in Figure 2.2. For each level of the profile, consider the type of assessments that might have been carried out, e.g. Level A: Audiometry. You may need to refer to Appendix 2 for help. Once you have considered each level of the profile, summarize Nicholas's areas of strength and areas of weakness. Now refer to the Key to Activity 2.1 at the end of this chapter to see what assessments we carried out with Nicholas to build his profile.

The Speech Processing Box-and-arrow Model

There are three broad aspects to speech and language processing: input, stored representations and output. These three essential components of speech and language processing were represented in the simple figure shown in Figure 1.1 from Stackhouse and Wells (1997) and shown in Figure 2.1 as they related to the speech processing profile. The psycholinguistic framework also contains a box-and-arrow model of speech processing. Stackhouse and Wells justify the need for such a model as follows:

> In order to have a greater understanding of children's speech and literacy difficulties from a psycholinguistic perspective, for research purposes, or to communicate with other professionals using a psycholinguistic approach, it is helpful to be more explicit about the levels of processing and processing routes that are being assumed by the

√ = age appropriate performance
X = 1 standard deviation below the expected mean for his age
XX = 2 standard deviations below the expected mean for his age

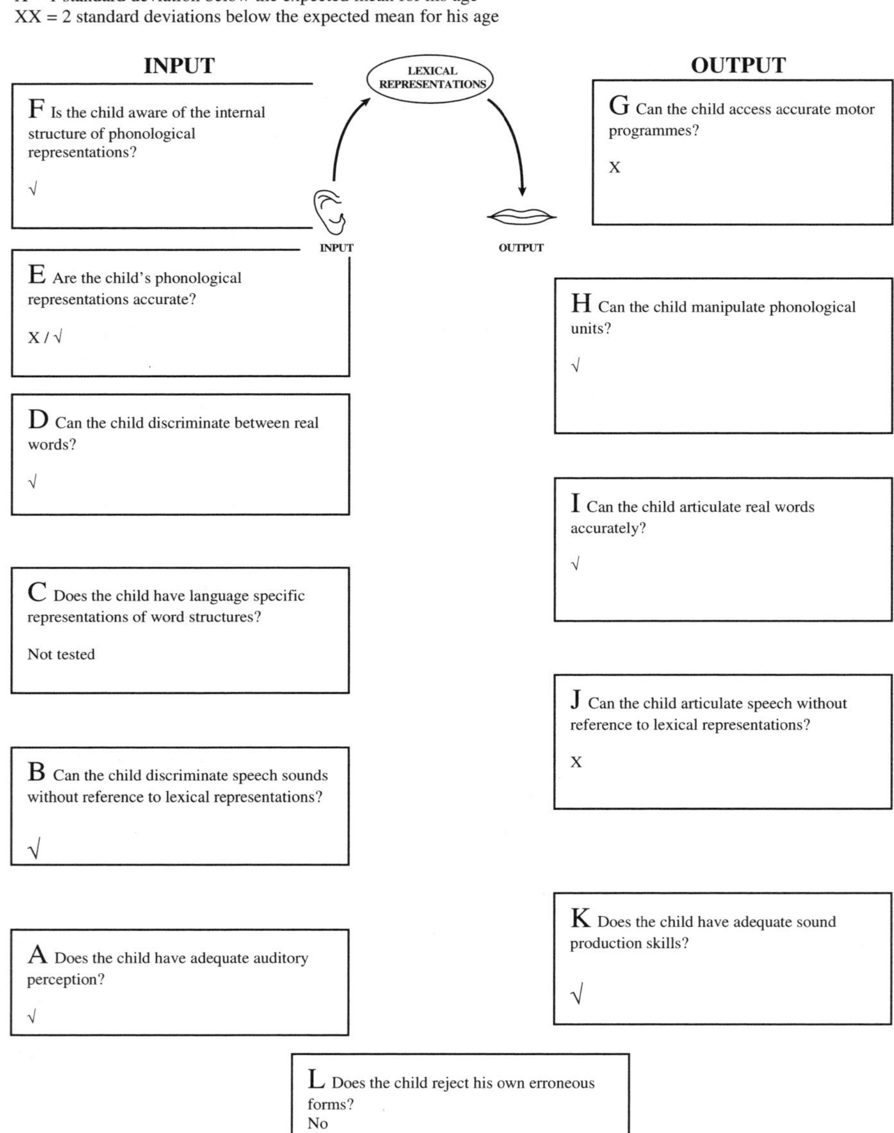

INPUT
LEXICAL REPRESENTATIONS
OUTPUT
F Is the child aware of the internal structure of phonological representations?
√
G Can the child access accurate motor programmes?
X
INPUT
OUTPUT
E Are the child's phonological representations accurate?
X / √
H Can the child manipulate phonological units?
√
D Can the child discriminate between real words?
√
I Can the child articulate real words accurately?
√
C Does the child have language specific representations of word structures?
Not tested
J Can the child articulate speech without reference to lexical representations?
X
B Can the child discriminate speech sounds without reference to lexical representations?
√
K Does the child have adequate sound production skills?
√
A Does the child have adequate auditory perception?
√
L Does the child reject his own erroneous forms?
No

Figure 2.2: Nicholas's speech processing profile at age 7;4.

> framework. The conventional way of representing levels of processing and routes between them is an information processing model in the form of a diagram consisting of boxes (levels of processing) and arrows (processing routes).
>
> (Stackhouse and Wells, 1997, p. 144)

This model, like other box-and-arrow models or information processing models, is a visual representation of the processes and components that are thought to be involved when children process and produce speech. Essentially, creators of box-and-arrow models take the simple speech processing chain, and develop it, breaking down each aspect, i.e. input, representations and output, into further levels usually based on observations and experimental evidence. The speech processing model from Stackhouse and Wells (1997) is presented in Figure 2.3, as well as Appendix 3 for photocopying purposes.

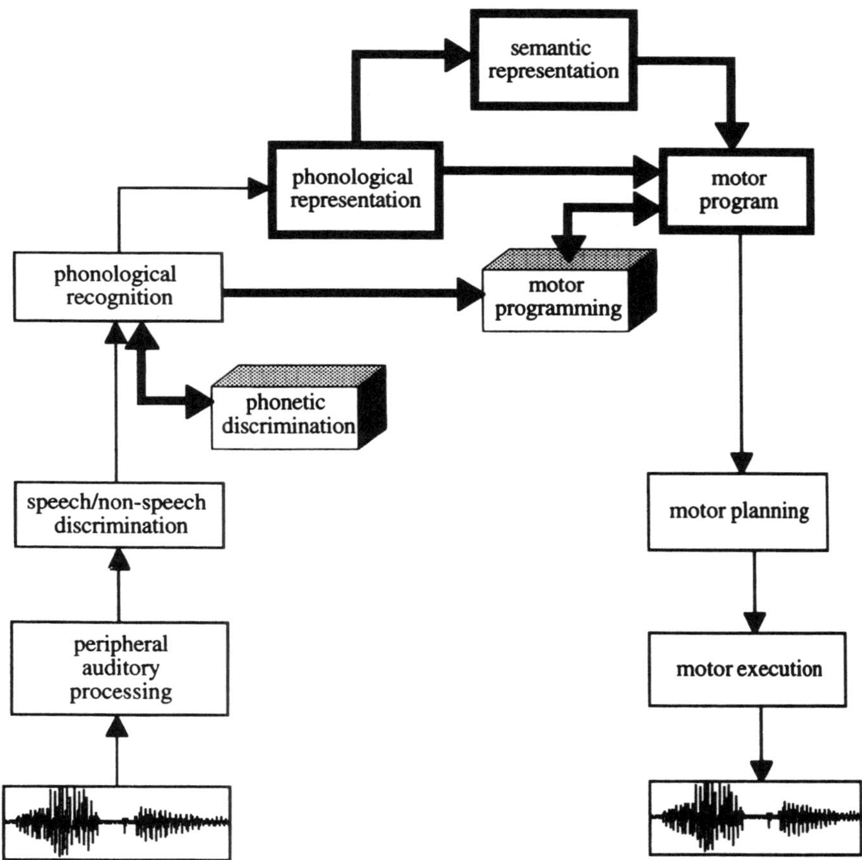

Figure 2.3: The speech processing model. (Reproduced by kind permission of Whurr Publishers from Stackhouse and Wells, 1997.)

In Book 1 of the series, the model shown in Figure 2.3 was built up gradually through reflection on the sub-processes involved in input processing, lexical representations and output processing. We provide a brief review of this information here, but readers are referred to Chapter 6 in Stackhouse and Wells (1997) for further details of the model and how it was devised. Plain boxes represent levels of processing, while those enclosed with a bold line represent stored knowledge. The shaded boxes – phonetic discrimination and motor programming – indicate 'off-line' processing. These boxes have a role to play in learning over time rather than in the 'on-line' processing of familiar input in real time. Similarly the bold arrows indicate the flow of knowledge between boxes as part of an ongoing learning process. Information processing models were originally used to help understand the speech and language processing of adults. Children differ from adults in that they are still learning language, and information processing models for children need to take that into account. Let us consider each of the processing levels on the model (i.e. the boxes) in turn.

Input Processing

Peripheral auditory processing

This level represents general auditory ability not specific to speech. This level would usually be tapped by means of hearing tests. It is the lowest level of the input side and is represented in the simple speech processing model by the ear.

Speech/non-speech discrimination

This level of processing represents normally developing children's ability to separate out speech input from other input, and then carry out further processing on the speech signal using the speech processing system. Most children we work with are able to do this perfectly well, but some children, e.g. those with acquired language difficulties following a road traffic accident or convulsions, maintain their hearing acuity but are unable to distinguish between speech and environmental noises.

Phonological recognition

The child has separated out speech input from other sounds. The next step in the processing chain is distinguishing between the child's own language/s and other languages. If English-speaking children receive input in English then through this level of processing they will recognize that further processing needs to occur. If the language is unknown to the children, then no further processing will take place, unless of course they are trying to learn a new language.

Phonetic discrimination

This shaded box indicates off-line processing. It indicates that phonetic processing can be drawn on as needed when circumstances demand. A typical case when it might be used is when processing unfamiliar accents. In order to understand speakers with different accents, an English-speaking child will need to draw on phonetic discrimination abilities much broader than those required by his or her own accent (see Nathan, Wells and Donlan, 1998, for further discussion of the development of children's accent processing).

Lexical representations

From a young age children store a great deal of information about words: knowledge of the word's sound structure (phonological knowledge); information about a word's meaning (semantic knowledge), grammatical knowledge (e.g. how to change a singular word such as CAT or FOOT into a plural form like CATS and FEET) and later, orthographic knowledge (e.g. that /kæt/ is spelt <cat> and /jɒt/ is spelt <yacht>. An underlying representation captures information stored about words that a child knows. Psycholinguistic models of information processing must account for lexical processing in some way. Chiat (2000, p. 15) notes, 'Each word . . . is a phonological-semantic-syntactic complex. To know words is to have stored such complexes in our minds, in what is termed our mental vocabulary or lexicon.'

Stackhouse and Wells (1997) describe early lexical representations as consisting of three essential parts: semantic information, a phonological (input) representation and a motor program (output representation). These are shown in Figure 2.3 with the bold boxes indicating that they are bodies of knowledge built up over time. As children develop, their knowledge of words expands to contain grammatical and orthographic information. Grammatical and orthographic representation stores do not yet appear in Figure 2.3 but are considered an important part of lexical knowledge. Pages 157–8 in Book 1 (Stackhouse and Wells, 1997) cover the content of lexical representations in greater detail.

Phonological representation

A phonological representation is the stored knowledge of the sound structure of a word. For a word to be correctly identified from spoken input, the appropriate phonological representation must be accessed. The representation must contain enough information for a specific word to be distinguished from other related items (e.g. CROWN as opposed to CLOWN), but at the same time it should not be so specific that the production of

CROWN by a range of speakers with different accents and voices would not be recognized.

Research into phonological acquisition has long been concerned with understanding the nature of children's underlying representations (e.g. see Dinnsen, O'Connor and Gierut, 2001). While it is certain that the lexicon in childhood is a dynamic entity, what is less certain is the nature of representations within the lexicon and the way in which these change over time. The term phonological lexicon is used to refer to a store (or dictionary) of phonological representations. Many theorists assume that the word or lexeme is the storage unit of the phonological lexicon (Treiman and Baron, 1981; Jusczyk, 1986; Waterson, 1987; Ingram and Ingram, 2001), but there may be some evidence for syllables (Ferguson and Farwell, 1975; Levelt, 1989, 1999; Gierut, 1999), or smaller units as the fundamental structure that is stored. Furthermore, the nature of children's representations is likely to be changing over time as development takes place. The lexical restructuring model proposed by Metsala and Walley (1998) claims that children's lexical representations are initially holistic (i.e. words) but gradually become more segmental (i.e. broken into segments) as more words are acquired. According to this model, children differentiate their earliest words based on overall phonetic shape rather than at a segmental level. As the lexicon grows the holistic representations are not sufficient for distinguishing between all words, and children must necessarily turn their attention to fine-grained phonetic detail.

Semantic representation

The semantic representation is the stored knowledge of the meaning of words. For example if asked to think of an animal that is hairy, has four legs and can bark most people would think of DOG. They have accessed their semantic knowledge of the word DOG. If asked to describe a CAT, you might use words like FURRY, PET, MAMMAL, MIAOWS, WHISKERS. Again, you would be drawing on your semantic representation of that particular word.

Motor programs

The motor program for a word consists of a series of gestural targets for the articulators, i.e. tongue, lips, soft palate, vocal folds. This is like a template for production that is designed to achieve an acceptable pronunciation of a word, one that is compatible with the phonological representation.

Output Processing

Motor programming

This level of processing is responsible for the creation of new motor programs. In our review of the lexical representation in the previous section, we described aspects of stored knowledge about words. One of the aspects of stored knowledge was that of the motor program – but how was that 'template' of gestural targets devised in the first place? Motor programming is called upon when speakers have to produce new words for the first time. It appears in Figure 2.3 as a shaded box because, as for phonetic discrimination, this box will not be needed if the child is producing familiar words that already have a stored motor program. Models such as Stackhouse and Wells' differentiate between online processing at a given moment in time, and also in terms of a child's general competence built up over time. Thus, for example in Figure 2.3 it can be seen how there are links between input and output representations. But, the model also accounts for how motor programs come to exist as stored representations. The online motor programming device creates new motor programs based on input. The model is thus able to account for repetition of non-words at a sub-lexical level, as well as children's learning of new words and production of familiar words.

Children give us ample opportunity to observe the different processing routes involving stored motor programs and online motor programming. This can account for variability in some children's speech when one compares their production of target words in therapy (i.e. the words have been produced online and in isolation using a phonological plan), and the same words spoken spontaneously in connected speech where they revert to a stored routine that reflects realization rules from an earlier phase of development. Our intervention with Joshua, CA 7;2 focused on his production of consonant clusters (see Chapters 5 and 6 of this volume). We were delighted to hear him using a new motor program for the word GLOVE, and producing it as [glʊv] in a picture naming game, which gave him ample opportunity for online production of a new motor program. However, towards the end of the session he told a story about events that had taken place at playtime earlier that day, and how he had lost his [gʊv]. In the spontaneous speech he reverted to his own stored, and inaccurate, representation of that word.

Motor planning

Once a motor program has been retrieved or created, it is now assembled for 'real-world' production bearing in mind the contextual influences that will affect production. While the motor program is a template or blueprint for how to say the word in an ideal world, motor planning involves processing for realization in the real-world. Pronunciation is influenced by how quickly the word or utterance is spoken; the intonation and rhythm that is used; the volume or emotion associated with the word; the influence of neighbouring sounds and words. This is the level of processing at which slips of the tongue can occur in otherwise normal speakers.

Hewlett's (1990) model provides an alternative conceptualization of motor planning. This speech processing model specifies two distinct levels of motor planning rather than the one described by Stackhouse and Wells (1997). Hewlett terms these 'motor processing' modules but the description of the modules is very similar to what is envisaged in Stackhouse and Wells's (1997) motor planning. Hewlett differentiates between his two boxes, with the one being 'motor processing at a syllabic level', followed at a lower level by 'motor processing at a segmental level'. Hewlett (1990, p. 31) notes:

> The task of the Motor Processing component is to assemble the motor plan of the sequence of gestures involved in pronouncing the word, and determine the precise values of the articulatory parameters involved. The output from the Motor Processing component contains all the information required to achieve the actual muscular contractions (motor execution).

The division of motor processing into the syllable and segmental level comes from a developmental perspective since it is thought that during development of motor control and when learning new words, there is more reliance at a syllable level. Later, more emphasis is placed on a segmental level. Hewlett conceptualizes a great deal of feedback taking place between each of the levels of output, so that if there is sufficient awareness of difficulties at a particular level of processing, then subtle modifications can be made to increase speech production accuracy. This model is a useful one particularly when focusing on levels of speech output and the interplay between phonetics and phonology.

Motor execution

This is the lowest level of the output side and represented in the simple speech processing model by the mouth. This level represents the vocal tract and its physical role in producing speech. If there are anatomical or functional difficulties with any part of the vocal tract then the execution of speech may be problematic, e.g. as in the case of cleft lip and palate. Motor execution gives rise to an acoustic signal of speech, and completes the speech processing chain.

The Developmental Phase Model

Box-and-arrow models are a useful way of looking at children's speech processing. In the previous section, we have seen how Stackhouse and Wells's psycholinguistic model conceptualizes children's speech processing and how some of the boxes and arrows indicate processing that

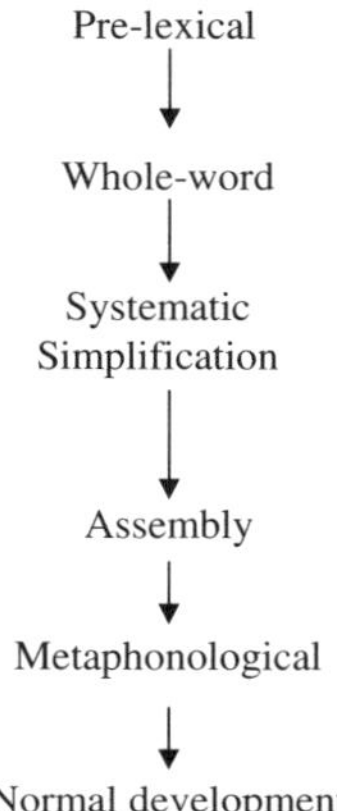

Figure 2.4: The developmental phase model. (Reproduced by kind permission of Whurr Publishers from Stackhouse and Wells, 1997.)

happens developmentally over time rather than at a specific moment in time. The third element of the psycholinguistic framework is the developmental phase model. This model outlines phases in the normal development of children's speech. It is presented in Figure 2.4.

The developmental phase model shows the phases that characterize children's speech. In the first year of a normally-developing child's life they will be in a pre-lexical phase: the elements of the speech processing system, i.e. input, stored representations and output, are coming together but the child has yet to produce recognizable speech. The next phase of development is the whole-word phase in which single words predominate during the second year of life. This is then followed by a systematic simplification phase in which phonological simplification processes are exhibited. We know that processes such as cluster reduction, fronting and stopping are characteristic of the speech of young normally-developing children and that most of them soon grow out of this phase. The assembly phase involves 'bringing it all together' with single words incorporated into connected speech and used to achieve a range of communicative ends. The metaphonological phase follows at early school-age. It is one in which children develop the ability to reflect on their own speech, and to manipulate and understand their own language in a more abstract way.

Difficulties can occur at any of the phases outlined in the developmental phase model. Potential difficulties linked to specific phases are shown in Figure 2.5.

If the individual components of a child's speech processing system, i.e. input, stored representations and output, do not come together in the

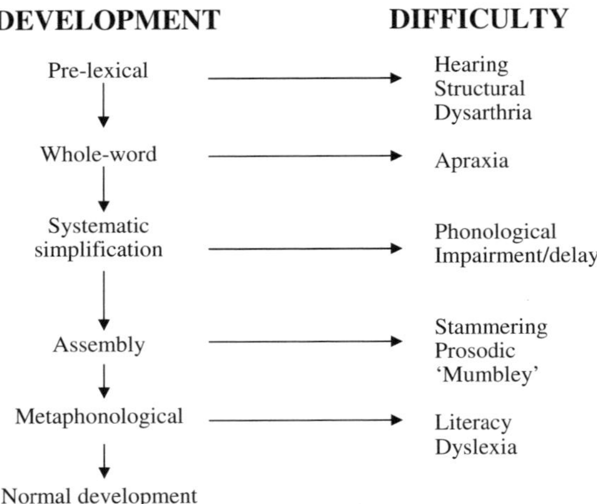

Figure 2.5: A developmental phase perspective on speech difficulties.

first stage of development in the normal way, difficulties at the pre-lexical level will be noted. These may include hearing impairment, structural difficulties such as cleft lip and palate, or dysarthria. Development becomes arrested for some children at the whole-word phase. These children may have problems with accurately storing and accessing motor programs for words. Such difficulties may be associated with apraxia. Some children do not move through the systematic simplification phase with the same ease as their normally-developing peers. These children may experience phonological impairment or phonological delays. The next phase of development is the assembly phase where children are required to bring together all aspects of their speech for successful communication. Some children will experience difficulties here with dysfluency, prosodic difficulties or simply sounding unclear and 'mumbley'. Children who experience difficulties with the metaphonological phase will find it hard to reflect on the sounds comprising their speech. These difficulties may give rise to literacy difficulties or dyslexia. Of course, it is possible for a child to become arrested at an early stage of development and present with marked delays in the skills associated with all successive phases when compared to their peers, e.g. consider some school-age children with PSDs who are described as 'apraxic', 'dyslexic' and 'mumbley'.

The phase model is an important component of the psycholinguistic framework since it is truly developmental in its perspective. Children's difficulties can be accounted for in terms of arrested development at a particular phase: a useful approach since this allows practitioners to move away from a deficit-based model and consider constructively how best to help children move forward to the next phase of development. The developmental phase model is probably the element of the Stackhouse and Wells framework that has been used least by practitioners and researchers. It has important perspectives to offer on children with PSDs and we refer to it as appropriate in our intervention cases.

The Psycholinguistic Approach to Intervention

Now that we have revised the three key elements of the psycholinguistic framework, let us consider the use of the psycholinguistic framework in therapy. A psycholinguistic understanding of assessment and therapy tasks is important if we are to confidently answer the question 'Why are you doing this?' Task analysis is vital in carrying out and interpreting assessment and intervention. In Books 1 and 2 of the series, the authors devoted chapters to the questions 'What do tests really test?' (see Chapters 2 and 3 in Book 1, Stackhouse and Wells, 1997) and 'What do tasks really tap?' (see Chapter 3, Book 2, Stackhouse and Wells, 2001) emphasizing the importance of these issues. Through a psycholinguistic approach we are able to maximize intervention success and isolate the level of the speech processing system that therapy tasks are tapping, then make appropriate revisions.

Rees (2001b, Volume 2 of the series) refers to tasks as being made up of materials, procedures, feedback and optionally the use of specific techniques. This can be written as an equation as follows:

TASK = Materials + Procedure + Feedback (+ Technique)

Materials might include pictures of stimuli and puppets. Procedures might include getting the child to listen and make judgments about the puppets' naming of the pictures. Feedback might entail stickers and verbal praise for correct judgments, while incorrect judgments would give opportunity for discussion and information-giving on a puppet's performance and another chance to listen. Specific techniques might involve the use of visual cueing, or using an amplifier to ensure that the stimuli are more clearly heard. Rees's way of analysing what is taking place at any given moment in intervention helps us to answer the question: 'Why are you doing this?' Further to Rees's suggestions for task analysis, one should be able to state which levels of the speech processing system are being tapped at any given time, and how this fits in with the overall plan for intervention. This type of analysis is the focus of Activity 2.2.

ACTIVITY 2.2

Aim:

1. To revise the task analysis presented in Book 2 ('What do tasks really tap?').
2. To reflect on the way in which this precise approach can improve our understanding of intervention, as well as our ability to carry out and communicate research.

Consider the simple intervention task that was carried out with Simon. Simon, aged 10;11 was asked to gather together some of his favourite toys from the therapy room. Each toy then had a turn to participate in a quiz. The therapist turned over a picture and the toy produced a word to describe that picture. Simon was required to judge whether the toy's production of the word was accurate or not. The stimuli used were single words containing /k/ and /g/ in word-initial position, e.g. CURL, GIRL, CARD, GUARD, COAT, GOAT. The therapist named some of the items correctly and for others produced the inappropriate minimal pair, e.g. saying 'curl' for GIRL, and 'goat' for COAT. If Simon judged the toy's production as accurate he was able to place a sticker on the toy. If the toy's production was inappropriate for the given picture, he was to throw the toy into a bin, and the toy was given a second chance in the quiz show later on in the session. The therapist gave verbal praise to Simon for correct judgments, and where incorrect judgments were made he was asked to listen again to an exaggerated production and encouraged to reflect on what he had heard. In some cases, Simon did not know whether the toy had been correct or not. He was reminded of earlier work that had been done on the concepts of 'noisy' and 'quiet' and given the opportunity to make his own productions and feel whether or not his larynx vibrated.

(a) Describe the task further in terms of the following formula

TASK = Materials + Procedure + Feedback (+ Technique)

(b) What aspects of the speech processing model (Figure 2.3) are being tapped?

(c) Given that this is an intervention task, suggest ways in which Simon's responses might be managed, i.e.
- If the task is easy for him, how might the task be made more challenging?
- If the task is too hard for him, how might he be supported to achieve success?

Compare your responses to the answers in Key to Activity 2.2 at the end of this chapter.

Methods in Intervention Studies

Approaches to intervention studies vary widely, from randomized control trials (RCTs) involving hundreds of participants to single case studies that focus in-depth on one child and his/her response to a specific intervention. RCTs are studies involving relatively large numbers of participants who are randomly assigned into two groups: one group receives a particular treatment or therapy, and another group receives no treatment. Assigning participants at random reduces the risk of bias (i.e. where individuals are aware that they are being treated and change in anticipation of the treatment) and increases the probability that differences between the groups can be attributed to the treatment.

There are relatively few RCTS that have been carried out in the field of speech and language therapy, and even fewer with children with speech difficulties. The randomized control trial carried out by Almost and Rosenbaum (1998) is one of the few to specifically address therapy for children with phonological difficulties, although it focused on preschoolers rather than school-aged children with PSDs. Thirty children with severe phonological disorders were randomly assigned to two treatment groups. Group 1 received treatment for four months followed by four months without treatment, while group 2 underwent four months without treatment followed by four months of treatment. The children were seen individually twice weekly for half hour sessions. A range of outcome measures were used to evaluate any changes in their speech. The term 'outcome measures' refers to assessments or measurements used to evaluate any changes arising as a result of intervention. Outcome measures are sometimes specifically created for a particular child, e.g. lists of words that relate to their difficulties and what is being treated in intervention. Standardized tests can also be used. Other indices of change commonly used for speech are measures such as percentage of consonants correct (PCC) in which a count is made of the child's accurate productions divided by the number of opportunities for consonant production.

In Almost and Rosenbaum's study outcome measures included a standardised test, the *Goldman-Fristoe Test of Articulation* (Goldman, Fristoe and Woodcock, 1972) and the speech severity index of percentage consonants correct (PCC) for single words and connected speech. Group 1 showed significant differences in phonological measures after the first four months of the study when they received treatment, when compared to Group 2, the untreated group of children. Following the eight-month assessment both groups had improved significantly from baseline in terms of their speech production. The severity index for conversational speech continued to be significantly different, with children in Group 1 scoring higher than those in Group 2. It was suggested that children in the earlier treatment group had had longer to generalize the new speech sounds into their connected speech. The expressive language measure (mean length of utterance or MLU) did not detect a difference between groups at any time suggesting that the benefits of phonological therapy were specific to speech and had no significant impact on language.

While RCTs have been described as the gold standard of intervention research, they are not without problems. Speech and language intervention is clearly very different from prescribing medication for an illness! Indeed, RCTs are well suited to medical studies in which participants are given active medication or placebos, but it is considerably more difficult to control for the effects of therapy. What exactly does the therapy entail? Who is delivering it? What are tasks really tapping? What else is going on in the child's environment, e.g. home and school, that might affect the outcome. Some studies have used terms like 'traditional articulation therapy' and 'phonological awareness therapy' to describe the interventions carried out. These labels can mean many different things depending on the nature of the tasks given and the stimuli used. In the RCT carried out by Glogowska, Roulstone, Enderby and Peters (2000) the effectiveness of speech and language therapy provision for pre-schoolers was evaluated. Although results suggested no significant difference between the children who received provision and those in a 'watchful-waiting' group, it is clear from the study that the amount and nature of intervention varied widely from child to child. As we do not know what intervention was taking place with which particular children, the RCT gives us an impression of the ineffectiveness of service provision generally but not of any specific intervention. This point is returned to in later chapters, but for now the key message is that RCTs are just one approach to intervention research and one that may not always be the most useful in providing the information that is needed on speech and language interventions (see Pring, 2004 and 2005 for further discussion of this point).

Robey and Schultz (1998) describe a five-phase outcome research model that we refer to throughout this book. It provides a step-by-step method for developing a treatment and testing its value. Specific research designs are appropriate for each phase in the model. Progression through the phases must occur in a sequential way with each phase building on the findings from the previous one. The first phase is about 'discovery', developing hypotheses about intervention to be tested in later phases. Single case study designs are appropriate at this level. In phase II single subject designs remain appropriate, but are used to more systematically investigate and review efficacy: does the intervention work in optimal circumstances? In phases III, effectiveness in real-life settings is evaluated. It is at Phases II and III at which many speech interventions take place. This is entirely appropriate given the relative youth of the profession. Pring in a paper entitled 'Ask a silly question: Two decades of troublesome trials' notes:

> Researchers in speech and language therapy have given too little attention to the basics of clinical outcome research. This requires that clinical and theoretical insights are used to identify specific therapies for well-defined groups of clients. These therapies must be tested first in efficacy, then in effectiveness studies, and their results should be disseminated to practitioners. Only then is it meaningful to carry out large-scale trials of the effectiveness of therapy provision for a client group or to conduct systematic reviews of existing research.
>
> (Pring, 2004, p. 285)

We need a great many more single case studies to give a solid foundation from which to move on to other aspects of Robey and Schultz's framework. Single subject designs or single case studies can be defined as studies in which intervention given to one, or a small number of participants, is considered in great detail in terms of the individual response to that intervention. Single case reports can be descriptive, simply outlining what took place with a specific child. Experimental single case designs are our focus here, since these will have specific research questions and be set up in such a way as to provide answers to them. In experimental case studies there will also be clear independent and dependent variables. A specific therapy is usually the independent variable and the dependent variable the outcome measure used to assess change.

The single-case methodology has been widely advocated by authors (such as Barlow and Hersen, 1984; Hegde, 1985; Howard, 1986; Attanasio, 1994; Enderby and Emerson, 1995; Seron, 1997; Millard, 1998; Adams, 2001) who suggest it is the method of choice for clinical sciences involving intensive interaction, such as speech and language therapy. This approach solves the problem of widely different participants in that subjects serve as their own control and treatment can be tailormade to their specific needs. By varying aspects such as the time treatment commenced, or the type of treatment given, it may be possible to identify change as being due to specific intervention, rather than the effects of treatment in general, or of external factors and maturation. The strength of single case and small group studies is in the detail of particular approaches to treatment. While results of case studies cannot be generalized to other cases, they have a role in establishing methods of treatment that can then be examined in larger scale studies (Adams, 2001). Single case research lacks the power associated with larger studies and randomized control trials, but such studies provide valuable information and have been widely used to explore the nature of individual difficulties, motivations for therapists' intervention and the effects of that intervention. In the following section we review some single case study research.

Children with PSDs: A Review of Single Case Studies

We carried out a literature search for intervention studies published in peer-review journals in which a single case methodology was used. In particular we looked for studies in which participants were school-age children aged 5 years or older, and in which these children's speech, language or literacy difficulties were addressed. We found 12 papers which met our criteria (see Appendix at the end of this chapter (pp. 60–1) for full details of the studies). Many investigations were found which (a) did not have an intervention component, or (b) were carried out with adults or younger children. The earliest papers that met the search criteria were from the early 1990s (e.g. Bryan and Howard, 1992; Broom and Doctor 1995a, b) with a steady increase of papers to the present time. Typically these studies focused on one child, with a participant mean age of 7;9 years. The paper by Spooner (2002) focused on two children, while Stiegler and Hoffman's (2001) work extended to three children, and Best (2005) carried out intervention with a case series of five children. As we have seen from the definition given above for single case studies, the term does not necessarily mean that only one child is studied, but rather that all children are treated as individuals in their own right and data are not pooled or averaged across cases.

The children in these studies experienced a full range of difficulties with many showing complex combinations of deficits, e.g. the child described by Crosbie and Dodd (2001) had severe speech and language difficulties affecting both input and output. The studies typically begin with a section devoted to investigation of the child's underlying difficulties, providing detailed information about the child's strengths and weaknesses. It is vital that this is done so that those reviewing the evidence and wishing to use it as a basis for their own evidence-based practice, can make decisions about whether it is appropriate for their particular client. An overview of participant characteristics in each of the papers is presented in Table 2.1.

The studies used a range of different theoretical models to guide their interventions, with some of these stated more explicitly and adhered to more closely than others. Developmental models such as those of Chiat (2000) and Stackhouse and Wells (1997) seemed to dominate in the more recent studies. These models developed specifically for use with children can be contrasted with some of the models borrowed from adult cognitive neuropsychology and adapted for work with children (e.g. Shallice, 1987; Ellis and Young, 1988; Rapp and Carramazza, 1991; Goldrick and Rapp, 2002). Bishop (1997b) cautions that such models may not be appropriate for use with the developmental group. Few of the papers gave an explicit

Table 2.1: Single-case interventions for school-age children: Participant characteristics

Author/s	N =	Ages (years)	Sex	Participants' main difficulties
Best (2005)	5	6	M	Word-finding difficulties
		8	F	
		9	F	
		9	F	
		10	M	
Broom and Doctor (1995a)	1	11	M	Surface dyslexia
Broom and Doctor (1995b)	1	11	M	Phonological dyslexia
Bryan and Howard (1992)	1	5	M	Deviant speech production and delayed vocabulary
Crosbie and Dodd (2001)	1	7	F	Severe language disorder
Gibbon and Wood (2003)	1	8	M	Longstanding articulation disorder
Norbury and Chiat (2000)	1	8	M	Specific language impairment and weak phonological skills
Pantelemidou, Herman and Thomas (2003)	1	8	F	Hearing impairment
Pascoe, Stackhouse and Wells (2005)	1	6	F	Unintelligible speech
Spooner (2002)	2	6	F	Severe expressive and receptive language delays
		9	F	
Stiegler and Hoffman (2001)	3	9	M	Word-finding difficulties
		9	M	
		9	M	
Waters, Hawkes and Burnett (1998)	1	5	M	Unintelligible speech

rationale for using a particular model, with the exception of Broom and Doctor (1995a, b), Norbury and Chiat (2000) and Best (2005). Many of the studies seemed to be attracted mainly by the clinical utility afforded by the models, e.g. the Stackhouse and Wells (1997) framework allows for explicit consideration of a child's strengths and weaknesses, which was important in the work described by Waters *et al.* (1998) and Pascoe *et al.* (2005).

Single case studies do not necessarily need to make explicit mention of the theoretical models employed – although we suggest that it can be helpful for readers if they do, and also helpful to those carrying out the study in evaluating and modifying intervention. Many of the studies introduced models that were used in combination to develop a rationale for intervention (e.g. Bryan and Howard, 1992; Broom and Doctor, 1995a, b). Other studies aimed to explicitly test out a particular model of language processing, for example Norbury and Chiat (2000) tested assumptions underlying Plaut's (1996) connectionist model. The studies by Spooner (2002) and Stiegler and Hoffman (2001) were studies that were carried out in the spirit of psycholinguistics, alluding to theoretical models rather than applying them explicitly or testing them through intervention. The studies by Gibbon and Wood (2003) and Pantelemidou, Herman and Thomas (2003) used instrumentation, in both cases electropalatography (EPG), to promote changes in their participants' speech, relying on more descriptive, linguistic approaches.

The children in the studies showed a range of difficulties and these were addressed using a variety of approaches. It is essential for single case studies to give clear and detailed descriptions of the intervention that took place, e.g.

- What stimuli were used, and why?
- How much intervention took place?
- Who delivered the intervention?

Outcome measures (i.e. the way in which success was measured) should also be clearly defined. Many studies will have a range of success indicators or outcomes measures. The term primary outcome measure refers to the key assessment or area used to evaluate outcome.

Single case interventions should be described in enough detail so that others reading the study would be able to replicate it. In Table 2.2 we summarize the intervention given in each of the studies, the primary outcome measures and the result. It can be seen that all the interventions were successful in achieving significant improvements in their primary outcomes measure. This is not surprising since many authors do not submit unsuccessful interventions for publication, and some editors are hesitant to publish interventions with negative results. Nevertheless

Table 2.2: Single-case interventions for school-age children: Interventions, outcomes and results

Study	Intervention	Primary outcome measure	Result
Best (2005)	A computerized aid to promote word-finding skills	Picture naming of single words	Significant improvement for all children
Broom and Doctor (1995a)	Reading: linking visual code and meaning	Reading of single words	Improvement on reading of treated words
Broom and Doctor (1995b)	Reading: building up phoneme–grapheme correspondence	Reading of single words	Significant improvement in phonological reading with generalization to untreated items, and an overall change in reading strategy
Bryan and Howard (1992)	Input tasks to shape phonological representations e.g. same/ different judgments and phoneme identification approach	Picture naming and repetition	Significant progress with real word speech production
Crosbie and Dodd (2001)	Input training: auditory discrimination using real and non-words	Real and non-word discrimination	Auditory discrimination improved, but gains did not generalize to other language processes
Gibbon and Wood (2003)	Electropalatography (EPG) focused on velar production	Velar production in single word speech	Significant progress in use of velars in single words

Table 2.2: *Continued*

Study	Intervention	Primary outcome measure	Result
Norbury and Chiat (2000)	Semantic intervention – making explicit links between orthography and meaning	Reading of single words	Reading improved for treated target words
Pantelemidou, Herman and Thomas (2003)	Electropalatography (EPG) focused on production of /k/ in single words	/k/ production in single word speech	Significant progress in use of /k/ in single words
Pascoe, Stackhouse and Wells (2005)	Minimal pair work focusing on final consonant production; Connected speech work using graded sentences	Single word and connected speech production of final consonants	Significant progress in use of final consonants in single word and connected speech
Spooner (2002)	Picture-based semantic therapy involving listening and production	Sentence production	Children made progress in the structure and content of their expressive language
Stiegler and Hoffman (2001)	Discourse contextual approach, e.g. narratives and story retelling	Overt word-finding behaviours in conversational speech	Overt word-finding behaviours decreased
Waters, Hawkes and Burnett (1998)	Input processing using a variety of listening and speaking tasks	Picture naming and spontaneous speech	Significant improvement in speech production

we suggest that studies that do not have positive outcomes can be extremely illuminating and are an important part of the evidence-base that should be shared.

Five of the studies in our review were concerned specifically with speech production (Bryan and Howard, 1992; Waters *et al.*, 1998; Gibbon and Wood, 2003; Pantelemidou *et al.*, 2003; Pascoe *et al.*, 2005). While Bryan and Howard worked on output (to improve output), Waters *et al.* (1998) focused on input as a means to improving output (see also the chapter by Daphne Waters in Stackhouse and Wells, 2001). Pascoe *et al.* (2005) worked on both single words and connected speech, and also evaluated changes occurring in the child's spelling of these words.

Both EPG studies (Gibbon and Wood, 2003; Pantelemidou *et al.*, 2003) focused on production of velars, and both demonstrated success in children who had made slow progress with other forms of therapy. Crosbie and Dodd (2001) addressed input and hoped to improve this aspect of speech processing (rather than speech production itself). Their intervention too was successful. The studies by Best (2005), Stiegler and Hoffman (2001) and Spooner (2002) were concerned with broader aspects of language processing. Best (2005), and Stiegler and Hoffman (2001) addressed word-finding difficulties, while Spooner focused on improving grammar. Three of the studies focused on remediation of reading difficulties (Broom and Doctor, 1995a, b; Norbury and Chiat, 2000).

All of the studies gave sufficient detail to enable replication. However, dosage, or amount of intervention, was one area in which full information was not always found. For example, many of the studies gave an indication of therapy frequency but not of the total duration of the child's involvement. This remains an important yet unresolved area in intervention research, and information about dosage must be considered as vital in intervention studies. Issues surrounding dosage are discussed further in Chapter 13. In terms of outcomes measures, most of the studies addressed the impairment level with a range of specific outcomes measures employed, and designed to be sensitive to the child/children in question (e.g. see Crosbie and Dodd, 2001). Standardized tests were sometimes used as a measure of more global functioning, e.g. Norbury and Chiat (2000) and Spooner (2002). Few socially valid measures were incorporated beyond the impairment level, e.g. self-esteem indicators. However, Waters *et al.* (1998) provided subjective insights into the improved behaviour of their participant, and Best (2005) gave a questionnaire to the participants in her study to ascertain their views about the therapy.

Intervention researchers often get asked the question, 'How do you know that the changes observed in the child are due to your intervention, and not something else, e.g. classroom environment, maturation of child?' It is a difficult question to answer, but controlling for as many other external variables as possible can make answering it a little easier. Let us consider how the studies we reviewed controlled for factors beyond their interventions. Broom and Doctor (1995a, b) employed a rigorous design using multiple baselines, and repeated pre- and post-therapy measures. Multiple-baseline designs are ones in which treatments are introduced in a stepped fashion. A simple design would start from a baseline point and then introduce treatment and observe the effects of this. A multiple baseline design starts by introducing treatment A (e.g. work on CV words), and observing its effect on the outcome measure of interest. Then treatment B is introduced (e.g. working on CVC words), and its effects observed, then treatment C is introduced (working on CCVC words) and so on. This gives the opportunity to repeatedly demonstrate the effects of an intervention, and also show the cumulative effects of interventions on related aspects of speech.

All the studies opted for designs which compared results before and after intervention (pre- and post-intervention design). The studies included control measures so that the authors could state with relative confidence that the results seen were due to the specific effects of intervention. Typically such control measures included incorporation of an unrelated language processing task, e.g. syntactic complexity as measured by MLU, so that it could be demonstrated that general developmental improvements were not responsible for the outcomes observed (e.g. Bryan and Howard, 1992; Crosbie and Dodd, 2001). Some of the studies attempted to achieve a stable baseline prior to intervention, either through carrying out specific assessments (Broom and Doctor, 1995a, b; Best, 2005; Pascoe *et al.*, 2005) or through documenting the child's earlier history of intervention and its outcomes (e.g. Gibbon and Wood, 2003). If it can be shown that the child was not improving on the selected outcomes measures prior to intervention starting, then there is good evidence that any changes observed post-intervention are due to the intervention. Long-term follow-up after a period with no intervention is also useful in demonstrating where children have maintained any gains made in therapy, e.g. as described in the study by Norbury and Chiat (2000). In many single case studies the person carrying out the intervention is also the person carrying out the assessments. Ideally, assessments should be carried out by a neutral third party so that there are no opportunities for bias. This is not always practical. As a compromise some studies use more than one rater to transcribe and score speech data. Where this is done, inter-rater reliability – the agreement between the two raters – can be calculated using statistical procedures.

In terms of generalization, studies were evaluated by noting the following.

(a) Across-item generalization. Whether generalization occurred from treated stimuli (i.e. the words or phrases worked on in intervention) to untreated items. The untreated items are usually matched to the treated items. They are similar words to the ones addressed in therapy but have not been used in intervention.
(b) Across-task generalization. Whether generalization has extended from the task treated in intervention (e.g. speech production of a particular set of words) to related tasks not specifically addressed in intervention (e.g. spelling of the same set of words).

While all the studies showed positive outcomes, generalization varied widely between them. Some studies did not achieve any significant generalization (e.g. Broom and Doctor, 1995a; Norbury and Chiat, 2000). Many of the studies were able to show across-item generalization, e.g. untreated word lists improved in the studies of Broom and Doctor (1995b), Crosbie and Dodd (2001), Spooner (2002) and Stiegler and Hoffman (2001). The studies by Bryan and Howard (1992), Waters *et al.* (1998) and Pascoe *et al.* (2005) were the most successful in terms of generalization, since they could demonstrate both across-item generalization as well as across-task generalization. In Bryan and Howard's study, the child's speech production as well as his auditory discrimination had improved beyond chance levels. Waters *et al.*'s child improved in terms of his speech production as well as his phonological awareness and literacy. The child described by Pascoe *et al.* (2005) improved in both her speech and her spelling. Table 2.3 summarizes the studies by design, controls and generalization observed.

We have described a small group of studies that have carried out specific interventions with school-aged children with persisting difficulties. Such studies have demonstrated the efficacy of intervention with each of the studies reporting positive results. Clearly there is a great need for further studies to be done, either replicating what has already been done or using other approaches to intervention. We need a large body of quality evidence as the first stage in the development of an outcomes database. The final activity in this chapter focuses on critical reviews of intervention studies.

Table 2.3: Single case interventions for school-age children: Design, controls and generalization

Author/s	Design	Controls	Generalization
Best (2005)	Pre- and post-therapy assessment	Unrelated language processing tasks Achieved stable baseline Long term follow-up	Across-item generalization (for two children) Across-task generalization for one child (reading)
Broom and Doctor (1995a)	Multiple-baseline design with repeated pre- and post-therapy assessment	Unrelated language processing task Achieved stable baseline	Not significant
Broom and Doctor (1995b)	Multiple-baseline design with repeated pre- and post-therapy assessment	Unrelated language processing task	Across-item generalization
Bryan and Howard (1992)	Pre- and post-therapy assessment	Unrelated language processing task	Across-item generalization Across-task generalization (for related language processing task)
Crosbie and Dodd (2001)	Pre- and post-therapy assessment	Unrelated language processing task Achieved stable baseline	Across-item generalization

Gibbon and Wood (2003)	Pre- and post-therapy assessment	Detailed history data prior to intervention Long-term follow-up post-intervention	Across-item generalization Across-task generalization (from single word speech to connected speech)
Norbury and Chiat (2000)	Pre- and post-therapy assessment	Long-term follow-up Unrelated language processing task	Not significant
Pantelemidou, Herman and Thomas (2003)	Pre- and post-therapy assessment	Detailed history data prior to intervention Long-term follow-up post-intervention	Across-item generalization
Pascoe, Stackhouse and Wells (2005)	Pre- and post-therapy assessment	Achieved stable baseline Long-term follow up Unrelated language tasks	Across-item generalization Across-task generalization (from speech to spelling)
Spooner (2002)	Pre- and post-therapy measures	None	Across-item generalization
Stiegler and Hoffman (2001)	Multiple baseline design with pre- and post-therapy measures	None	Across-item generalization
Waters, Hawkes and Burnett (1998)	Pre- and post-therapy measures	None	Across-item generalization Across-task generalization (for related language processing task)

ACTIVITY 2.3

Aim: To critically evaluate an intervention study.

Find and read one of the intervention case studies described in our review (listed in the appendix at the end of this chapter), or select another case study that you have read or want to read. Use the Critical Evaluation template below to structure your evaluation of the article and the evidence it presents about intervention. It may be helpful to carry out this activity with someone else or as a group activity. The template is also included in Appendix 4 at the end of the book for photocopying purposes.

Critical evaluation template

Title: Authors: Journal: Publication Date:	
Participant(s) details	
Theoretical framework used	
Research questions	
Intervention, e.g. tasks, dosage, stimuli	
Design	
Outcome measures used	
Changes noted in outcome measures	
Generalization observed	
Controls employed, e.g. stable baseline, inter-rater reliability; long-term follow-up	
Other Comments: Main messages	

Summary

This chapter has aimed to review the psycholinguistic framework, as well as related theoretical and methodological issues. The key points in this chapter are as follows.

- Working within an explicit theoretical framework helps us to answer the question: 'Why are you doing this?' and to continually revise and reformulate hypotheses about a child's difficulties.
- A psycholinguistic approach is one theoretical approach that we have found useful when working with children with PSDs.
- There are three key elements to the psycholinguistic framework introduced in Books 1 and 2 of this series: the speech processing profile, the speech processing model and the developmental phase model.
- The speech processing profile is a practical tool that can be used to organize assessment data into appropriate processing levels.
- The speech processing model is a box-and-arrow model that shows how children's speech processing can be conceptualized.
- The developmental phase model shows the phases through which children need to pass in order to develop normal speech processing skills.
- The psycholinguistic framework enables us to be specific about 'what tests are really testing' in assessment tasks.
- It can also be used to describe 'what tasks are really tapping' enabling us to better understand how our intervention is affecting the speech processing system.
- There are different methodological approaches that can be used in intervention studies.
- Randomized control trials are large-scale studies in which groups of clients and their responses to an intervention are contrasted.
- Single-case studies are smaller intervention studies in which one child (or a small number of children) are considered in terms of their own individual changes to intervention.
- There is a great need for more single-case research since this is the first stage in the hierarchical process of evidence building.
- Single-case studies should provide detail of the participant and his/her difficulties so that others can decide whether the intervention would be appropriate for their own clients.
- Intervention should be described in sufficient detail to enable replication to take place.
- Outcomes measures are the assessments, indices or evaluations used to determine whether intervention has brought about changes.
- Intervention studies need to employ some control measures to ensure that any changes observed can be attributed to the therapy.

KEY TO ACTIVITY 2.1

Nicholas's speech processing profile with the specific tests carried out at each level

√ = age-appropriate performance
X = 1 standard deviation below the expected mean for his age
XX = 2 standard deviations below the expected mean for his age

INPUT

F Is the child aware of the internal structure of phonological representations?
√ - PhAB picture alliteration subtest (supplementary test; examiner does not name pictures) (Frederikson *et al.*, 1997)
Obtained 100% on sorting tasks in which he was required to sort pictures by initial segments

E Are the child's phonological representations accurate?
X - Auditory lexical decision task (Constable *et al.*, 1997)

D Can the child discriminate between real words?
√ – Real word discrimination test (Bridgeman and Snowling, 1988)
√ - Aston index discrimination subtest (Newton and Thompson, 1982)
√- PhAB alliteration subtest (Frederikson *et al.*, 1997)
√ - Auditory discrimination test (Wepman and Reynolds, 1987)
√ - Auditory discrimination of own errors

C Does the child have language specific representations of word structures?

Not tested

B Can the child discriminate speech sounds without reference to lexical representations?
√ – Non-word discrimination test (Bridgeman and Snowling, 1988)

A Does the child have adequate auditory perception?
√ - audiometry

OUTPUT

G Can the child access accurate motor programmes?
X – Single word naming test (Constable *et al.*, 1997)
X – Word-finding vocabulary test (Renfrew, 1995)
X – Edinburgh articulation test (Anthony *et al.*, 1971)
XX – The Bus Story (Renfrew, 1969)

H Can the child manipulate phonological units?
√ - PhAB spoonerism subtest (Frederikson *et al.*, 1997)
√ - PAT rhyme fluency subtest (Muter *et al.*, 1997)

I Can the child articulate real words accurately?
X – Real word repetition subtest (Constable *et al.*, 1997)
√ - Aston index blending subtest – real Words (Newton and Thompson, 1982)

J Can the child articulate speech without reference to lexical representations?
X – Aston index blending subtest – nonwords (Newton and Thompson, 1982)
X – Non-word repetition subtest (Constable *et al.*, 1997)

K Does the child have adequate sound production skills?
Stimulable for all sounds
Oro-motor assessment (Nuffield Dyspraxia Programme, Williams and Stephens, 2004) – lateralizes /s/ on occasion

L Does the child reject his own erroneous forms?
No (based on observation)

Comments on Nicholas's speech processing profile

Nicholas has more difficulties with output than with input. Within each of the different levels, Nicholas performed variably: his difficulties were often item-specific rather than being a general problem with a particular level of processing.

Strengths

In terms of input, Nicholas has strengths towards the lower part of the profile: he performed in an age-appropriate way on all real word (Level D) and non-word (Level B) auditory discrimination tasks. His phonological representations (Level E) were found to be generally accurate - a relative strength - although for some of the longer, less familiar words they were less clear. He has knowledge of the internal structure of phonological representations of CVC and CCVC words, as tested by sorting tasks (Level F).

Weaknesses

Nicholas had widespread difficulties on the output side of the profile. These were weighted to the top of the profile as Nicholas had adequate lower level sound production skills (Level K), although he lateralizes [s] on occasion. He produces consistent speech errors in his repetition (Levels I, J) and naming (Level G). Nicholas's speech errors are generally like those of a younger child rather than being unusual or symptomatic of deviant development. His speech delay is in line with his language levels and cognitive skills. Longer words that Nicholas found hard to recognize on the Constable *et al.* (1997) auditory lexical task (Level E), e.g. ESCALATOR, were also harder for him to produce in an accurate way (Level G) suggesting that he has inaccurate phonological representations and thus motor programs for these items.

KEY TO ACTIVITY 2.2

(a) *Materials*: Toys, stickers, picture cards, bin.
Procedure: Each toy 'names' a picture. Simon is the judge of their success and is required to listen carefully to the toy's production and then either reward or dismiss the toy.
Feedback: If Simon inappropriately rewarded or dismissed a toy, the therapist cautioned him to listen carefully and repeated the toy's attempts in an exaggerated fashion.
Technique: When Simon had difficulty in discerning what was right and what was wrong. He was encouraged to name the picture and feel whether or not his larynx was vibrating to produce the noisy [g] or quiet [k].

(b) In terms of the speech processing model (Figure 2.3) what aspects are being tapped? Simon is presented with both visual and auditory information about the stimulus. Looking at the picture he is able to access semantic information and associated phonological information about the word, e.g. he recognizes that it's a picture of an animal, namely a GOAT, and has top-down access to his own phonological representation of GOAT. At the same time, he uses bottom-up auditory processing to make sense of what the therapist has said. He then needs to compare whether the therapist's production of the target matches his own phonological representation.

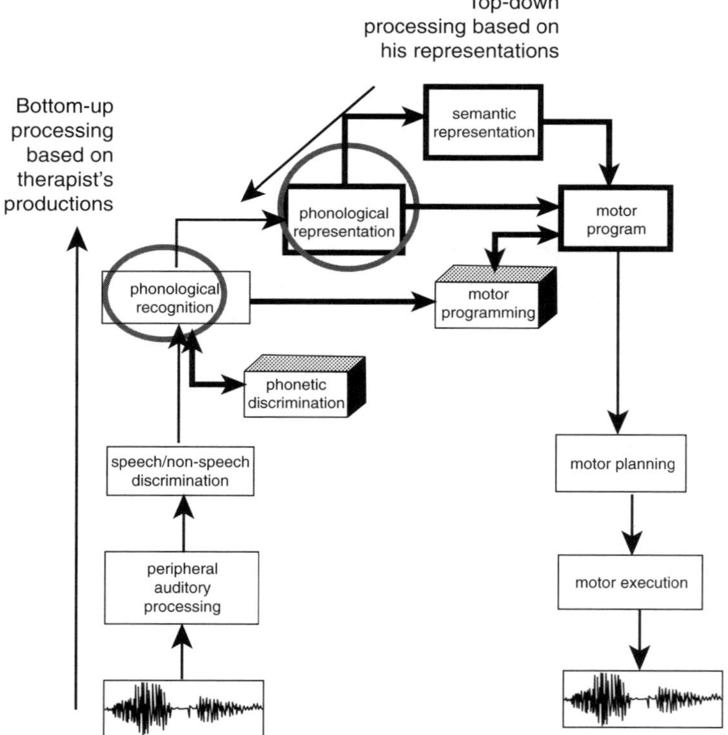

(c) The task could be made more challenging by using longer words (e.g. CARRIAGE, GARAGE); words with k/g in different word positions (e.g. word finally such as LOG, LOCK), or placing the words into sentences, e.g. She loves her GOAT/COAT. If the task had been too hard for Simon, it might have been made easier by getting him to listen to amplified speech, using written symbols to convey the difference between the words or having him place his hand on the therapist's larynx as she (or the toy) produced the word. On the other hand one might have reduced the phonetic complexity and number of words used, e.g. using only CV minimal pairs and just one pair to begin with.

Appendix of Papers Reviewed in this Chapter

Best, W. (2005) Investigation of a new intervention for children with word-finding problems. *International Journal of Language and Communication Disorders*, **40**(3), 279-318.

Broom, Y. and Doctor, E. (1995a) Developmental phonological dyslexia: A case study of the efficacy of a remediation programme. *Cognitive Neuropsychology*, **12**(7), 725-66.

Broom, Y. and Doctor, E. (1995b) Developmental surface dyslexia: A case study of the efficacy of a remediation programme. *Cognitive Neuropsychology*, **12**(1), 69-110.

Bryan, A. and Howard, D. (1992) Frozen phonology thawed: The analysis and remediation of a developmental disorder of real word phonology. *European Journal of Disorders of Communication*, **27**, 343-65.

Crosbie, S. and Dodd, B. (2001) Training auditory discrimination: A single case study. *Child Language Teaching and Therapy*, **17**(3), 173-94.

Gibbon, F. and Wood, S. (2003) Using electropalatography (EPG) to diagnose and treat articulation disorders associated with mild cerebral palsy: A case study. *Clinical Linguistics and Phonetics,* **17**, 365-74.

Norbury, C. F. and Chiat, S. (2000) Semantic intervention to support word recognition: A single-case study. *Child Language Teaching and Therapy*, **16**(2), 141-63.

Pantelemidou, V., Herman, R. and Thomas, J. (2003) Efficacy of speech intervention using electropalatography with a cochlear implant user. *Clinical Linguistics and Phonetics*, **17**, 383-92.

Pascoe, M., Stackhouse, J. and Wells, B. (2005) Phonological therapy within a psycholinguistic framework: Promoting change in a child with persisting speech difficulties. *International Journal of Language and Communication Disorders*, **40**, 189-220.

Spooner, L. (2002) Addressing expressive language disorder in children who also have severe receptive language disorder: A psycholinguistic approach. *Child Language Teaching and Therapy*, **18**(3), 289-313.

Stiegler, L. and Hoffman, P. (2001) Discourse-based intervention for word-finding in children. *Journal of Communication Disorders*, **34**(4), 277-304.

Waters, D., Hawkes, C. and Burnett, E. (1998) Targeting speech processing strengths to facilitate pronunciation change. *International Journal of Language and Communication Disorders*, **33**, 469-74.

Chapter 3
Stimuli Design: Segments in Single Words

The design and selection of appropriate stimuli for phonological intervention is an important issue. Stackhouse and Wells emphasize the importance of careful stimuli selection:

> The psycholinguistic framework . . . does not constitute a fixed and immutable set of procedures, and thus differs from a test battery. It suggests a way of thinking about, and organizing, tests and assessments that practitioners use – tests that are available in the public domain . . . and also assessments devised by the practitioner to meet the specific needs of a child.
>
> (Stackhouse and Wells, 1997, p. 307)

Time spent on appropriate stimuli selection is time well spent in intervention planning, particularly for children with PSDs. This chapter focuses on questions commonly asked when planning therapy such as the following.

- What level of stimuli will be addressed in intervention? Single sounds, single words or phrases may all be considered.
- Which specific single sounds / single words / phrases will be used in intervention?
- How many single sounds / single words / phrases will be used in intervention?
- What other factors need to be taken into account when compiling stimuli wordlists?

Chapters 1 and 2 of this book emphasized the importance of having an explicit theoretical rationale to account for what we do in therapy. The same applies for stimuli selection. Although our choices might not always result in the most effective intervention, if we have based our choices on a clear theoretical rationale, then we will be in a better position to return to our original hypothesis and revise our decisions. The ultimate aim of intervention is to encourage generalization throughout the speech processing system, and careful selection of targets may maximize the generalization achieved, ultimately increasing the efficiency of intervention.

This chapter starts with the level of segments, focusing on how these might be selected and incorporated into single words. In the first part we review approaches to stimuli design and selection, illustrating these with examples from research where possible. Stimuli selection within a psycholinguistic framework is the focus of the second part of the chapter. In the third section of the chapter we consider some do's and don'ts for best practice in the stimuli design and selection of segments in single words. In Chapter 4 we present a detailed intervention case which illustrates the approach we took with one child with PSDs. Generalization is the central focus of Chapter 9, but this chapter will introduce some of the key principles developed later in that chapter.

Approaches to Stimuli Design and Selection

Stimuli design and selection issues are controversial. This section explores what is known about target selection for intervention. Much has been written about stimuli selection in phonological therapy from a variety of perspectives. These perspectives typically include:

- a developmental perspective;
- a productive phonological knowledge or complexity perspective;
- a functional perspective;
- a systemic perspective.

Let us now consider each of these approaches in turn.

A Developmental Perspective

Stimuli design and selection is often based on a developmental perspective. The focus is on looking at the normal developmental sequence of sound acquisition and moving the child forward in a normal sequence of development. It is presumed that sounds acquired first are easier for children to master, and it seems quite logical to presume that children with difficulties should be taken through the hierarchy from easy sounds to harder ones. Grunwell (1987) grouped the segments of English into developmental stages, broadly delineated time periods in which children with normally-developing speech typically acquire the segments. These developmental norms are frequently used as guidelines for intervention planning. Table 3.1 outlines Grunwell's profile of phonological development.

Therapists using a developmental approach are likely to consider the child's current phonetic inventory, possibly circling the segments which

Table 3.1: Developmental phonological norms (Reproduced by kind permission of Grunwell, 1987)

Stage	Consonants	Processes	
Stage I (0;9–1;6)	LABIAL LINGUAL NASAL PLOSIVE FRICATIVE APPROXIMANT	*First Words* tend to show: - individual variation in consonants used; - phonetic variability in pronunciations; - all simplifying processes applicable.	
Stage II (1;6–2;0)	m n p b t d w	Reduplication Consonant Harmony FINAL CONSONANT DELETION CLUSTER REDUCTION	FRONTING of velars STOPPING GLIDING /r/ → [w] CONTEXT SENSITIVE VOICING
Stage III (2;0–2;6)	m n (ŋ) p b t d (k g) w h	Final Consonant Deletion CLUSTER REDUCTION	{FRONTING of velars} STOPPING GLIDING /r/ → [w] CONTEXT SENSITIVE VOICING

Stage	Segments		
Stage IV (2;6–3;0)	m n ŋ p b t d k g	Final Consonant Deletion CLUSTER REDUCTION	STOPPING /v ð z ʧ ʤ/ /θ/ → [f] FRONTING /ʃ/ → [s] GLIDING /r/ → [w] Context Sensitive Voicing
Stage V (3;0–3;6)	f s j h w (l)	Clusters appear: obs. + approx. used; /s/ clusters may occur	STOPPING /v ð/ (/z/) /θ/ → [f] FRONTING of /ʧ ʤ ʃ/ GLIDING /r/ → [w]
Stage VI (4;0–4;6) (3;6–4;0)	m ŋ p b t d ʧ ʤ k g f v s z ʃ h w l (r) j	Clusters established: obs. + approx.: approx. 'immature' /s/ clusters: /s/ → FRICATIVE obs. + approx. acceptable /s/ clusters: /s/ → type FRICATIVE	/θ/ → [ŋ] /ð/ → [d] or [v] (PALATALISATION of /ʧ ʤ ʃ/) GLIDING /r/ → [w]
Stage VII (4;6<)	m n ŋ p b t d ʧ ʤ k g f v θ ð s z ʃ ʒ h w l r j	(/θ/ → [ŋ]) (/ð/ → [d] or [v]) (/r/ → [w] or [ʋ])	

the child has acquired in Table 3.1 or the processes which appear to dominate the child's speech. The therapist might conclude that a particular child is currently at Stage V since he or she has most (but not all) of the segments expected by this level, and the processes outlined at that level are still predominating. Intervention needs to consolidate the child's skills at Stage V, and then move him or her forward into Stage VI. Selecting intervention targets would involve considering which sounds are missing from the child's current phonetic inventory and addressing these in intervention. The missing sounds would be sounds that are not yet acquired at Stage V, for example the child in question has yet to acquire /f/ or /h/. A slightly different approach would be to address the main processes characterizing a particular stage, although it is likely that the information from the phonetic inventory would also need to be used to supplement the process data. Rees (2001a) gives the example of a child who has not yet developed fricatives. She is realizing most fricatives as homorganic plosives, e.g. FOUR is realized as [pɔ], and SUN is realized as [tʌn], while most other aspects of the child's phonology are age-appropriate. In this case, a therapist, guided by developmental norms, might well choose to work on the process of stopping.

The age bands associated with Grunwell's stages remind us that normally-developing children will have mastered the basic sound system of their language by the age of approximately 5 years. Indeed, Lynch and Fox (1980) suggest that by age 3 children should be between 75% and 100% intelligible to their parents. For children with PSDs these milestones of normal communication may be achieved at far later ages - or in some cases, never at all. Nevertheless, developmental norms such as Grunwell's are useful when working with children with PSDs in reminding us of the sequence of normal development irrespective of the ages attached to each stage. Grunwell's norms apply to British children, but for readers in other countries, alternative sets of norms may also be available. Sharynne McLeod (2002) has compiled a set of norms for the typical development of speech in a variety of countries around the world and from a variety of theoretical perspectives.[1] These can be useful references to guide stimuli selection for intervention.

The principle of normal phonological development can be applied in other ways. Hodson and Paden (1991) devised a cycles approach to therapy. The cyclical approach to intervention involves a small set of carefully selected error sounds being targeted in therapy in a way which closely resembles the way in which children naturally acquire speech sounds. Target sounds (or processes) are individually addressed in terms of both input and output, in a successive way with each of the targets worked on for a limited amount of time before moving on to another target. When all targets have been addressed, the cycle begins again and continues for as many rotations as needed until a given segment has been acquired, at which point it drops out of the cycle. In this way, the child is exposed to more than one isolated sound over the course of intervention and has the opportunity for making rapid progress with some sounds and slower progress with more challenging targets. This type of approach may be particularly useful when working with children with severe and persisting difficulties.

Hodson (1997) describes four children, aged 3;6 to 5;11 and the way in which their targets were selected for their cycles intervention. She notes that the primary potential target patterns for beginning cycles for highly unintelligible children include:

- early developing patterns;
- anterior/posterior contrasts;
- /s/ clusters (see Chapters 5 and 6 of this book);
- liquids.

Early developing patterns might include:

- 'Syllableness', i.e. working on utterances restricted to monosyllables and working towards more appropriate 2 and 3 syllable targets. For example, Michael (aged 3;6) was noted to occasionally duplicate syllables but could not yet sequence varied syllables. Therefore being able to sequence two syllables was his first target pattern in the first cycle of intervention.
- CV, i.e. consonant vowel structures if the child is only producing V or VC structures. A typical target might be an initial labial in a CV structure such as MY. For example, Tim (aged 5;0) was found to be omitting word-initial voiceless obstruents, including stops. His first target in the first cycle of intervention was producing voiceless prevocalic obstruents.
- VC where final C is lacking. A typical target might include final /p/, /t/ or /k/, or final /m/ or /n/ if these are lacking. For example, Alan (aged 5;11) lacked word endings. Production of voiceless final stops became his first intervention target.

Hodson and Paden's (1991) cycles approach to therapy uses developmental perspectives to aid in stimuli selection, but it is an approach that has strong elements of our other stimuli selection categories, e.g. it is also a functional approach and a systemic approach. Practitioners will typically use more than just one approach to stimuli selection. Powell (1991) outlined 21 factors which affect target selection for therapy. Stimulability is one of these factors and is defined as the degree to which a misarticulated sound can be articulated correctly (Hodson, 1997). If children can physically produce a particular sound not normally used in their speech, e.g.

they can produce it when given specific instructions and modelling, it is described as stimulable. Stimulability is described by Elbert as 'an enduring concept . . . [that has] withstood the effects of time' (1997, p. 54). Indeed, it is a concept that most practitioners today will be familiar with, but that is also referred to in some of the earliest literature on speech difficulties. Some research evidence suggests that non-stimulable sounds, i.e. sounds which a child cannot physically produce, require direct treatment, but that stimulable sounds, i.e. the sounds that they can produce with support even if they do not normally appear in the phonological repertoire, may be acquired without direct treatment. In a traditional approach to target selection, sounds that are stimulable are chosen first because they are thought to be easier for the child to learn (e.g. Hodson and Paden, 1991). However, Miccio and Elbert (1996) have suggested the selection of non-stimulable targets since these are not likely to be spontaneously acquired and are therefore a greater priority for intervention.

ACTIVITY 3.1

Powell (1991) outlined 21 factors which need to be taken into account in the process of selecting targets for intervention with children with speech difficulties. We have already discussed stimulability. What do you think the other 20 factors might include? Write down your ideas, and then compare these with Powell's suggestions included at the end of this chapter in the Key to Activity 3.1.

Although the children described by authors such as Hodson (1997) and Miccio and Elbert (1996) are younger than children with PSDs discussed in this volume, the principles used to select their targets are still relevant. In general, the principles behind Hodson and Paden's cycles approach are developmental ones. They suggest that for normally-developing children phonological acquisition is a gradual process that comes about primarily through listening to the sound patterns of one's language. The cycles approach to intervention aims to replicate this approach in intervention with a focus on listening activities and exposure to a range of sounds and sound patterns that characterize the ambient language.

However, there are some problems with the developmental approach to target selection for children with PSDs. The use of developmental norms is based on the assumption that normally-developing children pass through a sequence of stages in their acquisition of sounds, and that acquisition of earlier sounds is a prerequisite for acquisition of later-developing sounds. Children with PSDs may not, however, be destined to follow the normal developmental sequence. Their difficulties may constitute more than a simple delay, with an entirely different path of acquisition taking place. Their difficulties are likely to be more severe and qualitatively different to those of younger children evidencing phonological lags in relation to their peers. If children with PSDs are inherently different to children with phonological delays, then it may be that they are not following a developmental sequence, and one might ask whether it is still logical to adhere to the developmental norms. Lof (2004) suggests that stimuli selection is not quite as simple as pulling out a set of norms and using these to determine what is worked on in therapy. Of Powell's (1991) 21 factors that need to be taken into account when considering stimuli or target selection, just three of these were related to developmental norms:

- the age of the child;
- the age-appropriateness of the child's errors;
- normative sequence of development;

Clearly these are important considerations - but they are not the only considerations. Let us now move on to other approaches useful in target selection.

Productive Phonological Knowledge or 'Complexity'

Developmental approaches to stimuli selection suggest that a child is slowly moved up the ladder of phonological development from lower rungs to more lofty heights. However, some authors have adopted the opposite approach suggesting that the lofty heights of later-acquired targets should be the immediate focus. These authors, unlike those who advocate a developmental approach, are assuming that earlier segments are not prerequisites for the acquisition of later segments, and therefore that children with speech sound difficulties do not necessarily need to follow one fixed route in their phonological acquisition. Such approaches are sometimes referred to as complexity accounts because they favour the targeting of more complex targets. This may at first seem counter-intuitive. However, the approach has been devised to maximize treatment efficacy, and it is this important objective that sets it apart from more traditional developmental approaches. The theory suggests that working on more complex stimuli results in downward generalization to less complex targets and thus that ultimately the approach can maximize the efficiency of intervention: a child's entire speech system is more rapidly changed than if a segment-by-segment approach was adopted using a developmental hierarchy. We know that working according to a developmental hierarchy on a segment-by-segment basis 'up the ladder' can work, but we also know that for children with PSDs it can take a long time. Hodson notes 'Highly unintelligible children with extensive omissions and limited repertoires of sounds . . . typically require 5 or 6 years (or more) to become intelligible via phoneme-oriented programs' (1997, p. 198).

For children with PSDs, focusing on just one target sound at a time may not be the most efficient way to approach therapy, and furthermore selecting the easy targets first may also not be the most efficient way of utilizing precious therapy time. Some research studies have been carried out in which complex, later-developing targets were chosen as intervention stimuli (e.g., Gierut and Dinnsen, 1987; Gierut, Elbert and Dinnsen, 1987; Gierut, Morrisette, Hughes and Rowland, 1996; Rvachew and Nowack, 2001). Many of these studies showed positive results, suggesting that working on these challenging targets can lead to more generalization throughout a child's system. However, the results are not without controversy. We describe some of these studies in greater detail in the following section.

In order to systematically quantify the knowledge that children possess about their native phonology, authors such as Gierut *et al.* (1987) use surface speech errors to infer a child's productive phonological knowledge (PPK) of individual segments. PPK can be defined as the degree to which a child has internalized a particular segment into their phonological system, and it is a key concept linked to complexity accounts of treatment efficacy. Gierut *et al.* (1987) devised a scale of productive phonological knowledge whereby each segment in a child's ambient language can be classified into one of six categories. The categories of productive phonological knowledge are summarized in Table 3.2.

Gierut *et al.* (1987) suggest that PPK should be determined by evaluating samples of children's spontaneous speech and single word productions. The PPK categories are based on output but use this information to make inferences about a child's phonological output lexicon or motor programs, to evaluate what the child knows about how to produce par-

Table 3.2: Description of types of productive phonological knowledge (from Gierut *et al.*, 1987)

Type	Description
1	Produced correctly in all word positions for all morphemes
2	Produced correctly in nearly all morphemes but alternations between the target and another sound observed for some morphemes (optional rule)
3	Produced correctly in nearly all morphemes but some 'fossilized' forms always produced incorrectly
4	Produced correctly in one or more word positions and consistently incorrect in other word positions
5	Inconsistently correct in one or more word positions and consistently incorrect in other word positions
6	Produced incorrectly in all word positions and all morphemes

ticular segments in single words and connected speech. PPK is a useful measure with potentially important clinical implications: the authors have shown that the less knowledge a child has about a particular segment, the greater the potential generalization that occurs to the rest of the segment system when that particular segment is targeted in therapy. This means that it may be more efficient to target segments with high PPK. Type 6 targets are favoured as they will result in more widespread generalization throughout the system, ultimately making intervention using these targets more efficient.

Intervention research has been carried out to evaluate the validity of PPK categories and claims about the differential responses of these to intervention. Williams (1991) studied the use of 'least phonological knowledge' (Type 6) by treating nine children (ages 3;8–5;9) with similar levels of knowledge on the same error. The level of phonological knowledge did not appear to be related to outcomes as children varied widely in the generalization achieved. A study carried out by Rvachew and Nowack (2001) suggested that the traditional approach to target selection (i.e. using developmental norms) may indeed be most effective. In their study, 48 children with moderate–severe phonological delays received therapy for four different targets. The segments were selected based on either developmental or PPK target selection criteria. Children who received treatment for segments that are early developing and associated with greater productive phonological knowledge showed more progress in their acquisition of target sounds than the participants who received therapy for later-developing segments that were associated with little or no productive phonological knowledge. No between-group differences in generalization were found. The children's enjoyment of therapy did not differ significantly between the two groups, but parental satisfaction with treatment progress was greater for children in the traditional (developmental) group than for those in the PPK group whose intervention targets were not based on traditional choices. This is in contrast to what has been predicted by Gierut *et al.* (1987), although the authors did acknowledge that in a longer study the impact of treating 'least knowledge' segments may have been seen. Although there is a body of evidence arguing strongly for the more complex, non-developmental targets, there remains evidence that refutes this and suggests a developmental approach may be more effective. These differences may be due to the individual differences of the children participating in the studies, and to the fact that effectiveness and efficiency are slightly different concepts. Effectiveness involves measure of outcomes in a particular (non-ideal or real-life) situation. Efficiency takes this concept further and considers cost and the time and effort needed to reach positive outcomes. The non-developmental targets may ultimately be more efficient in the long term, but in the short to medium term there may be more evidence for developmental targets.

A Functional Perspective

A functional approach to stimuli selection is based on practical rather than theoretical considerations. Although we have emphasized the importance of choosing a theory (or theories) to guide intervention, the functional perspective can be combined with more theoretical approaches to stimuli selection, and in its own right may have an important place in evidence-based practice. A functional approach to stimuli selection might involve selecting targets that appear in a child's name as the main focus of therapy. For some school-age children with PSDs, not being able to produce their own name accurately is a great source of distress and embarrassment. Other functional approaches to target selection will involve consideration of the sounds that occur most frequently in a given language, e.g. /s/ is often chosen as a target because of its widespread use in English. If a functional approach can be shown to be effective, then it will certainly have an important place in our theories of therapy.

Some functional approaches are less concerned with specific segments in single words and have single words as whole units as their focus. An example of this type of approach is the core vocabulary approach for children with speech difficulties (Dodd, 1995, 2005; Crosbie, Holm and Dodd, 2005). This is a good example of a functional approach that has been shown to be effective and can be couched within a broader theoretical framework.

In Chapter 1 we introduced Dodd's (1995, 2005) work in which children with speech difficulties are grouped into categories based on the nature and underlying cause of their speech problems. The sub-groups outlined by Dodd included:

- children with articulation difficulties;
- children with phonological delays;
- children with consistent deviant phonology;
- children with inconsistent deviant phonology.

This last sub-group of children is an interesting group thought to show delayed and non-developmental errors, but in addition the children show significant variability in their speech production that does not reflect a maturing system. Children are considered to be included in this category if they produce ten or more of 25 single words differently on two out of three occasions (Dodd, 1995 pp.56–7). The productions must not follow immediately, so typically the first naming task is carried out and then followed by some other activities, before returning to the naming task for a further set of productions. The *Diagnostic Evaluation of Articulation and Phonology* (DEAP) (Dodd *et al.*, 2002) provides specific stimuli to help in making this diagnosis. For example, Anna, aged 5;9 produced the following inconsistent realizations of target words taken from the diagnostic screen of the DEAP.

Target	Production 1	Production 2
WATCH	[wɔks]	[wɔks]
GLOVES	[klʊbz]	[plʊbz]
SPIDER	[ˈpaɪdə]	[ˈflaɪdə]
THANK YOU	[ˈtæŋkju]	[ˈkæŋku]
UMBRELLA	[ʌmˈbəpəʊ]	[ʌmˈbwɛlə]

Barbara Dodd and her colleagues have carried out research which demonstrates the most appropriate type of intervention for each of the different sub-groups (Dodd, 1995; Holm and Dodd, 1999; Dodd and Bradford, 2000; Crosbie, Holm and Dodd, 2005; Holm, Crosbie and Dodd, 2005a,b). It has been shown that for children with inconsistent and deviant phonology, a core vocabulary approach might be the most effective. This is an approach where a set of words, the core vocabulary, is selected and these addressed using a drill-type approach in therapy and at home. The aim is for the child to develop stable productions of these items, the first step in developing their phonological system. Dodd (1995) suggests that high frequency words that are motivating to the child should be selected, and thus the child and their carers/teachers will have an important role in suggesting these words. However, she also suggests that the therapist can manipulate the phonological structure of the words to reflect the child's specific speech difficulties.

We have been involved in interventions using a core vocabulary approach with school-age children with PSDs. For example, Townsend (2005) used a small set of core vocabulary items with an 8-year-old boy called Adrian with Down syndrome. Parents and teachers selected 12 words that were relevant and important for Adrian, e.g. SPIDERMAN. These words were worked on in six intervention sessions of one hour's duration each, carried out over a three-week period. A set of real words of matched frequency, semantics and length were also selected (e.g. SUPERMAN), as well as a set of matched non-words in order to probe generalization. The non-words were created by changing vowels in the target words while keeping consonants the same. Vowel length was kept the same so that short vowels were substituted with short vowels, long vowels with long vowels and diphthongs with diphthongs, e.g. [ˈspeɪdɪmɒn]. The matched words and non-words were not used in intervention. At the end of the intervention Adrian's speech production on all three wordlists was reassessed. He was found to have made improvements in the consistency of his production of the target words that was greater than what would be expected through chance alone. His accuracy of production had also improved although the level of change had not yet reached significance. Changes in consistency and accuracy were not significant for the control wordlists, although it was suggested that there had been insufficient time for generalization to occur given the short duration of the intervention programme. Similarly, Teal (2005) used the core vocabulary approach successfully with a girl called Ruth, aged 6;11 with PSDs and learning difficulties. The consistency of Ruth's production of target words improved significantly following 6 hours of intervention. As happened with Adrian, Ruth's speech accuracy as measured by PCC did not change significantly and minimal generalization was noted for the untreated control wordlists. Nevertheless, it was hypothesized that with further intervention changes in accuracy might be obtained and more generalization noted. In Appendix 5 we provide the complete lists of stimuli that were used with Ruth.

When using a core vocabulary approach the therapist should strive to encourage the child's best possible production of each word, aiming for consistency and accepting developmental errors as appropriate. The therapist needs to ensure that parents and teachers are aware of the desired productions, and that the child is given plenty of opportunities to produce and practise these. The core words we used with Anna, aged 5;9, diagnosed as having inconsistent speech difficulties, included names suggested by her and her parents such as her siblings' names, the names of her friends, favourite foods and television programmes. In addition, we included words that contained velars in a variety of positions, since although stimulable for /k/ and /g/, these were a particular challenge for Anna in spontaneous speech. Anna made rapid progress with the core vocabulary approach, which she found motivating and structured. Her parents and teachers found it easy to work on a small number of words each week. The stability achieved in Anna's phonology through this programme generalized to untreated words, and as a result her intelligibility improved. After using the core vocabulary approach for approximately six months of weekly, one-hour therapy, Anna seemed to have reached a plateau. At that point we carried out a full psycholinguistic and phonological assessment using the speech processing profile to organize the data and consider Anna's phonology within the context of that. New aims and hypotheses were then devised, moving away from a core vocabulary approach, which was no longer considered appropriate.

Intelligibility is a key concept when working with children with PSDs. The ultimate aim of many of our interventions is to improve intelligibility so that children are able to make themselves understood to both familiar and unfamiliar listeners. As such, intelligibility is an important functional consideration in stimuli selection. The core vocabulary approach outlined above is partly driven by the need to maximize intelligibility. Similarly, Hodson and Paden's cycles approach to therapy has the improvement of intelligibility as its ultimate aim. There is some intervention work that has been carried out with adults with dysarthria and which claims to be intelligibility-driven (Yorkston and Beukelman, 1981). There is further scope for developing our knowledge of intelligibility and how it may be used to drive intervention for children with PSDs. Grunwell's (1987) developmental norms were presented earlier in this chapter. These were taken from the *Phonological Assessment of Child Speech* (PACS) (Grunwell, 1985), a comprehensive linguistic assessment of a child's speech production. Grunwell describes her approach to target selection as functional rather than developmental since one of the ultimate aims of the assessment is to reveal where the child is having difficulties in conveying meaning and how a system of contrasts might be developed to improve this. For example, there is a section of the PACS that requires reflection on examples of homonymy in the child's speech. Homonymy means 'same name' and would involve cases where a child uses a particular word such as [dɒ] to mean DOG, DAD, GOT and SOCK. Intelligibility is the main theme of Chapter 11, and we return to develop some of these points in that section.

A Systemic Perspective

Many authors have argued that if we are to bring about long-lasting changes in a child's speech system then we need work on the entire speech system as a whole (e.g. Hodson and Paden, 1991; Rees, 2001a). Oppositions and contrasts between the stimuli used in intervention form the focus of this section as many authors have argued that children will only be able to bring about change in their phonology if we select stimuli that highlight contrasts between the different targets, e.g. Gierut, 1989; Gierut, 1990; Williams, 2000a,b; Rvachew and Nowack, 2001. How many stimuli should we select, and how should they be contrasted? The answer to these questions will vary depending on your theoretical orientation.

Most practitioners are familiar with the concept of minimal pairs where words are selected to highlight contrasts between relevant segments and their features. For example, Simon aged 10 years had an inaccurate motor program for the word GIRL which resulted in him producing 'curl'. He had clear semantic representations of both words: CURL and GIRL. In intervention we were able to use this semantic knowledge to help devise a new motor program for GIRL so that Simon was able to distinguish between the two. Meaningful minimal contrast therapy was described by Weiner (1981) and there are many published resources available which incorporate minimal pairs, e.g. *Metaphon* (Howell and Dean, 1994), and the *Nuffield Centre Dyspraxia Programme* (Williams and Stephens, 2004). Not all minimal pairs are constructed in the same way: some will differ in terms of one feature only (e.g. [k] and [g] in COAT and GOAT differ only in terms of voicing) and others will differ in three ways (e.g. PIN and GIN differ in the word-initial (WI) consonants in terms of place, manner and voicing). The selection of such stimuli words and the extent to which segments in these words differ has become an increasingly important issue in phonological intervention. Hilary Gardner's (1997) paper entitled 'Are your minimal pairs too neat? The dangers of phonemicisation in phonology therapy' highlights the importance of careful selection and usage of minimal pairs in therapy. In Appendix 6 we include some sample lists for minimal pair contrasts which practitioners may find helpful as a starting point in their stimuli selection. However, it is also important to remember that stimuli should ideally be tailor-made for individual children and based on the child's own errors.

Recent work into multiple oppositions (e.g. Williams 2000a,b) has shown that this may be an effective and efficient way of bringing about reorganization of children's phonological systems. The principle of multiple oppositions therapy is to create a set of contrasting words and to focus on these all at one time. Rather like Hodson and Paden's (1991) cycles approach to intervention, these authors consider that phonology is about learning patterns, and that children will make more progress if they are exposed to a fairly wide, but carefully constrained, range of patterns in therapy. It has been noted (Flipsen, 2002) in particular that this may be an effective way of remediating the phonology of children with very limited repertoires. The concept of homonymy is important in designing stimuli for multiple oppositions therapy. In our earlier example of homonymy we described a child who uses a particular word such as [dɒ] to mean DOG, DAD, GOT and SOCK. These words, DOG, DAD, GOT and SOCK might form a set of therapy stimuli with the child being encouraged to differentiate between his or her productions in order to realize the distinct meanings. This type of approach to therapy may thus be more suitable for children with good semantic awareness.

A traditional minimal opposition approach targets contrasts with the fewest differences between target and error, e.g. [f] and [v] differ only on voicing in FAN and VAN. A maximal oppositions approach, on the other hand, is based on the idea that error sounds should be contrasted with very different sounds as this makes the error sound more noticeable. Some studies (e.g. Gierut, 1989) have suggested that generalization may be faster with this approach where the child's attention is focused on more than one distinction along the broad multiple dimensions of voice, place and manner. In Chapter 4 we show how we varied stimuli selection with a 5-year-old boy to include both minimal and maximal differences between words. In the following Activity, we provide the opportunity to experiment with stimuli.

ACTIVITY 3.2

Consider the following small data set from Elizabeth, aged 7;4. The words were produced in a naming task.

Target	Production
CAN	[tæn]
CUP	[dʌp/tʌp]
KEY	[ti]
DOG	[dɒd]
CAMEL	['tæmɪl]
COMPASS	['tʌmpə]
MAGNET	['mædɪt]
GUITAR	['bɪtɑ:]
HANGER	['ændə]
ESKIMO	['ɛtɪməʊ]

1. What aspects of Elizabeth's speech would you want to change in intervention and why?
2. Bearing in mind your answer to (1) above, imagine you are going to carry out meaningful minimal contrast therapy. Choose five word pairs that you might use in intervention.
3. Returning to a psycholinguistic perspective, what further questions would you want to ask about Elizabeth's speech?

Now turn to the Key to Activity 3.2 at the end of this chapter and check how your responses compare with ours.

Psycholinguistic and Phonological Approaches Combined

In this chapter, and successive ones, we focus on the design and selection of stimuli. While our focus is phonological, we consider this complementary to the psycholinguistic approach that was reviewed in Chapter 2. For children with PSDs, the psycholinguistic approach is best combined with a phonological approach. While psycholinguistic approaches inform the process of intervention, knowledge from phonology enables one to focus on the content of intervention, answering the question: 'What stimuli will be used in the activities?' All too often in the history of speech and language intervention 'old' approaches have been discarded in favour of new approaches without consideration of how the best parts of old and new can be combined. Psycholinguistic approaches have become increasingly popular over recent years (e.g. see Baker *et al.*, 2001), but the use of such an approach with children with speech difficulties does not mean that more traditional approaches to phonological analysis should be forgotten! Speech and language therapists are uniquely skilled in their abilities to transcribe and analyse speech, and these skills are compatible with a psycholinguistic approach to intervention.

Ebbels (2000) provides an excellent example of how the two approaches can be combined. She used a psycholinguistic approach to evaluate the speech processing skills of a girl, TG aged 10;4 with PSDs and hearing impairment, and then focused on the way in which specific segments were affected at different levels of the speech processing profile. TG had a moderate to severe bilateral sensori-neural hearing loss. It was unclear whether the hearing impairment was the main cause of her speech and language difficulties, or whether she had a specific speech and language impairment in addition to her hearing impairment. Certainly TG's speech and language difficulties seemed greater than what might be expected given her degree of hearing loss. In terms of educational placement she had been in both language units and units for children with hearing difficulties.

TG had already been investigated using traditional speech and language assessments. Ebbels suggests that while these assessments are important they did not reveal TG's precise difficulties. She carried out further psycholinguistically-oriented assessment in three phases. First, naming tests were carried out. TG fared poorly with these. However, difficulties with naming could mean breakdown at many levels such as auditory discrimination, inaccurate/fuzzy phonological representations, 'frozen' motor programs that had not been updated to match the phonological representations, or output difficulties (see Book 1, Stackhouse and Wells, 1997, pp. 115–18). Thus, the second stage of the assessment involved more output tasks, the results of which were compared with the naming tests. These involved repetition of real and non-words, and reading of single words. Comparisons of these allowed inferences to be made about phonological processing strengths and weaknesses since each task uses different processing routes through the speech processing system. For example, Figure 3.1 shows the processing route through the speech processing system for naming (see Book 1, Stackhouse and Wells, 1997, Chapter 6 for further examples of processing routes through the model).

Here it can be seen that a semantic representation is triggered by the picture, and this in turn triggers the associated motor program. The motor program is the blueprint for the production of the word and this is followed by further steps on the output side of the model until the acoustic signal is produced by the vocal apparatus. In contrast, Figure 3.2 shows the processing route through the system for non-word repetition.

Here it can be seen that input processing is also involved as the child needs to hear the examiner's production of the word in order to produce it. Because the word is a nonsense one, the child will not have heard it before and therefore will have no stored phonological representation of the item. This is the reason for the arrow moving from phonological recognition to phonological representation: there is no stored phonological representation already existing and thus no associated semantic informa-

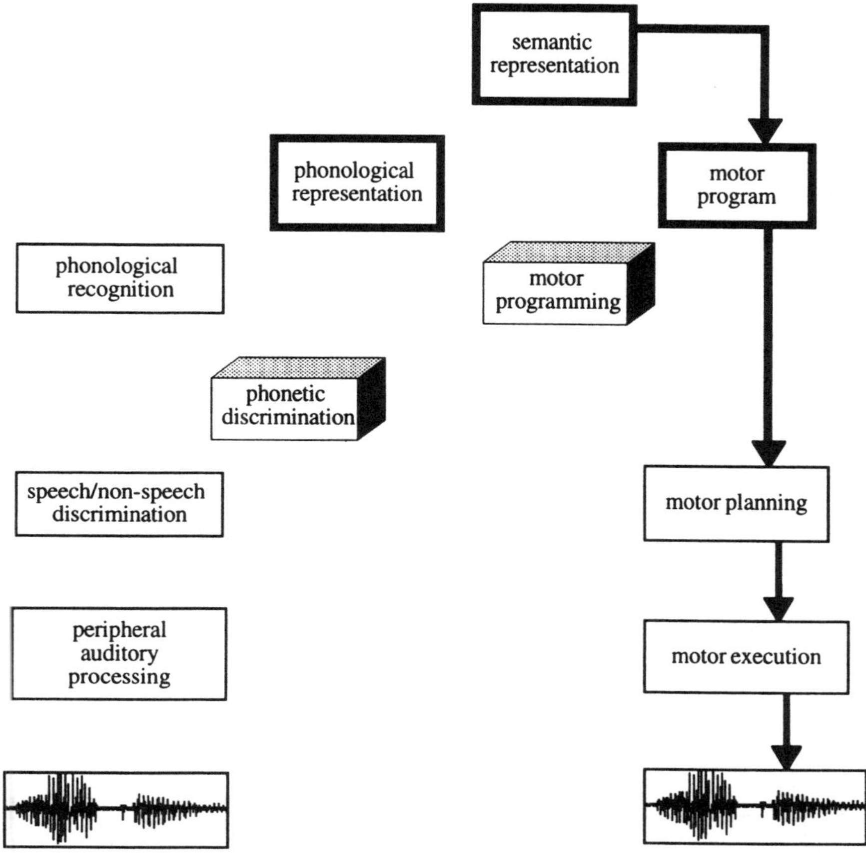

Figure 3.1: Speech processing route for naming. (Reproduced by kind permission of Whurr Publishers from Stackhouse and Wells, 1997, p. 179.)

tion or stored motor program. A new motor program must be created through online motor programming.

Comparison of the different processing routes involved in picture naming and non-word repetition shows how there are aspects of processing that are common to the two tasks: both involve access of a motor program, motor planning and motor execution. Where the tasks differ is that non-word repetition involves input processing (e.g. peripheral auditory processing and phonological recognition) and the online creation of a new motor program based on phonological recognition. If a child has greater difficulties with non-word repetition than with picture naming, one might hypothesize that this is due to:

(a) difficulties on the input side with peripheral auditory processing, and/or phonological recognition;

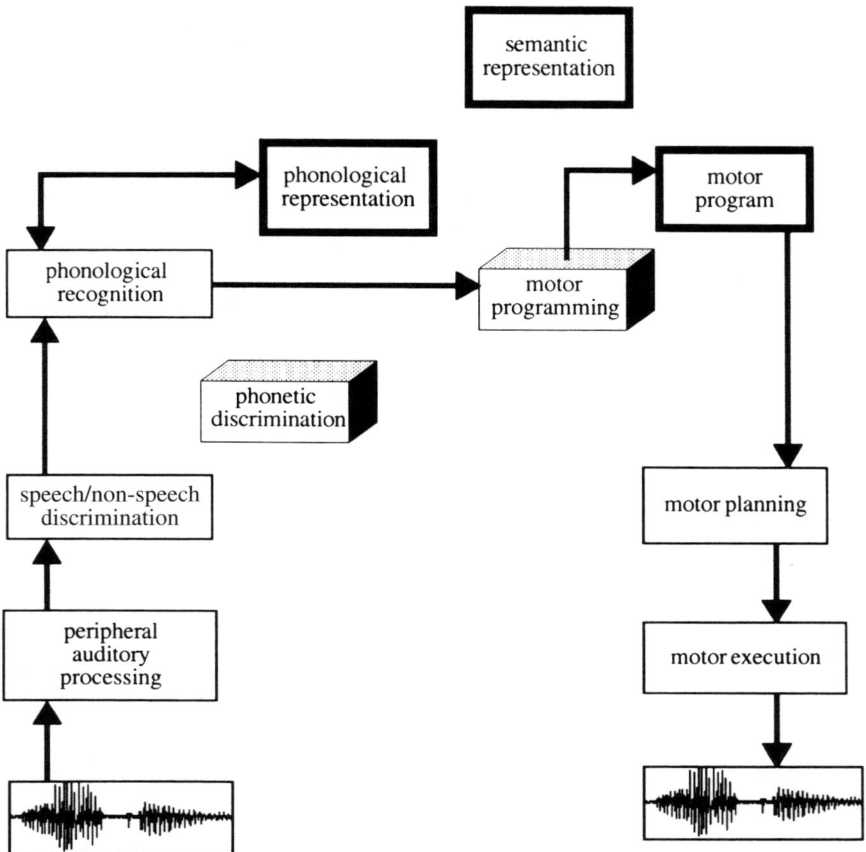

Figure 3.2: Speech processing route for non-word repetition. (Reproduced by kind permission of Whurr Publishers from Stackhouse and Wells, 1997, p. 180.)

(b) difficulties with online motor programming;
(c) difficulties with both (a) and (b).

Indeed, TG was found to perform significantly better with naming than with non-word repetition. Similar comparisons were made between other tasks and it was found that real word repetition was better than non-word repetition. There was no significant difference between reading of single words and naming of the same items.

In the third phase of the assessment, input processing was the main focus. To test the integrity of TG's phonological representations, she was presented with her own speech errors and asked to judge whether or not the words were correctly produced. Table 3.3 (adapted from Ebbels, 2000) shows examples of some of the realizations of the target segments which

Table 3.3: Realization of segments in target words pronounced wrongly by the tester but accepted as correct by the child (TG) (adapted from Ebbels, 2000)

Word-initial		Within-word		Word-final	
Target	accepted	Target	accepted	Target	accepted
θ	θ, f	k	k, t	p	p, ʔ
s	s, st, ts, d, dz	g	g, d	b	b, d
z	z, dz, d	s	s, ts, d	d	d, n, g, dg, ʔ
		z	z, d	k	k, t, s, ts, ʔ
				n	n, m, gh, l
				s	s, ts, t

TG considered correct. This means that TG was accepting words such as [dæn] for SAND, suggesting that her own phonological representations for these words were fuzzy and inaccurate. However, this was not the case for all words since TG was able to reject many of the tester's incorrect productions. Up to this point the psycholinguistic assessments had focused on whole words, but at this point we see how Ebbels zooms in at a segmental level: all the incorrect words that TG accepted as correct were found to share certain affected segments shown in Table 3.3.

Some of TG's 'wrong' answers in the phonological judgment task may have been because of auditory discrimination difficulties, i.e. TG may have said that 'elebint' was acceptable for ELEPHANT because she is not able to auditorily distinguish between /b/ and /f/. Thus, a further auditory discrimination test was conducted in which TG was required to make same/different judgments about closely-related word pairs that her previous errors had suggested might pose trouble for her at this level. TG achieved 75% accuracy on this task suggesting that while some of the errors in the auditory lexical decision task described above may be due to her hearing impairment, it is not enough to be causing all the difficulties observed at a higher level.

Ebbels concluded by suggesting that TG had fuzzy phonological representations for many words, which had led to imprecise motor programs and output errors beyond what would be expected from her hearing impairment. The fuzzy representations did not affect all words but in particular involved those containing segments in the word positions outlined in Table 3.3. These could be used as the basis of stimuli design for intervention.

Ideas for Stimuli Design

In this chapter we have highlighted four approaches to stimuli selection:

- developmental approaches;
- complexity approaches;
- functional approaches;
- systemic approaches.

We have emphasized through examples that approaches to designing and selecting stimuli may very often draw on several of these areas. In this section we try to pull together the information that has been presented in this chapter into a series of practical ideas for designing and selecting stimuli for intervention. We have also included examples of stimuli lists where possible, and these have been collated into stimuli reference lists in Appendices 5 and 6. As noted at the start of the chapter, the key aspects of good stimuli design are (a) knowing what theoretical rationale you are following, and (b) spending time in the design of the stimuli since this time may well make intervention more effective (see Stackhouse and Wells, 1997, Chapter 11, for further discussion of stimuli design).

The following guidelines may be useful when designing and selecting stimuli for intervention with children with PSDs.

1. Carry out detailed psycholinguistic and phonological assessment since these data are the foundation of our decision making about stimuli for intervention.
2. Give careful consideration to the stimuli used in assessment as well as intervention. For example, Ebbels (2000) used the same words in her naming and real-word repetition tasks. This can be helpful since it allows us to rule out the influence of any lexical factors, such as words on the naming task being semantically or phonologically more challenging than the words used in the repetition task.
3. Use non-words as these provide useful information about how children deal with new words, and the online abilities of their speech processing system as opposed to the stored knowledge they have built up over time. Non-words should ideally be matched to real words by using the following principles:
   (a) Maintain the same number of syllables in the new word.
   (b) Maintain the same phonotactic structure in the new word, e.g. CVC or CCVC.
   (c) Keep consonants the same, but substitute new vowels.
   (d) Maintain the same vowel length in the new word, e.g. short vowel, long vowel or diphthong.
   (e) Ensure that non-words really are non-words!
   (f) Produce the words using the same stress patterns as the original.

ACTIVITY 3.3

Teal (2005) created a preliminary set of non-words matched to core vocabulary words used with Ruth, aged 6;11 as follows:

Core-vocabulary words	Matched non-words
1. CHIP	ʧʊp
2. JUICE	ʤis
3. BATH	bʌθ
4. MILK	mʊlk
5. TEA	teɪ
6. PINK	pʌŋk
7. CAR	kɜ
8. CAT	kaʊt
9. PIZZA	ˈputsə
10. BALLET	ˈbɒlaʊ

Work through the principles given for non-word stimuli selection in (3) above, checking each matched word pair in turn. Are these difficulties or problems with any of the items, and what alternatives would you suggest? Turn to the Key to Activity 3.3 at the end of this chapter to see which items were changed/discarded.

4. Decide whether you will follow a functional approach in which whole words will be selected that are of relevance to the child. Indications from the evidence base suggest that children with deviant and inconsistent phonology will benefit from a core-vocabulary approach. If using a core-vocabulary approach remember that the word items can be selected to fit with particular phonological aims, e.g. selecting words with velars since the child has particular difficulties with these, or in the case of older children choosing multisyllabic words. Activity 3.3 above shows 10 examples of core-vocabulary words used with a 6 year old child with inconsistent and unintelligible speech.
5. Decide whether you will select segments to be used in single words, and the basis for this decision. Single segments may be selected based on developmental norms (e.g. using Grunwell's norms shown in Table 3.1), or complexity accounts which hope to achieve maximum generalization throughout the system, or functional perspectives (e.g. working on the sounds in a child's name or on the most commonly-used sounds in the child's language).
6. Consider the child's speech processing system as a whole by considering how selected stimuli will be contrasted in intervention,

e.g. through minimal pairs based on the child's homonymy, or using multiple oppositions or a cycles approach.

7. Use matched words not only in assessment but also to monitor effects of intervention. This is discussed in greater detail in Chapter 12. The aim is to create wordlists that are as identical as possible so that if improvement is shown on one list we are able to make fair comparisons between the two lists without having to take into account semantic or phonological differences. In Activity 3.3 we showed examples of 10 core vocabulary words used with a child with inconsistent speech. We also showed 10 non-words matched to these core words. These non-words were not worked on in intervention but were used to monitor the effects of intervention on other parts of the child's speech processing system. The hypothesis was that by revising Ruth's stored motor programs for commonly-used words we might shake-up her online motor programming too. One way of testing this was to get her to repeat non-words, and make comparisons between her performance before and after intervention. In this same intervention programme, a third set of words was created. These were real words also matched to the treated core-vocabulary words in terms of semantics and frequency, i.e. they were also words that Ruth was likely to have stored representations of and use on a regular basis. Again, the aim with these words was not to use them in intervention but evaluate if Ruth was able to generalize any of the progress made with the treated words to these words. Matches from these lists included the following:

Core-vocabulary words	**Matched words**
JUICE	COKE
MILK	BREAD
CAT	DOG
PIZZA	PASTA

(See Appendix 5 for the full list of matched words.)

Creating matching wordlists is a challenging and time-consuming task. In some cases it may be impossible to meet all criteria. In the examples above, the main focus was on semantic matching but attempts were also made to control for phonological differences, e.g. the word final consonant cluster in MILK is balanced by the word initial cluster in BREAD.

8. Use phonetic context as a support. As noted in Activity 3.2 phonetic context should not complicate the task for the child. Where possible avoid using items which contain the child's favoured substitution in addition to the target sound, e.g. in the case of a child who substitutes /t/ for /k/ avoid using e.g. CAT, GATE in the early stages of intervention since these will all too easily be produced as /tæt/ and

/teɪt/. Supportive phonetic contexts include using stressed syllables (Kent, 1982), combining front consonants with front vowels (e.g. TEA) and back consonants with back vowels (e.g. CAR) (Grunwell, 1992). Many fricatives may be easier for children to say in word-final position (Edwards, 1983).

9. Carefully consider how you will score stimuli – both in assessment and as you evaluate intervention. Many practitioners will use a right or wrong approach, but in cases of children with severe and persisting speech difficulties it may be more helpful to use a more fine-grained approach. Scoring on a segment-by-segment basis can yield a more specific picture of any gains that a child makes over therapy. Bryan and Howard's (1992) approach was to score each consonant out of a potential three points, with one point assigned for each correct feature, i.e. place, manner and voicing. This was the same method used by Ebbels (2000) in her case study. Scoring methods form the focus of the final activity in this chapter.

ACTIVITY 3.4

Aim: To practise different scoring methods.

Consider the following data from Anna, aged 5;9.

Target	Pre-intervention	Post-intervention
WATER	[ˈwɔwə]	[ˈwɔtə]
GLOVES	[plʊbz]	[klʊfz]
SPIDER	[ˈpaɪdə]	[ˈflaɪdə]
THANK YOU	[ˈtæŋkju]	[ˈfæŋku]
UMBRELLA	[ʌmˈbwɛlə]	[ʌmˈbwɛlə]

1. Use a right/wrong scoring method to compare Anna's pre- and post-intervention productions.
2. Now rescore her results using a segment-by-segment approach.
3. Now score all her consonants on a three-feature basis: 1 point for correct voicing; 1 point for correct place of articulation; and 1 point for correct manner of articulation.
4. Comment on the different impressions these scoring methods give of Anna's progress.

Now turn to the Key to Activity to 3.4 at the end of this chapter and check your responses against ours.

This chapter has covered some issues related to the design, selection and scoring of stimuli for assessment and intervention purposes. Our focus in this chapter has been on segments in single words. In the following chapter we describe the intervention that took place with Oliver, aged 5;6. The presentation of his case gives many opportunities to discuss and exemplify principles of stimuli selection at a single word level. But segments and single words are not the only levels that might be addressed in intervention. Chapters 5 and 6 focus on consonant clusters in single words, and Chapters 7 and 8 on the use of connected speech stimuli in intervention.

Summary

The key points are as follows.

- Choosing segments in single words as assessment and intervention stimuli is not a straightforward task.
- Powell (1991) suggested that there are at least 21 factors that might influence this decision, including stimulability and developmental factors.
- Having a well thought out rationale for our stimuli design and selection is important.
- Developmental norms can be helpful for selecting individual sounds or processes to be addressed in intervention.
- The cycles approach from Hodson and Paden (1991) is based around developmental principles in the way in which children are exposed to many targets in both input and output. This approach also draws on other more functional perspectives.
- Developmental norms may not always be helpful for older children with PSDs whose speech is disordered rather than delayed.
- Productive phonological knowledge (PPK) and complexity theories provide an alternative approach to target selection and strive to maximize the efficiency of intervention.
- A child's knowledge of individual segments can be classified into six types based on surface speech errors. There is some research to suggest that working on sounds with low PPK brings about more generalization through the child's speech processing system than working in a developmental segment-by-segment way.
- Functional approaches to stimuli design include the core vocabulary approach (Dodd, 1995, 2005) which helps children with inconsistent speech to stabilize their productions of high-frequency words.
- When working on children's speech it is important to consider the speech processing system as a whole.
- Systemic approaches focus particularly on the contrasts made explicit in intervention, e.g. using minimal or maximal pairs.
- Phonological approaches ('What stimuli?') can be combined with psycholinguistic approaches ('How to address?'). The psycholinguistic approach informs us about levels of breakdown, but within each level we need to investigate further regarding the individual segments affected.

- Phonetic context is important; manipulation of the phonetic context can optimize a child's chance of success in therapy, e.g. by not including the child's own favoured substitution in the target word in the early phases of intervention.
- Scoring approaches can vary widely from right/wrong approaches that give a broad overview of a child's performance to more specific segment-by-segment, and feature approaches that can allow one to account for any changes made over the course of intervention in a more specific way.

KEY TO ACTIVITY 3.1

Powell (1991) suggested that the following factors will affect stimuli selection:

1. age of child;
2. age appropriateness of error(s);
3. normative order;
4. ease of production;
5. effect on intelligibility (See Chapter 11);
6. error consistency;
7. frequency of sound occurrence;
8. homonymy: where two (or more) different target words (e.g. CAT, DOG) are pronounced in the same way resulting in one label (e.g. [beʊ]) being used to refer to multiple referents;
9. markedness: the degree of 'unusualness' of an error;
10. morphological status: some segments have additional important roles in word morphology, e.g. /s/ in indicating plurals;
11. number of errors;
12. perceptual saliency: how obvious and noticeable is the 'error'?;
13. phonetic inventory: what is the range of sounds that the child can currently use?;
14. phonetic error type: details of the child's articulation and degree of deviation from the norm;
15. phonological error type: details of the child's phonology and degree of deviation from the norm;
16. phonotactic constraints: some children may be able to produce specific segments in one word position only, e.g. <u>C</u>VC but not C<u>C</u>VC;
17. phonological knowledge (see section on productive phonological knowledge or complexity)
18. relevance to child (see section on functional perspective)
19. resources available;
20. severity of disorder;
21. stimulability.

KEY TO ACTIVITY 3.2

1. What aspects of Elizabeth's speech would you want to change in intervention, and why?

From the small speech sample given, it can be seen that Elizabeth demonstrates the following phonological processes: fronting of velars; inappropriate voicing (on one occasion, i.e. CUP → dʌp); cluster reduction (i.e. in ESKIMO) and final consonant deletion (e.g. in COMPASS). We chose to address her fronting of velars for the following two reasons: (a) It appears to be the most dominant process of her speech affecting intelligibility (a functional reason); and (b) by the age of seven normally-developing children should have acquired [k] and [g] and be using these consistently in their speech (a developmental reason).

2. Bearing in mind your answer to (1) above, imagine you are going to carry out meaningful minimal contrast therapy. Choose five word pairs that you might use in intervention.

Selected word pairs should meet the following criteria:

- Elements of a pair should be matched for phonotactic structure, either both CVs or CVCs, etc.
- Real words should be selected in all examples for the meaningful therapy, although names familiar to the child could be used.
- Phonetic context should be used to support the child, not complicate the task. Where possible avoid using
   i. more than one velar per item, e.g. CAKE
   ii. items with velars embedded in clusters, e.g. MASK
   iii. items which contain both velars and Elizabeth's favoured frontal plosives, e.g. CAT, GATE.

Examples of minimal pair stimuli for the fronting target might be:

CV	CVC
key/tea	cool/tool
car/tar	can/tan
core/tore	call/tall
go/dough	gum/dumb
gear/dear	gull/dull

3. Returning to a psycholinguistic perspective, what further questions would you want to ask about Elizabeth's speech?

Having carried out a phonological analysis of Elizabeth's speech, we may have developed clear ideas of what aspects of her phonology need to be addressed. However, our analysis has only been based on surface error analysis. Using a psycholinguistic framework, we would want to find out more about the underlying causes of her difficulties:

why is Elizabeth realizing velars in this way? The following questions would need to be addressed before we could determine whether in fact the 'meaningful minimal contrast therapy' is the most appropriate intervention for Elizabeth, or even if it is, how we would administer it:

- Does Elizabeth have difficulties in detecting the differences between [k] and [t], and [d] and [g] on an auditory discrimination task, i.e. does she have input difficulties?
- Does Elizabeth have inaccurate or fuzzy phonological representations for all or some of the words containing velars?
- Does Elizabeth have inaccurate motor programs for all or some of the words containing velars?
- Does Elizabeth have difficulty in the physical production of velars?

The way in which the phonological and psycholinguistic approaches can be combined is discussed in greater detail in the text.

KEY TO ACTIVITY 3.3

Items 5, 6 and 8 violate the principles for a good list of matched non-words.

Item 5: /teɪ/ for TEA – A diphthong is included in non-word /teɪ/, but should be matched to a long vowel in TEA. Using another long vowel such as [ɜː] to give /tɜː/ would be preferable.

Item 6: /pʌŋk/ for PINK – One would need to check whether /pʌŋk/ is in fact a non-word for Ruth since many people will have this word in their lexicons. /pæŋk/ may be a preferable choice.

Item 8: /kaʊt/ for CAT – Again, there is a mismatch here between the short vowel in CAT and the diphthong in /kaʊt/. It would be preferable to change /kaʊt/ to /kɛt/.

KEY TO ACTIVITY 3.4

1. Use a right/wrong scoring method to compare Anna's pre- and post-intervention productions. X = INCORRECT, √ = CORRECT

WATER	['wɔwə] X	['wɔtə] √
GLOVES	[plʊbz] X	[klʊfs] X
SPIDER	['paɪdə] X	['flaɪdə] X
THANK YOU	['tæŋkju] X	['fæŋku] X
UMBRELLA	[ʌm'bwɛlə] X	[ʌm'bwɛlə]X

pre-intervention 0/5 post-intervention 1/5

2. Now re-score her results using a segment-by-segment approach, i.e. score 1 point for each correct segment.

WATER (['wɔtə] 4 potential segments)	['wɔwə] (3)	[wɔtə] (4)
GLOVES ([glʊvz] 5 potential segments)	[plʊbz](3)	[klʊfs] (3)
SPIDER (['spaɪdə] 5 potential segments)	['paɪdə] (4)	[flaɪdə] (3)
THANK YOU (['θæŋkju] 6 potential segments)	['tæŋkju] (5)	[fæŋku] (5)
UMBRELLA ([ʌm'brɛlə] 7 potential segments)	[ʌm'bwɛlə](6)	[ʌmbwɛlə](6)

27 potential segments

pre-intervention 21/27 post-intervention 21/27

3. Now score all her consonants on a three-feature basis: 1 point for correct voicing; 1 point for correct place of articulation; and 1 point for correct manner of articulation.

Pre-intervention

WATER ['wɔwə]:
- w for w = 3/3 as place, manner and voicing are all correct
- w for t = 0/3 as place, manner and voicing all differ

GLOVES [plʊbz]:
- p for g = 1/3 for manner and place; both are stops
- l for l = 3/3 as place, manner and voicing are all correct
- b for v = 1/3 as both are voiced
- z for z = 3/3 as place, manner and voicing are all correct

SPIDER ['paɪdə]:
- s omitted 0/3
- p for p = 3/3
- d for d = 3/3

THANK YOU ['fæŋkju]:
- f for θ = 2/3 as both are voiceless fricatives
- ŋ for ŋ = 3/3
- k for k = 3/3
- j for j = 3/3

UMBRELLA [ʌm'bwɛlə]:
- m for m = 3/3
- b for b = 3/3

r for w = 2/3 for voicing and manner
l for l = 3/3

Total potential features correct: 51
Features correct: 39

Post-intervention

WATER ['wɔtə]: w for w = 3/3 as place, manner and voicing are all correct
t for t = 3/3 as place, manner and voicing are all correct

GLOVES [klʊfs]: k for g = 2/3 for manner and place
l for l = 3/3 as place, manner and voicing are all correct
f for v = 2/3 for manner and place
s for z = 2/3 as place and manner are the same

SPIDER ['flaɪdə]: f for s = 2/3, share manner and voicing; both voiceless fricatives
l for p = 0/3
d for d = 3/3

THANK YOU ['tæŋkju]: t for θ = 1/3 as both are voiceless
ŋ for ŋ = 3/3
k for k = 3/3
j for j = 3/3

UMBRELLA [ʌm'bwɛlə]: m for m = 3/3
b for b = 3/3
r for w = 2/3 for voicing and manner
l for l = 3/3

Total potential features correct: 51
Features correct: 41

4. Comment on the different impressions these scoring methods give of Anna's progress.

The right/wrong method gives a quick overview of Anna's progress, but does not give her any credit for improvements that were made towards the adult target. Method 2, the segment-by-segment approach is potentially a more sensitive method but here it revealed no difference in Anna's performance. Her speech is inconsistent and although some aspects of her speech had changed as a result of intervention, some aspects of her speech were less accurate at the post-intervention assessment, and the two effectively cancelled each other out. The final method of scoring is the most sensitive method and allows us to detail changes in a very specific way. Credit is given for all changes towards the adult target. The method is, however, time-consuming, and one would need to modify it to include scoring of vowels.

Note

1. http://members.tripod.com/Caroline_Bowen/acquisition.html

Chapter 4
Working on Segments in Single Words

Chapter 3 introduced some principles used in the design and selection of segments in single word stimuli. In this chapter we present a case study of Oliver, a boy aged 5;6, which will illustrate some of these principles. Our intervention with Oliver could have taken many different paths and many different stimuli might have been used. We present the process that we undertook for Oliver's stimuli selection with opportunities throughout the chapter for reflection on aspects which might have been done differently. A key message throughout the chapter is that one should always aim for stimuli selection to be theoretically guided with an explicit rationale for each choice made.

In Chapter 3, we presented Ebbels's (2000) case study of a girl with hearing impairment and PSDs. This case study illustrated how a phonological approach, concerned with individual segments, can be combined with a psycholinguistic approach to understanding a child's difficulties. Both have an important role to play in intervention planning since the psycholinguistic approach informs our knowledge of levels of breakdown (the 'how' of intervention) and the phonological approach provides further information about the particular sounds, or words, affected at each level (the 'what' of intervention). Oliver's intervention also demonstrates the way in which psycholinguistic and phonological approaches can be combined. In addition, some of our plans for intervention were affected by Oliver's own social-emotional needs, a third very important strand that should not be forgotten when planning intervention for children.

Case Study: Oliver Aged 5;6

We first met Oliver when he was 5 years of age, his speech was understood by few people and he already had some difficulties with literacy acquisition in the classroom. Oliver had a severe expressive language impairment, and a mild impairment of comprehension of language. At CA 5;6

he had an extremely limited repertoire of vowels and consonants. A history of middle ear infections and fluctuating hearing loss has almost certainly contributed to this. Speech delay due to otitis media with effusion (SD-OME) is one of the aetiological categories suggested by Shriberg *et al.* (1997); see also Roberts and Burchinal (2001) and Nittrouer and Burton (2005) for further discussion of the effects of middle ear infections on speech and literacy development. However, Oliver had also been labelled as having 'developmental verbal dyspraxia' or 'childhood apraxia of speech'. Oliver appeared to be a socially-skilled child who, at that stage was able to make most of his needs known and who was not sensitive about his speech problem. In the classroom situation, he was popular and coping adequately with numeracy. He was not able to fully contribute to oral language activities. He had received approximately 30 hours of therapy in the past and continued to receive intensive input delivered primarily by his classroom learning support assistant (LSA). He had made some progress with his speech and language, but had a way to go in producing intelligible speech appropriate for a child of his age. Oliver was not always cooperative in therapy. He found speech output tasks a great challenge and sometimes refused to try tasks, knowing perhaps that he might be misunderstood or would not succeed. An important psychosocial consideration in our assessment and intervention planning was to consider ways into his speech processing system without putting him under pressure to produce speech.

Assessment Data

Severity indices are useful measures which can encapsulate the degree of difficulty children experience with their speech in a single number. Most typically used are indices such as percentage of consonants correct (PCC), or percentage of vowels correct (PVC). To obtain these indices, one typically takes a sample of a child's speech, either single words or spontaneous speech – although using spontaneous speech may not be practical in cases where children's speech is unintelligible and the target words are not known. Based on the speech sample of about 50 to 100 words, a count is made of all the possible consonants (or vowels) that would have been realized in an adult production of the words. A second count is then made of the number of consonants (or vowels) realized correctly by the child. The child's number of correct productions is divided by the number of possible adult productions and multiplied by 100 to give a percentage, i.e. PCC or PVC. PVC and PCC may also be combined to yield another index, that of PPC or percentage of phonemes correct. For example, if one were scoring the single word DAISY for PCC, one would first determine the number of possible consonants. There are two in this word, i.e. /d, z/. If the child produced DAISY → [eɪzi], the second count would involve the actual consonants used by the child, i.e. only /z/. The number of consonants correct (n = 1) divided by the possible number of consonants (= 2) would yield a PCC of 50%. The same process could be carried out on the word DAISY for vowels to give PVC, and then combining consonants and vowels to give PPC. Clearly, however one would need to do this for many more words than just the one given in this example. Typically 50–100 words are used to generate meaningful indices. The following guidelines are commonly used when describing PCC:

Severity level	**PCC**
Mild	90% +
Mild to Moderate	65–89%
Moderate to Severe	50–64%
Severe	49% or lower

The segments most well-established in Oliver's consonant inventory were the voiced plosives ([b], [d] and [g]) and nasals ([m], [n] and [ŋ]). He was able to use these in all appropriate word positions, although not consistently, e.g. DUCK → [dɑ], and DICE → [ɑɪ]. Voiceless plosives were starting to emerge but remained inconsistently used, e.g. KEY → [ki], CAR → [ɑ]. Fricatives [s] and [f] were used on occasion, e.g. ICE → [ɑɪs], FEATHER → [fɪ]. Oliver used a range of systematic simplifications in his speech, including processes such as:

- final consonant deletion. This was used in 43% of possible instances, e.g. BATH → [bɑ].
- reduplication. This appeared in 12% of possible instances, e.g. WATER → ['wɑwʊ].
- cluster reduction. This process was noted in 94% of possible instances, e.g. SPOON → [bʊ].
- stopping. This occurred in 32% of possible instances, e.g. LEAF → [it].
- pre-vocalic voicing. It was observed in 39% of possible instances, e.g. PENCIL → ['bɛnu].

These are all processes that one would expect to find in the speech of a younger child. Oliver also used initial consonant deletion (e.g. BLUE → [u], TEA → [i]) in 34% of possible instances, a process considered atypical or unusual by many authors (e.g. Dodd *et al.*, 2002). Some vowel distortion was also noted. At a syllable structure level, Oliver generally managed to preserve the correct number of syllables. He favoured syllable structure types of V, CV, VC, and CVCV (where V = vowel; C = consonant). Some isolated instances of closed CVC syllables were noted. [w] was well established in his phonetic inventory (e.g. WATCH → [wɑ], WATER → ['wɑwʊ]) with other approximants being used in an inconsistent way. Clusters did not yet occur in Oliver's inventory with the exception of [br] → [bw] and [fr] → [fw] which were noted in two isolated instances (e.g. BRIDGE →

[bwɪdʒ]). Table 4.1 provides a summary of Oliver's speech data at CA 5;6.

Oliver's speech processing profile showed difficulties throughout the system (see Figure 4.1). On the input side, he had some strengths towards the top level of the profile, e.g. he performed age-appropriately on the alliteration task which involved no speech but only picture identification (Level F, Phonological Assessment Battery (PhAB) picture alliteration subtest, Frederikson, Frith and Reason, 1997). On the output side, the pattern was reversed with Oliver having relative strengths towards the lower levels at Level K. However, generally he has a pervasive speech processing difficulty affecting input and output.

Oliver was aided by pictures and found having semantic knowledge to draw on useful. In terms of output, motor execution (Level K) was a relative strength for Oliver. He could produce almost all sounds in

Table 4.1: Summary of Oliver's speech data at CA 5;6

Assessment	Comments	
Severity indices	Percentage of consonants correct (PCC): 23.4% Percentage of vowels correct (PVC): 68.2% Percentage of phonemes correct (PPC): 39.7%	
Phonetic inventory	Word-initial position: [m, n, b, d, g, w, j] Word-medial position: [m, n, b, w] Word-final position: [m n, ŋ, ʤ]	
Stimulability	All segments stimulable except [v], [z], [θ], [ð], [ʒ]	
Phonological processes analysis (% use)	Developmental processes: cluster reduction (94%); final consonant deletion (43%); prevocalic voicing (39%); stopping of fricatives and affricates (32%); reduplication (12%) Non-developmental processes: vowel distortion (27%); initial consonant deletion (34%)	
Single word speech sample	DICE → [ɑɪ] DUCK → [dɑ] KEY → [ki] CAR → [ɑ] ICE → [ɑɪs] PENCIL → [ˈbɛnu] BLUE → [u] CROCODILE → [æ]	BATH → [bɑ] WATER → [ˈwɑwʊ] SPOON → [bʊ] LEAF → [it] WATCH → [wɑ] FEATHER → [fɪ] TEA → [ɪ] HELICOPTER → [eʔɑʔɑ]
Connected speech sample	RUN AWAY → [ˈbɑpɛwɛ] I WANT TO → [ɑɪˈwænʊ] MY BED → [ˈmɑɪbɛd] WHAT'S THAT NOISE? → [ˈwɑʔ æʔ ʊ] WHO BOUGHT THEM? → [ʊ bʊ ˈɛm]	

√ = age appropriate performance
X = 1 standard deviation below the expected mean for his age
XX = 2 standard deviations below the expected mean for his age

INPUT

F Is the child aware of the internal structure of phonological representations?
X – Picture rhyme detection (Vance *et al.*, 1994)
√ – Picture onset detection (PhAB picture alliteration subtest, Frederikson *et al.*, 1997)

E Are the child's phonological representations accurate?
X – Auditory detection of speech errors (Constable *et al.*, 1997).

D Can the child discriminate between real words?
X – Minimal pair auditory discrimination of clusters (Bridgeman and Snowling, 1988)
X – Aston Index discrimination subtest (Newton and Thompson, 1982)
X – Wepman's Auditory Discrimination (Wepman and Reynolds, 1987)
X – Own error discrimination test (Locke, 1980a, b)

C Does the child have language specific representations of word structures?

Not tested

B Can the child discriminate speech sounds without reference to lexical representations?
X – Minimal pair auditory discrimination of clusters in non-words (Bridgeman and Snowling, 1988)

A Does the child have adequate auditory perception?
X / √ – audiometry – has had problems in the past although these now seem to be resolved

OUTPUT

G Can the child access accurate motor programmes?

X – Word-finding vocabulary test (Renfrew, 1995)
XX – Edinburgh Articulation Test (Anthony *et al.*, 1971)
XX – The Bus Story (Renfrew, 1969)

H Can the child manipulate phonological units?
X – PAT rhyme fluency subtest (Muter *et al.*, 1997)

I Can the child articulate real words accurately?
X – Real word repetition subtest (Constable *et al.*, 1997)
X – Aston Index blending subtest – real Words (Newton and Thompson, 1982)

J Can the child articulate speech without reference to lexical representations?
X – Aston Index blending subtest – Non-words (Newton and Thompson, 1982)
X – Non-word repetition subtest (Constable *et al.*, 1997)

K Does the child have adequate sound production skills?
Can copy all phonemes except [v], [z] [θ], [ð], [ʒ]
Can't sequence sounds on a DDK task

L Does the child reject his own erroneous forms?
Informal observation – no.

Figure 4.1: Oliver's speech processing profile at CA 5;6.

isolation with the exception of [v], [z], [θ], [ð] and [ʒ]. In terms of input, discrimination of non-words was the most challenging task for Oliver. The lower levels of the input side of the profile were more challenging for Oliver, and this may give some indication of the way in which his middle-ear problems and his speech output difficulties are likely to have impacted on the entire speech processing system.

For output, Oliver's problems increased as one moved up the output side. He found repetition of real and non-word tasks difficult (levels I and J), and had major difficulty in accessing the accurate motor programs (level G) required in naming tasks and spontaneous speech. The fact that his performance did not improve from spontaneous naming to repetition suggested that he had difficulties with stored motor programs as well as with online motor programming. His phonological manipulation skills (level H) were surprisingly good - and this may be due to the effects of training and previous therapy.

ACTIVITY 4.1

Oliver has a range of difficulties with his speech. Consider the data presented in Oliver's speech processing profile shown in Figure 4.1. Make notes about the following questions based on the profile data.

(a) Compare the input and output sides (left and right) of the speech processing profile. Comment on Oliver's areas of weakness, and also his areas of relative strength.

(b) Compare the higher versus lower levels (top and bottom) of the speech processing profile. Identify any areas of relative strength and areas of weakness.

(c) Bearing in mind that Oliver's difficulties are widespread throughout most levels of the speech processing profile, what areas of relative strength would you use as a way into his speech processing system? Think of examples of tasks that might be used as a starting point in consolidating his relative strengths.

Now, turn to the Key to Activity 4.1 at the end of this chapter for our responses to these questions. These points are also discussed further in the section that follows.

Intervention Planning: A Psycholinguistic Perspective

The speech processing profile (Figure 4.1) revealed difficulties on both sides of the profile affecting input and output. From the profile, it was clear that Oliver's main areas of relative strength were at the top part of the input side of the profile (i.e., level F) and at the bottom part of the output side (i.e. level K). Level F poses the question: Is the child aware of the internal structure of phonological representations? We carried out two tests at this level. First, we used the supplementary alliteration test from the *Phonological Assessment Battery* (PhAB) (Frederikson *et al.*, 1997). In this test the child is presented with three pictures (e.g. CAT, DOG, CABBAGE) and asked to indicate the two pictures which start with the same sound (i.e. CAT, CABBAGE). The examiner does not name the pictures, so that the child is required to access his own phonological representation and then make a judgment based on these representations about the similarity of the pictures. Oliver performed in an age-appropriate way on this subtest. Second, we carried out a similar test (from Vance *et al.*, 1994) which involved identifying which two pictures rhymed out of the three presented (e.g. WHALE, NAIL, HAMMER). Oliver performed below the expected level for his age on this test, suggesting that his relative strength lies with onset rather than rime knowledge. It is important to refer to *relative* strengths, since these areas may not necessarily be age-appropriate skills, but in terms of a child's overall abilities, they are relative strengths.

Oliver had multiple difficulties in his speech processing system making it challenging to decide which parts of the system should be addressed. Evidence of some skills at the level of phonological representations (level F in the speech processing profile shown in Figure 4.1) suggested that this might be a way into his speech processing system. Bearing in mind our psychosocial aim of not putting Oliver under pressure to speak, we decided that Oliver's intervention should aim to target the input levels of phonological representation and phonological recognition. This knowledge might be a starting point in bringing about changes in his speech processing system. Carrying out, for example, tasks involving auditory lexical decision would help to develop his phonological representations and ultimately his mapping onto more accurate motor programs. Modifying input should have the effect of ultimately modifying output as input maps onto output. Because Oliver's auditory discrimination was weak we needed to control carefully the presentation of items and be sure that he was hearing the appropriate productions from the therapist.

The relationship between input and output skills is a controversial one. Some authors have suggested that input should always be addressed prior to output (e.g. Evershed Martin, 1991; Jamieson and Rvachew, 1992). Corrin (2001a, b) notes that as a general principle input should be addressed first, and this then used to strengthen output skills. However, authors such as Williams and McReynolds (1975) questioned the value of input therapy. A tenet of the psycholinguistic approach is that one should target specific underlying difficulties, and that whatever aspects are targeted should be done by means of appropriate stimuli that reflect a child's errors (Rees, 2001a). Input work may be irrelevant in cases where, following a detailed assessment no input problems can be found, or in cases where the input stimuli are not carefully chosen to reflect the child's specific problems. For some children both input and output therapy may be appropriate. Clearly Oliver has difficulties with both sides of the profile. The issue may thus be one of readiness, with input/output work both appropriate at different developmental phases.

Waters, Hawkes and Burnett (1998) and Waters (2001) used input work successfully with a child with severe speech output problems in the presence of relatively good input skills. The child's strengths were used as a way of modifying the speech processing system as a whole. In Oliver's case it was hypothesized that working on his input would be the first step in modifying his speech processing. By using his relative strength of onset awareness in phonological representations, we might be able to gain access to other aspects of his speech processing system such as motor programs, a particular area of difficulty for him (see Figure 4.1; level G). Corrin (2001a, b) describes a therapy programme in which individual segments inserted into onset position of single words are taken 'on tour' through the speech processing system, in a systematic, cyclical way. This approach was successful in the case of the child described, a 7-year-old girl with PSDs and severe speech processing problems throughout her profile. Drawing on this evidence, a similar principle was adopted for Oliver. Individual segments were selected, inserted into word-initial position in single word exemplars and used in a carefully devised series of tasks.

In devising tasks we need to be clear about exactly what aspects of the speech processing system are being tapped and why this will be helpful for the child. We devised five tasks which we ordered into a task hierarchy shown in Table 4.2.

The five tasks are ordered from 1, a task thought to be fairly easy for Oliver and based on his strengths, through to 5, a task that is judged to be challenging for him. Tasks outlined in the hierarchy were designed to tap one particular area, e.g. Task 1, the auditory lexical decision task was designed primarily to tap phonological representations. However, it is important to consider that all tasks will involve the stimulation of other related areas, e.g. Task 1 also allows for the downward flow of semantic knowledge and the bottom-up flow of auditory input. This is the principle of the therapy programme and allows for transitions to be made from one task in the hierarchy to the next. Tasks 1 and 2 gave Oliver the optional support of semantic knowledge, while tapping his phonological knowledge (Task 1) and his auditory discrimination abilities (Task 2). Oliver benefits from presentation of visual material, and giving him pictures of stimuli would allow him to use his semantic knowledge to support his less strong auditory skills without relying solely on the auditory information. Tasks 3–5 are more demanding, requiring careful listening as he moves from real word to non-word tasks. The final task was considered to be the most challenging for Oliver. This intra-personal judgment task required him to listen carefully to his own speech – as opposed to the

Table 4.2: Outline of Oliver's intervention task hierarchy

Task		Description	Aspect of speech processing system tapped
1 = easy; 5 = hard			
1	Auditory lexical decision task	Oliver is presented with a picture (e.g. COW) and asked to respond 'yes' or 'no' to questions such as: Is it a [zaʊ]? Is it a COW?	Primarily phonological representations but can access top-down support of semantic knowledge. Involves all levels of input as he hears the stimuli
2	Discrimination and onset segmentation (with picture)	Oliver is given a picture of a COW and hears the therapist produce that word at the same time. He is required to post the item into the relevant [k] post box	Phonological representations, phonological recognition and phonetic discrimination. Can access top-down semantic support, and involves all levels of input as he listens to the stimuli
3	Discrimination and onset segmentation (no picture)	As for Task 2, but for this task Oliver is not given the picture. He listens to the word and then, depending on the initial segment perceived (e.g. DOG or LOG), posts a token into the appropriate box (e.g. [d] or [l] box)	As for task 2 but must trigger own semantic support as picture not provided
4	Non-word discrimination	As for Task 3 but uses non-words	Primarily phonological recognition, but will also involve peripheral auditory processing
5	Intra-personal judgment	Oliver names a picture. He then listens to an audio-recording of himself and judges whether what he hears is correct or incorrect	Taps entire system starting from semantic representation and placing demands on both output and input

therapist's - and to make judgments regarding the accuracy of his own speech. Evershed-Martin (1991) notes that perception of others' speech seems to be ahead of self-perception, and this is thus considered a final but important stage of the hierarchy. Our intra-personal judgment task did not involve online monitoring, i.e. it was not truly intra-personal, but it aimed to move Oliver a way towards it.

With a clear idea of the tasks to be used in intervention and the ultimate changes that we were aiming to bring about in Oliver's speech processing system, the question still remained: Which segments should we address and in what phonetic/phonological context?

Intervention Planning: A Phonological Perspective

We chose to apply a combination of principles in our selection of targets.

Principle 1: Select targets at different levels of the developmental hierarchy in order to answer questions about Oliver's developmental progression. Table 3.1 in Chapter 3 shows Grunwell's developmental outline of phonological acquisition.

Principle 2: Select targets from different productive phonological knowledge (PPK) categories in order to answer questions about PPK and efficiency. Guidelines from Gierut *et al.* (1987) (see Table 3.2 in Chapter 3) were used. Oliver's intervention programme centred on input, but aimed to ultimately improve the entire speech processing system and Oliver's speech intelligibility. It was thus felt that the concept of PPK could be usefully invoked in the target selection for his intervention programme.

Principle 3: Select segments that require intervention at both input and output levels.

Principle 4: Once the main stimuli have been selected, devise further stimuli using a maximal opposition approach. Create contrasts that move from maximal oppositions (i.e. a big difference between sounds) to a minimal contrast between segments.

Principle 5: Confront child with own errors wherever possible. In addition to principle 4 (above) we wanted to contrast Oliver's own errors with the correct productions. Children such as Oliver with inaccurate phonological representations are more likely to respond to presentation of their own errors and error words than to words for which they have accurate representations. This is a point emphasized by Rees (2001a) and by other authors (e.g. Locke, 1980a, b; Jamieson and Rvachew, 1992; Rvachew, 1994) who suggest that auditory perception as a general approach to intervention is not successful: only if stimuli relevant to the child are used, will change occur.

ACTIVITY 4.2

Consider Oliver's speech data presented in Table 4.1 in the light of the target selection principles outlined above. Focusing specifically on principles 1 and 2, carry out the following tasks:

(a) **Principle 1:** Using your knowledge of normally-developing children's phonological acquisition or with reference to Grunwell's developmental chart in Table 3.1 (Chapter 3), make a note of segments that might be treated next using a traditional developmental hierarchy.
(b) **Principle 2:** Using Table 3.2 in Chapter 3, identify segments in each of the PPK categories for Oliver.

Now refer to the Key to Activity 4.2 at the end of this Chapter, and read on for further details of how we selected stimuli for Oliver.

Applying the principles

Principle 1: Select targets at different levels of the developmental hierarchy to investigate this issue. Table 3.1 in Chapter 3 shows Grunwell's developmental outline of phonological acquisition.

We considered all English consonants from a developmental perspective, in terms of Oliver's productive phonological knowledge, perception skills and segment oppositions. For each of these areas, a particular rationale was adopted, e.g. for normal development each consonant was grouped into categories of acquisition (from Grunwell, 1987) and the rationale adopted was that stimuli selected should cover a range of these to allow comparison of therapy outcomes. According to Grunwell (1987) /t/ is an early acquired segment associated with Stage 2 of phonological development. /k/ is an example of a segment that normally starts to appear in Stage 3, and becomes more established in Stages 4, and 5. /s/ is typically associated with Stage 5, and /dʒ/ with Stage 6.

Principle 2: Select targets from different PPK categories to investigate this issue. Guidelines from Gierut *et al.* (1987) (see Table 3.2 in Chapter 3) were used.

The four consonants /t/, /k/, /s/ and /dʒ/ also fit in well with our second principle of choosing segments from PPK categories 4–6. Segments from categories 4–6 have not yet been acquired and therefore it is logical to work on these, rather than segments from categories 1–3. We considered /t/ and /dʒ/ as examples of segments from PPK type 6 about which there is no knowledge. We considered /k/ and /s/ to be segments from PPK type 5 about which there is more, but still minimal, knowledge.

We posed the following questions about Oliver's intervention.

Question 1: Would early acquired segments be easier for Oliver to acquire than the later ones?
Question 2: Would sounds with minimal PPK bring about more changes in Oliver's speech?

Principle 3: Select segments that require intervention at both input and output levels.

This was not difficult to do as Oliver had such widespread auditory perception difficulties.

We now discuss the target segments and the context in which they were used, before continuing with consideration of principles 4 and 5.

The Target Segments in Context: Stimuli Design

Having selected the target segments /t/, /k/, /s/ and /dʒ/ based on a set of explicit principles, it remained for us to consider how to address these in intervention. Would we work on these segments in single words, phrases or in isolation? In order to answer these questions, we again returned to the theory. It is important to consider the effects of word position since some children will find it easier to produce their targets in specific positions. Research (e.g. Ferguson, 1978; Edwards, 1983; Grunwell, 1985; Redford, MacNeilage and Davis, 1997) has suggested that some segments emerge first in word-final position before becoming established in word-initial position, and in other cases the reverse is true. In Oliver's case there was no major difference in terms of his output production of segments in different word positions, although we had demonstrated that he had some relatively good knowledge of onsets, e.g. see Figure 4.1, Level F, *PhAB* picture alliteration subtest. Thus segments in word-initial position were targeted and the positional focus of all work – both input and output – was on the onset position.

Sets of stimuli words were then created for each of the four segments. These lists were devised using the following criteria.

1. For each segment, 5 CV and 5 CVC words with the target segment in word-initial (WI) position were created.
2. When selecting the target CVC words to be used in intervention, an attempt was made to avoid having the target stimuli ([t], [k], [s], [dʒ],) in word-final position as well. As noted in Chapter 3, phonetic context should be used to support – not hinder – the child's production, thus words like CAKE, and SAUCE were avoided.
3. Words were selected which were familiar to Oliver, as determined by picture naming tasks.

4. The words were matched across sets in terms of age of acquisition and spoken language frequency using the MRC psycholinguistic database.[1] Age of acquisition refers to the average age at which children are thought to acquire particular words. Spoken language frequency refers to how often a particular word occurs in the language. The MRC psycholinguistic database is an online resource that is freely available for all to use. By ensuring that age of acquisition and spoken language frequency are balanced across the lists, any differences in the changes occurring from list-to-list will be attributed to the target itself rather than the words chosen.

Table 4.3 shows these four target wordlists.

Principle 4: Once the main stimuli have been selected, devise further stimuli using a maximal opposition approach. Create contrasts that move from maximal oppositions (i.e. a big difference between sounds) to a minimal contrast between segments.

Principle 5: Confront child with own errors wherever possible.

Each of Oliver's stimuli words shown in Table 4.3 were used as the starting point in following principles 4 and 5. We started by contrasting each /k/ stimulus with a very different word initial segment, e.g., /z/ which differs from /k/ in terms of place, manner and voicing. Thus, it should be easy for Oliver to hear the difference between the two. Slightly less different is the contrast between /k/ and /d/: these segments differ in two features only. Moving towards minimal pairs, we then have /k/ contrasted with /g/ which differs only in voicing. We then get more specific, contrasting the target stimuli with Oliver's own production and/or auditory discrimination errors, e.g. in the case of /k/, we made further contrasts with /b/ and /p/ (Oliver's favoured substitutions), and no contrast at all, i.e. /k/

Table 4.3: Oliver's wordlists for intervention

[k]	[ʤ]	[s]	[t]
COW	JAR	SEA	TOE
CAR	JOE	SAW	TWO
KEY	JAW	SEW	TIE
KAY	JAY	SUE	TAR
CORE	JEE	SIR	TEA
CAGE	JAYNE	SAD	TEACH
CAT	JEEP	SWORD	TALK
CALL	JET	SEAL	TAIL
CARD	JAIL	SUN	TEN
CAN	JUICE	SOCK	TOUGH

Table 4.4: Oliver's single word stimuli with contrasts used in the intervention

Stimuli words for [k]	Maximal	→	Contrast segments Minimal Opposition			
	Differs on 3 features	Differs on 2 features	Differs on 1 feature		Own errors	
[k]	[z]	[d]	[g]	[b]	[p]	#
COW	[zaʊ]	[daʊ]	[gaʊ]	[baʊ]	[paʊ]	[aʊ]
CAR	[zɑ]	[dɑ]	[gɑ]	[bɑ]	[pɑ]	[ɑ]
KEY	[zi]	[di]	[gi]	[bi]	[pi]	[i]
KAY	[zeɪ]	[deɪ]	[geɪ]	[beɪ]	[peɪ]	[eɪ]
CORE	[zɔ]	[dɔ]	[gɔ]	[bɔ]	[pɔ]	[ɔ]
CAGE	[zeɪʤ]	[deɪʤ]	[geɪʤ]	[beɪʤ]	[peɪʤ]	[eɪʤ]
CAT	[zæt]	[dæt]	[gæt]	[bæt]	[pæt]	[æt]
CALL	[zɔl]	[dɔl]	[gɔl]	[bɔl]	[pɔl]	[ɔl]
CARD	[zɑd]	[dɑd]	[gɑd]	[bɑd]	[pɑd]	[ɑd]
CAN	[zæn]	[dæn]	[gæn]	[bæn]	[pæn]	[æn]

vs. silence/omission. With the onset contrast segments selected we then created both real and non-words by combining these with the existing rime of the target stimuli, e.g. the first target item COW was contrasted with [zaʊ] and [daʊ] (maximal oppositions), then with [gaʊ] (minimal opposition) and each of Oliver's own productions in turn.

Table 4.4 shows the way in which the stimuli words were contrasted with segments in other words moving from maximal to minimal contrasts, as well as making contrasts with Oliver's own errors. The example is limited to showing how oppositions were structured at the beginning of Oliver's intervention programme, focusing on [k] but similar principles were used for the selection of the /t/, /s/ and /dʒ/ stimuli.

Phases of Intervention

Intervention consisted of four consecutive phases with each phase consisting of seven sessions: A total of 28 hours of intervention took place. The sessions were carried out on a twice-weekly basis in Oliver's school in a quiet room with only Oliver and the therapist present. Oliver was 5;11 at the start of the intervention itself and was 6;5 on completion of the final phase of intervention. Each phase centred round one segment: either /k/, or /dʒ/ or /s/ or /t/. The design of the intervention is outlined in Figure 4.2.

The intervention programme followed the hierarchy of tasks outlined in Table 4.2 using each of the selected stimuli in turn. For example, in

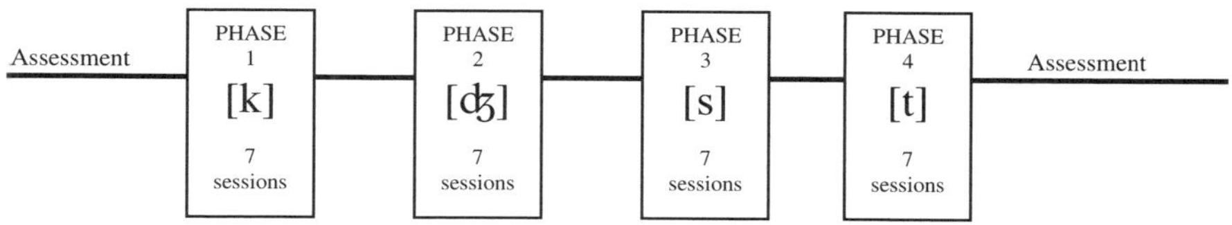

Figure 4.2: The design of Oliver's intervention programme.

Phase 1 of intervention, all the /k/ stimuli and contrasted stimuli were required (see Table 4.4). Each of the five tasks in the task hierarchy (see Table 4.2) formed a session of intervention, with the two extra sessions of intervention being used for addressing any of the tasks that required further work, giving a total of seven hours of intervention per phase. Thus, Task 1 involved the 'easy' auditory lexical decision task described in Table 4.2 using the stimuli outlined in Tables 4.3 and 4.4. Oliver was presented with a picture (e.g. COW) and asked to respond 'yes' or 'no' to questions such as: Is it a [zaʊ]? Is it a COW? Is it a [daʊ]? Is it a [gaʊ]? For Task 2, the discrimination and onset segmentation task (with pictures) which took place in session 2, Oliver was given a picture of, for example, a COW. He would hear the therapist produce that word at the same time and was then required to post the item into the relevant onset post box. This task was limited to the picturable real words, e.g. COW and POW with the latter represented by a toy gun. Task 3 took place in the third session and was the same as the previous task. However, it was made more challenging by not using picture stimuli. Oliver simply heard a word, and then depending on the perceived onset (e.g. COW or POW) posted a token into the appropriate box (e.g. [k] or [p] box). Task 4, in session 4, was non-word discrimination, and again was the same task as the preceding one but this time incorporating all the non-word contrasts, e.g. COW contrasted with [zaʊ]. Each of the tasks described was carried out using the 10 /k/ stimuli shown in Table 4.3 and the appropriate associated stimuli in Table 4.4. Thus a task was done several times in one session using all the stimuli described. In session 2, Task 2 would be worked through in the same way and so on.

The final task was the intrapersonal judgment task where Oliver agreed to be audiotaped naming a picture of one of his 10 /k/ stimuli. He then made a judgment about whether what he had said was correct or incorrect. In this task there was no pressure on him to produce the targets appropriately, rather he was rewarded for making the right listening judgments. After this phase of intervention addressing all the /k/ stimuli, we moved on to the next set of stimuli for /dʒ/, carrying out the same tasks as for the first phase but with different stimuli. This phase of intervention was then followed by the therapy phases for the other two segments. A range of motivating materials (e.g. stickers, toy cars, action people) and supports (e.g. tape recorder, computer activities) were used to make the activities exciting and enjoyable for Oliver.

Outcomes

Oliver's production of the four targeted segments improved significantly over the course of the intervention programme. This means that he made greater improvements with his speech production of these sounds than would otherwise be expected through chance or maturation. He made significant improvements with his ability to produce /t/ ($t(29) = -2.340$, $p < 0.05$); /k/ ($t(29) = -4.397$, $p < 0.001$) and /s/ ($t(29) = -2.626$, $p < 0.05$) when pre- and post-intervention results were compared, and statistical analysis carried out. We carried out paired samples t-tests to compare the difference in the accuracy of his speech production on the wordlists (see Pallant (2001) and Pring (2005) for further details of how to select statistical procedures and carry them out using computer software such as SPSS). There were no changes in his production of [dʒ] from pre- to post-intervention evaluation. Oliver found this segment challenging to produce. In Chapter 3 we considered the scoring of children's responses. In Oliver's case we scored his speech productions by considering only his production of the target segments, not of the whole words. If target segments were perceived as accurately produced we gave him 1 point, if target segments were not accurately perceived he received 0 points.

In addition to this quantitative analysis, we carried out a qualitative analysis examining the changes that had occurred in Oliver's speech over the course of the intervention (see Table 4.5). Some stimuli words were

Table 4.5: Examples of qualitative changes in Oliver's speech production

Target	Wordlist	Pre-intervention assessment	Post-intervention assessment
No change			
CAT	Treated	[æ]	[æ]
JOT	Treated	[ɒ]	[ɒ]
Increased accuracy			
JEWEL	Untreated	[u]	[dul]
JOE	Treated	[əʊ]	[gəʊ]
SOCK	Treated	[ɒ]	[dɒ]
Accuracy achieved			
COW	Treated	[aʊ]	[kaʊ]
TAIL	Treated	[teɪ]	[taɪjɪl]
SAT	Untreated	[æ]	[sæ]
SEA	Treated	[ɪ]	[si]
TEA	Treated	[ɪ]	[ti]

shown not to have changed over the course of the intervention programme, and these included both treated and untreated control words. Other words became more accurate as a result of intervention (e.g. see JOE and SOCK in Table 4.5), although the segments in question have not yet been acquired. The final category of words included those where the target sounds were accurately produced, although in some cases difficulties with the remainder of the word would still render it unintelligible, e.g. SAT in Table 4.5 still evidences final consonant deletion.

Addressing the Questions about Oliver's Intervention

Let us return to the questions posed about Oliver's intervention.

Question 1: Would early acquired segments be easier for Oliver to acquire than the later ones?

According to Grunwell (1987) /t/ is an early acquired segment associated with Stage 2 of phonological development. /k/ is an example of a segment that normally starts to appear in Stage 3, and becomes more established in Stages 4 and 5. /s/ is typically associated with Stage 5, and /dʒ/ with Stage 6. Oliver's response to intervention supported the use of traditional developmental hierarchies. He made the least progress with the latest developing sound: /dʒ/ from Stage 6. From a qualitative point of view, Oliver did make the most gains in his /t/ production and found many of the listening judgments involving /t/ stimuli relatively straightforward to make. It seemed as if he was developmentally ready to acquire this sound.

Question 2: Would sounds with minimal PPK bring about more changes in Oliver's speech?

We considered /t/ and /dʒ/ as examples of segments from PPK type 6 about which Oliver had no knowledge. We considered /k/ and /s/ to be segments from PPK type 5 about which Oliver knows more, but still has minimal knowledge. It has been suggested that segments from type 6 should be targeted to bring about greatest system-wide changes in intervention. In Oliver's case PPK did not seem to be an important consideration for intervention planning since /dʒ/, one of the type 6 segments, did not make more significant gains than the other segments. There are some methodological difficulties in measuring the effectiveness of PPK categorization in intervention. Our study with Oliver was not ideally designed to do so. Gierut (1992, 1998b) suggested that working on PPK type 6 targets maximally promotes generalization to other categories (i.e. it is most efficient) rather than stating that work on type 6 segments is more effective. This is an important distinction and reminds us that her claims are probably best investigated using groups of children, as has been done by authors such as Williams (1991). The results of the present work suggested that within the given timescales for intervention, greater change seemed to be brought about by working on developmental targets. It is, however, difficult to make any firm conclusions about this issue because the methodology does not allow for direct comparison of the two approaches, and if the children had received intervention over a longer period of time then the overall efficiency of the programme might have been shown to be different to that noted in the shorter term.

There are some difficulties with the concept of PPK. It does not give an indication of the child's ability to recognize and process segments in input. The notion of phonological knowledge as presented by Gierut *et al.* (1987) may be too broad to characterize the precise level of knowledge. There may be levels of partial knowledge with different categories of knowledge for different children, and the path through these more complex than has been proposed (Williams, 1991). Work on stimulability (e.g. Powell, Elbert and Dinnsen, 1991; Powell and Miccio, 1996) supports the notion that phonological competence is not all or nothing. The child necessarily passes through intermediate states in which knowledge of all aspects of perceiving and producing is built incrementally.

Oliver's intervention was aimed at developing his input processing in order to ultimately improve his speech output. The intervention focused mainly on input, although speech output skills were addressed in the final stages of the task hierarchy. This is an unusual approach to intervention for a child with apraxia of speech since traditionally drills and output work have been used, e.g. the *Nuffield Centre Dyspraxia Programme* (Williams and Stephens, 2004) is a programme of graded sessions to teach basic articulatory placement and coordination of motor speech sequences. Oliver's intervention was inspired largely by the work of Waters *et al.* (1998), as well as concerns about Oliver's self-esteem and the fact that he was under increasing pressure to talk and had had little success in previous speech therapy focusing on production. However, the child described by Waters was very different from Oliver, with many positive strengths in input processing that could be successfully brought to bear in intervention. Oliver showed one limited example of age-appropriate input processing in his speech processing profile (Level F in Figure 4.1). The intervention aimed to boost his input processing and phonological representations, enabling him to map representations from input to output. However, he may have benefited from a programme more balanced in terms of input and output, giving him more opportunity to put the mapping skills into practice. Gillon (2000) carried out programmes of phonological awareness in the hopes of improving the speech of children (ages 5;6–7;6) with spoken language impairments and matched controls. Children with spoken language impairment were allocated to three different treatment groups:

(a) an integrated phonological awareness programme, (b) a traditional programme, that focused on improving articulation and language skills, and (c) a minimal intervention control group. The phonological awareness tasks in this study aimed generally to improve children's awareness of sound structure in spoken language and to develop explicit knowledge of the links between spoken word forms and written representations. The traditional therapy involved a segment-oriented, articulatory approach and, in some severe cases, activities from the *Nuffield Centre Dyspraxia Programme* were used. The study found that children who received phonological awareness training obtained age-appropriate levels of literacy performance, and in addition their speech articulation improved, suggesting that speech output can be addressed by targeting other areas of the speech processing system. Thus, now we might question the traditional drillwork approach and focus more on input or at least input and output together.

In contrast to Gillon's study however, intervention studies by Harbers, Paden and Halle (1999) and Hesketh, Adams and Hall (2000) have been more cautious in their interpretation of the benefits of phonological awareness training on speech output performance. Harbers *et al.* found that the rate and degree of change in phonological awareness did not always parallel production performance. Hesketh *et al.* contrasted phonological awareness therapy and articulatory training approaches for children (aged 3;6–5;0) with phonological disorders. They found both types of therapy effective in enhancing phonological awareness skills and speech output, when contrasted with speech and phonological awareness gains made in a control group of normally developing children over the same period. However, no effect of therapy type was found in this study. Such comparisons of articulation vs. metaphonological therapies are problematic in that conventional articulation therapy can often be seen to require and encourage metaphonological awareness, although to a lesser extent than the pure phonological awareness training condition. This reminds us to always be explicit about what our tasks are really tapping.

Our primary outcome measure for the intervention with Oliver was his speech production of single words containing the target segments. However, other outcome measures were also used to evaluate changes in Oliver's speech processing. His auditory discrimination skills and his spelling of the single word stimuli were evaluated pre- and post-intervention in addition to his speech. Significant improvement was noted in both these areas with a greater effect noted for spelling than for speech. These improvements provided further evidence of the changes in Oliver's speech processing and the relationship between speech and spelling. Chapter 10 has the links between speech processing and literacy as its focus, and we return to this theme there.

Summary

This chapter described the assessment and intervention that took place with Oliver, a boy aged 5;6 with severe speech difficulties. The key points are as follows.

- Severity indices such as PCC and PVC are useful ways of encapsulating a child's degree of difficulty in a single number.
- Intervention planning with Oliver drew on psycholinguistic, phonological and psychosocial considerations.
- Psycholinguistic assessments suggested that Oliver had a pervasive speech processing difficulty but relative strengths at Level F of the speech processing profile in his phonological knowledge of onsets.
- Intervention aimed to use this area of strength as a way into his speech processing system.
- A task hierarchy was devised with each task aimed at tapping a different, but related part of the speech processing system.
- Stimuli selection was theoretically guided by an explicit rationale for each choice.
- Our target selection for Oliver was guided by five explicit principles, but a smaller number could also have been used.
- Four segments /t, k, s, dʒ/ were addressed as onsets in single CV and CVC words.
- These words were carefully selected based on stimuli selection principles introduced in Chapter 3.
- The main stimuli words were contrasted with a range of other single words moving Oliver from maximal contrasts to minimal contrasts, and contrasts with his own errors.
- The use of developmental principles was supported in the intervention study as Oliver made minimal gains with the latest-acquired segment.
- Segments were also classified into PPK categories, but these were found to have little bearing on the outcome of intervention.

KEY TO ACTIVITY 4.1

(a) Compare the input and output sides (left and right) of the speech processing profile. Comment on Oliver's areas of weakness, and also his areas of relative strength.

Oliver's speech processing profile shown in Figure 4.1 reveals difficulties on both sides of the profile affecting input and output. His speech input is affected at all levels tested, although he seems to have some relative strengths at Level F: Internal structure of phonological representations as assessed by the alliteration task using pictures only. Oliver's output is affected at all levels of the speech processing profile, with some possible strengths at Level K where he is stimulable for most sounds.

(b) Compare the higher versus lower levels (top and bottom) of the speech processing profile. Identify any areas of relative strength and areas of weakness.

In terms of input, Oliver has relative strengths with the top part of the profile as he performed in an age-appropriate way on the alliteration task (see above). If his hearing is now normal, he could also be seen to have strengths at Level A, the peripheral auditory level, although this certainly has not always been the case for him. In terms of output, his relative strengths lie towards the bottom of the profile as he was stimulable for many speech sounds at Level K.

(c) Bearing in mind that Oliver's difficulties are widespread throughout most levels of the speech processing profile, what areas of relative strength would you use as a way into his speech processing system? Think of examples of tasks that might be used as a starting point in consolidating his relative strengths.

Oliver's age-appropriate performance on one of the assessments at Level F is encouraging, suggesting that he has some accurate phonological knowledge. We suggest that this knowledge might be a starting point in bringing about changes in speech processing. We carried out tasks involving auditory lexical decisions in an effort to help develop his phonological representations and ultimately his mapping onto more accurate motor programs. Because his auditory discrimination is weak we need to control carefully the presentation of items and be sure that he is hearing the appropriate productions from the tester.

KEY TO ACTIVITY 4.2

(a) **Principle 1:** Using your knowledge of normally-developing children's phonological acquisition or with reference to Grunwell's developmental chart in Table 3.1 (Chapter 3), make a note of segments that might be treated next using a traditional developmental hierarchy.

Oliver does not yet have all consonants from Grunwell's (1987) Stage 2. The segments yet to be acquired include /p/, and /t/ and /d/. Oliver has acquired /b/ and owing to his voicing process finds it hard to realize /p/. It may be more helpful therefore to introduce a new place of articulation in the production of /d/. Oliver does produce /t/ in one instance of the speech sample when he says [it] for LEAF suggesting that he may be ready to make progress with alveolar stops.

(b) **Principle 2**: Using Table 3.2 in Chapter 3, identify segments in each of the PPK categories for Oliver.

This task needs to be carried out by looking at the data examples in Table 4.1. Data given in the phonetic inventory can also be a guide, but remember that PPK is based on the child's knowledge relative to the adult target. In many instances Oliver is noted to have particular segments in his inventory, but these are not actually used appropriately when considering the adult target. For example, Oliver uses /b/ as a substitute for many other segments in his speech, but when working out his PPK we need to scan the data for words that have /b/ in the adult realization, and then comment on what Oliver does in terms of his speech for each of those targets. The limited data provided make this activity challenging but the table below shows our classification based on the data given.

PPK type	Description of segment	Segments. Key: WI = word initial; WW = within word; WF =word final
1.	Produced correctly in all word positions for all morphemes.	• /m/. According to phonetic inventory this segment has been acquired in all word positions. The data reveal appropriate /m/ productions in Oliver's realization of phrases such as MY BED. • /w/. The phonetic inventory suggests that this segment has been acquired in WI and WW positions. The data show examples of appropriate usage in these positions.
2.	Produced correctly in nearly all morphemes but alternations between the target and another sound observed for some morphemes (optional rule).	No examples of this type.
3.	Produced correctly in nearly all morphemes but some 'fossilized' forms always produced incorrectly.	No examples of this type.
4.	Produced correctly in one or more word positions and consistently incorrect in other word positions.	No examples of this type.
5.	Inconsistently correct in one or more word positions and consistently incorrect in other word positions.	• /n/. Oliver's use of /n/ within words seems consistently accurate from the limited data, e.g. PENCIL → [bɛnu], but inconsistent in other word positions.

PPK type	Description of segment	Segments. Key: WI = word initial; WW = within-word; WF =word final
		• /d/. The phonetic inventory suggests /d/ is used WI and WW, but the data reveal inconsistent accurate productions. • /b/. The phonetic inventory suggests /b/ is used in WI and WW positions, but the data reveal that many of these are inappropriate production and there are few consistent and appropriate usages. • /k/. Appears to be used consistently in WI position, but not in other positions. • /f/. The data suggest that /f/ is used correctly in WI position, and that this is not the case for WF. • /s/. Appears inconsistently for WF targets, e.g. consider ICE → [ɑɪs] and DICE → [ɑɪ]. Appears consistently incorrect for WI and WW.
6.	Produced incorrectly in all word positions and all morphemes.	• /t/. No evidence of correct production of this segment in the data. When he produces LEAF → [it] this suggests he has /t/ in his phonetic inventory, but there is no evidence of knowledge of how to use the segment appropriately. • /p, z, h, tʃ, l, r, θ, ð/. No evidence of correct production of these segments from the limited data provided. • /g/ and /j/. The phonetic inventory suggests that these have been acquired in WI position, however there is no evidence of accurate and appropriate production in the data. • /dʒ/. Noted as being acquired in phonetic inventory but no evidence of this from the speech sample given.

Note

1. http://www.psy.uwa.edu.au/mrcdatabase/uwa_mrc.htm

Chapter 5 Stimuli Design: Consonant Clusters in Single Words

Much of the research into children's phonological development has centred on the production of individual segments, and many intervention programmes have individual segments as their focus. Yet consonant clusters (e.g. /bl/ in BLUE and /sn/ in SNAIL) are an important aspect of speech development for English-speaking children, and a frequent source of difficulty for them (e.g. Smit, 1993; McLeod, van Doorn and Reed, 1997). Many therapists working with school-age children with persisting speech difficulties will be addressing these children's difficulties in producing consonant clusters – possibly in both the children's speech and their spelling. The previous chapters had singleton segments as their focus, and emphasized some of the general issues associated with stimuli design and selection in phonological intervention. This chapter continues with the theme of stimuli design, but has consonant clusters and their place in intervention as its specific concern.

In this chapter the term consonant cluster is used to refer to adjacent consonant segments in the same syllable. These consonants might occur together in word initial position (e.g. **BR**OOM), word final position (e.g. PO**ST**) or within words (e.g. BA**SK**ET). Most research into clusters has focused on word-initial and word-final clusters, but there is increasingly more interest in investigating clusters within words (e.g. BA**SK**ET) and those occurring across word boundaries, e.g. in phrases such as BU**S T**IME (e.g. Ohala, 1999) – although whether or not abutting consonants can truly be considered consonant clusters is open to debate. Grunwell (1992, pp. 14–19) provides a concise overview of the structure of consonant clusters and the positional constraints which govern them.

To avoid confusion about terminology we refer to consonant clusters throughout this chapter, though some texts use the term 'blend' to refer to such adjacent consonant sequences. More importantly, the term adjunct is sometimes used to refer to [s] clusters because these consonants are thought to be more loosely adjoined to a word than a true cluster (Barlow, 2001; Velleman, 2002). This point is discussed in greater detail in subsequent sections but for now the important point to note is that we use the term consonant cluster in this chapter to refer to all sequences of two or more consonants, with awareness that this may not be strictly correct from a linguistic point of view.

The acquisition of consonant clusters is one of the longest lasting phases of speech acquisition observed in normally developing children. While children as young as 2 years of age produce some consonant clusters correctly, some 8–9-year-olds are still mastering this aspect of speech (McLeod, van Doorn and Reed, 2001). Consonant clusters are acquired relatively late in development and have been described as being 'extremely vulnerable in the acquisition course' (Gierut, 1999, p. 709).

This vulnerability makes clusters theoretically interesting, and practically important in terms of intervention. However, there are relatively few studies that have investigated children's development of consonant clusters. Some researchers have focused on the phonetic properties and substitution errors made by children with phonological difficulties, contrasting them with those developing normally (e.g. Allerton, 1976; Smit, 1993; McLeod *et al.*, 1997). Others have explored children's underlying knowledge about consonant clusters without requiring explicit productions (Lance, Swanson and Peterson, 1997). There is also a small group of studies that has investigated children's cluster development by manipulating clusters in intervention for children with phonological difficulties (e.g. Gierut, 1999; Gierut and Champion, 1999). Together these studies have contributed to the body of knowledge about consonant clusters, specifically with regard to theories about learning and language. For example, authors such as Elbert and McReynolds (1975) and Williams (2000a, b) focused on generalization and the patterns of generalization that occur within the sound class of clusters (see Chapter 9 for further discussion of generalization). Within-class generalization is a term used to refer to patterns of change that take place within a family of sounds, e.g. consonant clusters. Linguistic theories used to account for the development of consonant clusters are discussed in greater detail in the sections that follow.

There remains a great deal of uncertainty regarding consonant clusters and their acquisition both by children with normal phonological development and those with difficulties. This chapter reviews what is known about consonant clusters, especially in relation to children with PSDs. In the following chapter, Chapter 6, we describe the intervention that took place with a school-age boy: Joshua aged 6;10. Joshua's intervention focused specifically on clusters with all his initial consonant clusters being addressed. But, before focusing on this specific case in Chapter 6, let us consider what is known about the normal development of consonant clusters; what is known about intervention and consonant clusters, and the links between spoken and written production of consonant clusters.

ACTIVITY 5.1

1. Write down as many word-initial consonant clusters as you can think of in English.
2. Consider which of these can also occur word-finally.
3. Now list any other word-final consonant clusters you can think of.

Now turn to the Key to Activity 5.1 at the end of this chapter, before reading the following.

What Do We Know about the Normal Development of Consonant Clusters?

The reduction of clusters is a commonly occurring phonological simplification in children's speech. Children acquire word-initial clusters in a typical sequence:

1. initially omitting one part of the cluster, e.g. BLUE → [bu];
2. later, substituting for one part of the cluster e.g. BLUE → [bwu];
3. ultimately, correctly producing the entire cluster [blu].

In addition to cluster reduction, children can also process clusters in other ways, especially in their early development as they attempt to master them. Table 5.1 summarizes some of the developmental processes which affect consonant clusters.

Consonant clusters emerge later than singleton consonants, and therefore they are assumed to be more challenging to master. Accurate realizations of consonant clusters typically emerge slowly in children's speech between the ages of 3;6 and 8;0 (McLeod *et al.*, 2001). When children reduce clusters to singletons, they are usually systematic in terms of which consonant from the cluster they retain. Two linguistic theories have been used to account for the patterns observed in young children's production of consonant clusters:

- markedness theories
- sonority sequencing theories.

Markedness Theories

Markedness theories, also known as sequential markedness theories (e.g. Powell and Elbert, 1984; Clements and Hume, 1995) suggest that we can account for the way in which children realize part of a consonant cluster in early development. Children typically delete the more marked elements. In general linguistics, markedness refers to the way segments or

Table 5.1: Examples of phonological processes affecting consonant clusters (based on Kirk and Demuth, in press)

Phonological process	Target word	Response
Cluster reduction	FLOWER	['faʊwə]
Substitution	SWING	['fwɪŋ]
Coalescence	SPOON	['fun]
Metathesis	GHOST	['geʊts]
Deletion	BEST	['bɛ]

words are changed or added to, to give a special meaning. An unmarked segment or word (e.g. CAT) may be considered normal, but if something is added to it (e.g. plural 's'), it becomes special or marked (e.g. CATS). In terms of segments it is helpful to consider marked sounds as segments that are most challenging to produce. A typical developmental pattern would be for the consonant that is most difficult to produce (i.e. most marked) to be deleted. For example, young children typically produce /bun/ or /pun/ for SPOON. Markedness theories suggest that /p/ is an easier sound, acquired earlier in development than /s/, and hence /s/ is the deleted element in the consonant cluster.

Sonority Sequencing Theories

Sonority sequencing is another example of a linguistic theory often cited in relation to consonant clusters (e.g. Gierut, 1999; Pater and Barlow, 2003). Sonority is related to the openness of the vocal tract when a sound is spoken: vowels are most sonorous, stop consonants least sonorous, e.g. /p, b, t, d, k, g/. The sonority sequencing principle is a rule that governs the way in which consonants are combined within syllables (Clements, 1990), and may have important implications for our understanding of the place of complex onsets or codas (i.e. word initial or final consonant clusters) in the syllable. In order to account for their distribution, the components of the syllable are placed on a continuum ranging from most sonorous to least sonorous. The principle regulates the sequencing of segments in phonological constituents. This means that the syllable has to have a sonorous peak, i.e. a vowel, and sonority must decrease towards the edges. A simple sonority scale is shown in Figure 5.1 arranged from the most to least sonorous segment type.

Although the sonority sequencing principle can account for the structure of many English syllables, there are some exceptions to the rule. For example, in words with initial /sp, st, sk/ consonant clusters the principle is not adhered to as the more sonorous fricative precedes the less sonorous stop, e.g. consider words like SPOT and SPOON. The vowel forms the sonorous peak but the /p/ in the onset cluster is the lowest point, rising again for the /s/ that precedes it. It is for this reason that /s/ clusters have some-

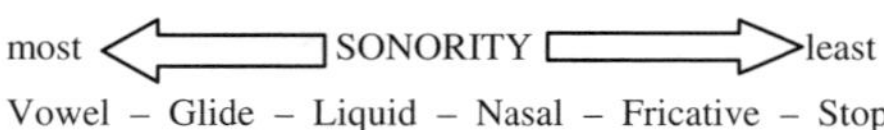

Figure 5.1a: Simple sonority scale.

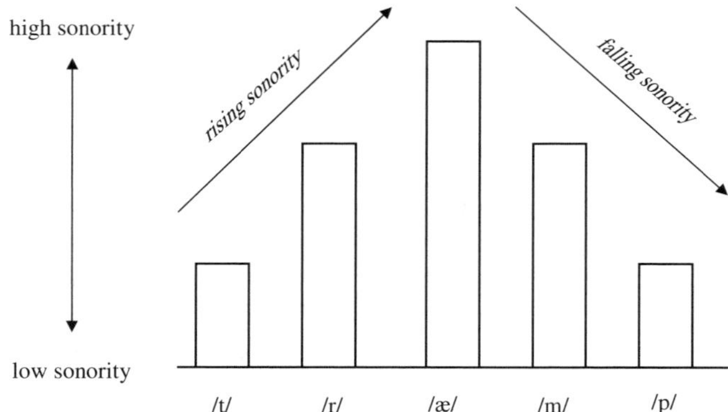

Figure 5.1b: Example of the sonority sequencing principle in a word with complex onset /tr/ and coda /mp/ (based on Wyllie-Smith and McLeod, 2001).

times not been considered true clusters but rather adjunct clusters where /s/ is regarded as an adjunct (or attachment) to the rest of the syllable which will then follow the rules of sonority.

A common pattern in children's production of consonant clusters is for the least sonorous member of the adult target cluster to surface (Ohala, 1999; Barlow, 2001). In cluster reduction, stops are the most readily maintained component, e.g. consider normally-developing children who typically reduce the onset in the adult target SPIDER as [paɪdə] or [baɪdə] thus preserving the stop element and deleting the more sonorous fricative. However, this so-called sonority sequencing principle is not always able to account for normal patterns of cluster reduction. Children favour deletion of fricatives and velars, which, in some circumstances, will conflict with a sonority-based choice. For example, for the target CLAP most normally-developing children will produce 'lap' rather than 'cap' favouring the more sonorous liquid and deleting the less sonorous fricative.

Table 5.2 provides guidelines of norms for the age of acquisition of word-initial consonant clusters in English. As noted in Chapter 3, one might use tables such as these as a guide in determining which targets to address in therapy. However, as noted in that chapter there are many other factors that need to be considered too - developmental tables should be considered in the light of factors relating to the child, as well as research evidence.

For most normally-developing children consonant clusters emerge with no specific intervention, and gradually come to be produced in adult-

Table 5.2: Word-initial consonant clusters and norms for acquisition (from McLeod, van Doorn and Reed, 2001)

Consonant cluster	Age of acquisition
[tw]	3;6
[kw]	3;6
[sp]	5;0-6;0
[st]	5;0-6;0
[sk]	5;0-6;0
[sm]	5;0-7;0
[sn]	5;0-7;0
[sw]	6;0
[sl]	7;0
[pl]	4;0-5;6
[bl]	4;0-5;6
[kl]	4;0-5;6
[gl]	4;0-5;6
[fl]	4;0-5;6
[pr]	5;0-6;0
[br]	5;0-6;0
[tr]	5;0-6;0
[dr]	5;0-6;0
[kr]	5;0-6;0
[gr]	5;0-6;0
[fr]	5;0-6;0
[θr]	7;0
[skw]	7;0
[spl]	7;0
[spr]	8;0
[str]	8;0
[skr]	8;0

like ways. In general it is agreed that there is a developmental pattern of consonant cluster acquisition, but that this can vary considerably from child to child (see McLeod, van Doorn and Reed, 2001). Two part consonant clusters (e.g. [sp], [pr]) are usually acquired between the ages of 3;6 and 7;0, and before three part ones (e.g. [spl] or [spr]) which are typically acquired between 6;0 and 8;0 years of age. Word-initial consonant clusters are sometimes acquired before and sometimes after word-final consonant clusters. Stop clusters are not necessarily easier than fricative ones.

Barlow (2001) notes that [s] clusters may be considered special cases, which according to some authors are acquired later than others, and earlier according to other authors. Exactly how they are exceptional has not yet been agreed! McLeod *et al.* (1997) have reported that there is no clear developmental hierarchy for the development of [s] clusters word-initially or finally, although it is known that [s] production may be easier for children acquiring this sound in word-final position (Grunwell, 1985; Redford *et al.*, 1997). In terms of the specific [s] + stop clusters, there is some evidence that [sk] may be slightly later in acquisition on average, when compared to [sp] and [st]. Consonant glide (e.g. [tr]) sequences are thought to emerge before consonant liquid (e.g. [fl]) sequences (Smit, 1993) and this liquid/glide difference is thought by some to be key to understanding cluster development (Powell and Elbert, 1984).

Studies of children's development of consonant clusters have focused largely on word-initial clusters (e.g. Allerton, 1976; Powell and Elbert, 1984; Smit, 1993; Gierut, 1999; Gierut and O'Connor, 2002). However in English, consonant clusters also occur in word-final position as well as within words. There remains a great deal of uncertainty regarding the development of these clusters by children with both normal and atypical phonological development. Most research that has focused on final consonant clusters has done so by looking at children's spelling rather than focusing on speech production. The normative tables given above make no mention of the use of word-final consonant clusters in words such as MASK and WISP. In terms of a developmental sequence, word-initial consonant clusters are sometimes acquired before and sometimes after word-final consonant clusters (McLeod *et al.*, 2001). Word-final clusters may emerge sooner than word-initial clusters as they are aided by morphology, e.g. past tense such as in /mɛst/ for MESSED, and plurals such as ROCKS.

The psycholinguistic framework encourages us to consider a child's speech processing system as a whole: input, stored representations and output are important. In terms of consonant clusters, it is therefore interesting and potentially illuminating to ask about the normal development of consonant cluster perception and how the ability to discriminate between closely related clusters ties in with their production. Bridgeman and Snowling (1988) did just that: comparing the perception of consonant sequences by children aged 7–11 years with apraxia of speech with those with normally-developing speech. Their research focused on children's auditory discrimination of word-final clusters [st] and [ts] using a same/different paradigm. The children were presented with word pairs such as FITS and FIST and asked to say whether each pair was the same or different. Stimuli words were selected to include both real and non-words, and words which differed in their consonant cluster sequence and words which differed in terms of segments only, not with clusters. Examples of the stimuli are shown in Table 5.3 below.

Bridgeman and Snowling (1988) found that both groups of children could discriminate real words equally well, but that the children with apraxia had problems with non-word discrimination. They had particular difficulty discriminating cluster sequences in non-words compared to the controls. The authors suggested that this difficulty is due to children having problems with sequential aspects of phonological processing.

Table 5.3: Examples of stimuli used in Bridgeman and Snowling's (1988) auditory discrimination task

	Real words	Non-words
Cluster contrast	LOST/LOTS	VOST/VOTS
Segment contrast	LOSS/LOT	VOS/VOT

Producing accurate consonant clusters often poses particular challenges for children with speech difficulties such as apraxia of speech.

What Do We Know about Intervention and Consonant Clusters?

The results of intervention studies addressing consonant clusters are not clear-cut, but such studies have the potential to offer important insights. It has been found that treating three-part consonant clusters, e.g. /spl/ in SPLASH, can result in widespread generalization to two-part consonant clusters, e.g. /sp/ and /sl/. This hypothesis is part of the complexity account of treatment efficacy (sometimes referred to as CATE, see Chapter 3), which states that working on more complex or marked structures typically acquired later in development can result in more widespread overall change than if adhering to a more standard step-by-step target selection process (Gierut and Dinnsen, 1987). It has also been demonstrated that working on consonant clusters (e.g. [pl]) improves singleton production (e.g. [p]), but the reverse has not been found (Gierut, 1999). This pattern of change fits with the ideas surrounding productive phonological knowledge (PPK) introduced in Chapter 3. There it was suggested that sounds classed as Level 6, i.e. sounds about which the child has no productive phonological knowledge, have the potential to be the best therapy targets leading to the greatest generalization.

It is known that [s] + stop clusters are different to other clusters, and require specific intervention to promote their accurate production (Barlow, 2001). Barbara Hodson (1997) suggests that /s/ clusters be incorporated as primary potential targets in her cycles approach for children with highly unintelligible speech. She suggests that /s/ clusters should be targeted before singleton stridents such as /s,f/ because working on the /s/ clusters will involve working on stridency – the forceful airflow striking the back of the teeth – and may have greater overall effects on a child's intelligibility.

Other authors have cautioned about the need to distinguish between the different /s/ clusters and how these are selected for intervention. Gierut (1999) carried out intervention with five children aged 3;5 to 4;8

years with phonological delays in order to investigate the emergence of /s/ clusters. Children were taught different /s/ clusters based on their differing phonological repertoires. They received intervention three times a week in 1-hour sessions. Intervention continued until a child achieved 90% accuracy over two consecutive sessions or until 12 sessions of intervention had been completed, whichever happened first. It was found that treatment of [s] + stop clusters, i.e. /st, sp, sk/ – the consonant clusters that violate the sonority sequencing principle – does not promote widespread change across all consonant sequences. From an intervention point of view working on these specific clusters does not seem to give rise to widespread generalization and should be avoided if the overall aim is to address all onset consonant clusters. However, this does not seem to apply for all consonant clusters, e.g. /sm, sn/ and treatment of other consonant sequences (e.g. /bl/) can promote change in [s] clusters.

An important message is that we need to select consonant clusters with care. Choosing /s/ clusters as an entire group of sounds may be confusing to the child given that /sp, st, sk/ have been shown to be inherently different to other clusters. Our choice of target consonant clusters will depend on our aims in intervention, and as emphasized in Chapter 3, the theoretical principles to which we are subscribing. Following a developmental principle may lead us to consider the tables of normal development shown in, for example, Table 5.2, making choices based on the child's current phonology and where he or she might be expected to progress to next in a developmental sequence. On the other hand, following principles of CATE and looking for least PPK might lead us to consider clusters about which the child has little knowledge in the hopes that working on such structures will result in widespread generalization throughout their system.

The psycholinguistic approach suggests that we consider an individual child's speech processing system as a whole, and determine the level/s of breakdown whether they be in input, output or stored representations. Once we have considered this, we should then focus more specifically on phonology and the way in which particular phonological units are implicated at each of these levels. We may find that a child is unable to perceive the difference between words such as POT and SPOT, or to perceive the difference between similar clusters such as those in words like SPLAY and PLAY. The psycholinguistic approach reminds us of the importance of individual variation since two children presenting with difficulties in their production of consonant clusters may have different underlying strengths and weaknesses. For example, child A may be unable to produce consonant clusters due to motor programming problems, while child B may be unable to discriminate between closely related consonant clusters as well as having difficulties producing these. Many of the studies about consonant clusters have speech output as their focus. The psycholinguistic approach asks, 'Why can't a child produce consonant clusters?' and checks input either by using general procedures (e.g. Bridgeman and Snowling's test on page 122), or more importantly through individually designed procedures for the child in question. In the following activity we focus on the question, 'Why can't a child produce consonant clusters?' and the individually designed procedures that might help us to answer this question.

ACTIVITY 5.2

Consider the following data for Anna, aged 6;5.

Speech output: Naming task.

Target	*Production*
SMOKE	[sməʊk]
SNAKE	[snəɪk]
STOP	[tɒp]
SKY	[gaɪ]
SPOON	[pun]
SLIDE	[slaɪd]
VEST	[vɛst]
DESK	[dɛsk]
GLOVES	[glʊbs]
SWEETS	[swits]

Speech input: Auditory discrimination task (Bridgeman and Snowling, 1988).

Anna was presented with pairs of closely-related words and non-words and required to judge whether these sounded the same or different. Examples of the stimuli are shown in Table 5.3 and involved a contrast of word-final clusters (e.g. LOST/LOTS) or word-final segments such as LOSS/LOT.

Anna's test results:

Real words: 18/18
Non-words: 17/18

Now answer the following questions:

1. Focusing on the small sample of Anna's single word speech output, what difficulties do you observe in her production of consonant clusters?
2. How do the speech input results from the Bridgeman and Snowling task inform our knowledge of Anna's speech processing system? What further testing would you carry out to find out more about Anna's auditory discrimination skills?
3. How would you test whether Anna has accurate representations of the words with which she has difficulties in her speech output? Give examples of the stimuli you would use.

Now turn to the Key to Activity 5.2 at the end of this chapter and check how your responses compare with ours.

Consonant clusters are frequently addressed in therapy. They often become the focus once singleton sounds have been mastered, i.e. working on singletons before moving on to /s/ clusters, in accordance with developmental norms for acquisition. This chapter has suggested that there is in fact some evidence for addressing consonant clusters earlier in development. Techniques used by therapists vary widely but often involve the visual presentation of multiple consonants, e.g. a child is encouraged to produce /t/ in isolation with this sound represented by a picture of a TAP. The child is then encouraged to produce /t/ in a simple CV or CVC word such as TIE or TOP. Following this, they are reminded of the /s/ sound often represented by a picture of a SNAKE. This additional picture is then placed to the left of the /t/ picture card and the child encouraged to 'glue the two sounds together' thus creating new words STY or STOP. Children need to be encouraged to produce a relaxed, smoothly flowing 'sssss' that gently leads into 'top'. Meaningful minimal pair work, and the use of written forms for older children, can also be useful in encouraging children's awareness of the difference between words such as STOP and TOP. These are some general techniques widely used by therapists, e.g. see the *Nuffield Centre Dyspraxia Programme* (Williams and Stephens, 2004). When working on consonant clusters in word-final position, morphology and phonology can often be linked, e.g. working on regular plurals will involve discussion about adding /s/ to the ends of words, e.g. CAT + S = many CATS. This can also afford an opportunity to work on final clusters such as /ts/. Simple activities like this can be contextualized within a psycholinguistic framework. Knowing exactly which segments are involved, and the level of speech processing that is being targeted will enable us to plan intervention that has the greatest chance of being effective.

ACTIVITY 5.3

In Book 2 of the series, Rachel Rees described therapy tasks as being made up of materials, procedures, feedback and optionally the use of specific techniques. She used the following equation to represent a therapy task (see also Chapter 2):

TASK = Materials + Procedure + Feedback (+ Technique)

Read the following description of a therapy activity where the focus was on consonant clusters.

Session with Anna (A) and Therapist (T)
A is presented with two pictures: TABLE and STABLE. These words are also written below the pictures.

T: Now have a look at these, Anna. Which one do you like best? Which one do you want?
A: I love horsies. I want the TABLE.
T: I know you love horses! But look the horse is here in the ssssstable. Are you sure you want the boring old TABLE? (gives Anna the TABLE)
A: No, silly! I want the SSSSSSSTABLE.
T: Oh, great. Here you are! You said that beautifully.
I'll have to have the TABLE then.
Now, look at these two, Anna.
(presents pictures of a TOOL and a STOOL)
Which one do you want this time?
A: umm. TOOL
T: OK – this one. For helping Dad in the garage
A: No. That's boring. I want this one (takes STOOL)
T: Oh, Anna – I'm sorry I never heard your snakey ssssss
Look at the word, how it's written, can you see that big 's' in front? Don't forget it or Mr Snakey will be sad.
So, what have you got?
A: SSSSSTOOL.
T: And what have I got?
A: TOOL

Now, describe the therapy task in terms of Rees's equation by completing Table 5.4.

Turn to the Key to Activity 5.3 at the end of this chapter and compare your completed pro-forma with ours. You may wish to reflect on how this task might have been improved in all or specific areas. Using a table like

Table 5.4: Pro-forma for describing therapy tasks (based on Rees, 2001a, b)

Task description Write a general description of the task	
Materials Note the materials used	
Procedures Outline what took place	
Feedback What feedback was given to the child?	
(Techniques) Were any supporting techniques used?	

this provides a very structured way of looking at therapy activities, and can form the basis of a discussion between therapists working on similar targets. Such a table is also helpful when evaluating therapy outcomes and sharing evidence of good practice with colleagues. A larger version of Table 5.4 is included in Appendix 7 for photocopying purposes.

Links between Speech and Spelling of Consonant Clusters

Investigation of children's spellings provides a way of gaining further insight into the phonological processes underlying literacy development. Research into children's speech and spelling development suggests that consonant clusters can pose particular difficulties for many children. During the early school years, children demonstrate an increased understanding of the grapheme to phoneme correspondence that underlies the alphabetic phase of literacy development (see Chapter 10 for further information about this phase of children's literacy development). However, the spellings produced by children at this age typically reveal that children are still unable to analyse words at the phonemic level. They often produce spellings in which groups of segments, e.g. word-initial and word-final consonant clusters are incorrectly represented by single letters. In initial consonant clusters, young children typically fail to spell the second or third elements of these clusters, e.g. 5-year-olds have been observed to spell PLAY as <pa>, and STREET as <set> (Treiman, 1993). In the case of final consonant clusters children often fail to represent the penultimate consonants of these clusters. For example, 5-year-old children often fail to mark the nasal /ŋ/ in DRINK writing <grak> instead, or do not represent the /s/ of POST writing <pot>.

Spelling errors are sometimes a reflection of speech errors. Children with speech difficulties or inconsistent speech may find it hard to use their own lexical representations or verbal rehearsal to help support their spelling. However, this is not always the case as children are often heard segmenting a word into onset and rime units correctly, e.g. saying 'pr-ince' but then writing <pince>. Treiman (1993) argues that the children's omission of initial and final consonant clusters reflects how young children persist in grouping together segments that adults represent using individual graphemes. For instance, the writing of POST as <pot> suggests that the child may believe that POST only contains three units of sound, i.e. initial /p/ followed by /əʊ/ followed by /t/. Children appear to be incorrectly grouping /əʊ/ and /s/ together, treating the segments as a single unit rather than a sequence of two segments. Similarly, children treat syllable initial consonant clusters as a cohesive unit. Thus, young children typically spell the word PLAY as <pay>. Here, the children appear to have analysed the cluster onset as containing a single segment, and have represented the two segment onset of the word <pl> with a single letter <p>. Treiman's proposal is supported by several studies investigating phonological awareness which have also shown that syllable initial consonant cluster onsets form a cohesive unit for children and adults. Several studies have demonstrated that preschool and kindergarten children have difficulties in tasks that require them to subdivide complex onsets (e.g. /fl/) and rimes (/aʊwə/) in FLOWER (Treiman 1985, 1993). Treiman (1985) found that beginning readers had greater difficulty recognizing that /flo/ begins with /f/ than that /fo/ or /fol/ begins with /f/. Based on these findings Treiman concluded that children find a segment harder to segment out when it is part of a cluster onset than when it is an onset on its own. However, it is important to note that most normally developing children can auditorily detect differences between singletons and clusters. What seems important is that they don't know how to write clusters until explicitly taught how to do so. It is hard for children to segment a cluster into its component sounds until basic reading skills have been acquired.

Treiman and Zukowski (1991) re-tested preschool children who had participated in an earlier study. The children were now 6 years of age and tested using the same phoneme comparison task as before. All of the children were found to be successful in the phoneme comparison task. On the basis of these findings the authors argued that the 6-year-old children had acquired the ability to analyse consonant clusters into their constituent phones. A number of other studies have found that children's ability to analyse cluster onsets and rimes is not mastered at 6 years of age, and in particular that children have persistent difficulties with tasks that require them to focus on the second consonant of a consonant cluster. Bruck and Treiman (1990) tested a group of children at first and second grade (age 6–7 years) on an auditory deletion task. This task required the children to listen to a non-word, e.g. /floi/, spoken by the experimenter. The child was then asked to remove the first sound and produce the remaining non-word. Each child was given numerous demonstrations and attempted several practice trials, during which they were shown that the correct response was /loi/. However, when the children attempted the task on their own, they frequently produced an incorrect response. The children demonstrated a tendency to remove the entire onset and produce /oi/, as opposed to removing just the first consonant of the onset and producing the correct response /loi/. A high proportion of the responses given by the children was incorrect, with children producing errors 62% of the time. Treiman (1994) argued that these findings illustrate how even children as old as 7 and 8 years tend to treat onset clusters as units. Furthermore, Treiman (1994) suggests that the second consonant of a two-consonant initial cluster is less salient than the first, as demonstrated by the greater difficulty experienced by the children when asked to preserve only the second consonant of the cluster. However, again it may be that there are differences between the participants in these studies depending on when and how they have received literacy instruction. Reading instruction may be the crucial factor that determines when children begin to use consonant clusters in their spelling rather than children's age per se.

It is clear that omissions of the interior consonants of word initial (e.g. <cene> for CLEAN) and final clusters (e.g. <wap> for WASP) are common among children beginning to spell. These sounds are less salient with children focusing on beginning, middle and end sounds as they sound out words. Bourassa and Treiman (2003) also describe the frequent insertion of vowels between cluster elements, e.g. writing <duripe> for DRIP, is a normal developmental spelling error made by children. Errors such as the omission of interior elements of clusters and the insertion of vowels between cluster elements are not significantly more frequent among children with dyslexia than among normally developing children of the same spelling level (Bourassa and Treiman, 2003). However, for many children with persisting speech difficulties these developmental spelling errors will persist as they are unable to sound out or in some cases perceive the consonant clusters that they need to write.

Many of the spelling difficulties with consonant clusters described in this section occur in normally-developing children. However, the challenges facing children with speech processing difficulties are even greater. The relationship between an individual child's spoken and written production of clusters is unlikely to be predictable: there are children who have difficulties in producing consonant clusters in their speech but show good written representation of consonant clusters in their writing. Other children are able to accurately realize consonant clusters in their speech but experience difficulties with their spelling, and others will have difficulties that affect both speech and spelling. What is clear is that young children's sound based errors reveal that spelling is predominantly 'a process of symbolising the linguistic structure of spoken words, and not simply a process of reproducing memorised letter sequences' (Treiman and Bourassa, 2000, p.11).

In Chapter 10 we return to issues of literacy for further consideration of the links between spoken and written forms.

Summary

This chapter has aimed to provide a review of consonant clusters in phonological theories and what is known about the development of clusters in children's speech and spelling. We have also considered the use of consonant clusters in intervention for children with persisting speech difficulties. In the following chapter, Chapter 6, we describe the intervention that took place with a school-age boy: Joshua aged 6;10. Joshua's intervention focused specifically on clusters with all his initial consonant clusters being addressed.

The key points of this chapter are as follows.

- Children with PSDs often experience difficulties in their spoken and written production of consonant clusters.
- Consonant clusters are acquired relatively late in development.
- In normal development, children acquire word-initial clusters in a typical sequence that involves initially omitting one part of the cluster, later substituting one part of the cluster with another element and ultimately producing the entire cluster correctly.
- Linguistic theories (e.g. markedness theories and sonority sequencing theories) attempt to account for the way in which children develop consonant clusters.
- Consonant clusters have traditionally been chosen as fairly late therapy targets following work addressing singleton sounds. However, choosing clusters as early intervention targets may result in more widespread generalization throughout the child's system as well as greater intelligibility gains.
- Clusters should be selected with care since studies show that different clusters have different generalization effects.
- Many of the target selection issues outlined in Chapter 3 also apply to the selection of consonant clusters, e.g. it is important to have a clear theoretical rationale for the clusters selected.
- /s/ clusters appear to be different to other clusters in their response to intervention. In particular, treatment of /s/ + stop clusters (i.e. /st, sp, sk/) has been shown to result in little generalization to other clusters suggesting that they may not be a good starting point if hoping to affect all clusters through intervention.
- As for speech, the spelling of consonant clusters is a challenge for young children, but developmental errors are predictable (e.g. omission of interior elements of clusters) and for most children are soon overcome in normal acquisition.
- The relationship between the spoken and written production of consonant clusters in children with PSDs is not a predictable one, but consideration of spelling can provide valuable insights into the phonological processing of these children.

KEY TO ACTIVITY 5.1

English contains 29 word-initial consonant clusters which are listed below. The clusters marked with an asterisk (*) can also occur in word-final position.

Consonant cluster
[tw]
[kw]
[sp]*
[st]*
[sk]*
[sm]
[sn]
[sw]
[sl]
[sf]
[pl]
[bl]
[kl]
[gl]
[fl]
[pr]
[br]
[tr]
[dr]
[kr]
[gr]
[fr]
[θr]
[ʃr]
[skw]
[spl]
[spr]
[str]
[skr]

Word-final consonant clusters - not permissible in word-initial position in English - include, e.g.

/kt/ in PACT
/ft/ in LEFT
/pt/ in OPT
/mp/ in RAMP
/nk/ in THINK
/ts/ in RATS
/ks/ in BOX
/ps/ in LIPS
/dz/ in BIDS
/gz/ in DOGS

KEY TO ACTIVITY 5.2

1. Focusing on the small sample of Anna's single word speech output, what difficulties do you observe in her production of consonant clusters?

Anna appears to have mastered most of her consonant clusters, e.g. /sm, sn, sl, sw, gl/, with the exception of the /s/ + stop clusters in word-initial position, e.g. producing STOP → [tɒp]; SKY → [gaɪ]; SPOON → [pun]. There are two words which give an opportunity to observe Anna's production of /s/ + stop clusters in word-final position: VEST and DESK. She appears to have no difficulty in producing the clusters in this position. From the limited evidence we would conclude that she has no difficulties with /sp/, /st/ and /sk/ in word final position - only initial position - although it would be helpful to see if she could also name words such as WASP accurately.

2. How do the speech input results from the Bridgeman and Snowling task inform our knowledge of Anna's speech processing system? What further testing would you carry out to find out more about Anna's auditory discrimination skills?

Anna's performance was at ceiling for the auditory discrimination task. We can deduce that she is able to accurately discriminate between closely related familiar and unfamiliar words which vary in terms of final segments. However, Anna's difficulties in speech production are with word-initial clusters not with word-final clusters. It would therefore be helpful to determine whether she can discriminate between words that reflect her own output errors, e.g. are these the same or different: TOP/STOP? SPOON/POON? When devising such a task we would use the child's own error productions in contrast with correct adult targets. We would need to randomly select about one third of the words and then present these as same items, e.g. SPOON/SPOON.

3. How would you test whether Anna has accurate representations of the words with which she has difficulties in her speech output? Give examples of the stimuli you would use.

In order to tap Anna's internal representations, we would choose words that she has difficulty in producing, e.g. SPOON. We would present Anna with a picture of a SPOON, and ask her to tell us whether we are right or wrong in how we name the picture. We would produce a variety of accurate and inaccurate productions of the word, e.g. Is this a 'poon'? Is this a 'boon'? Is this a 'SPOON'? Is this a 'moon'? Anna would be asked to indicate right or wrong (or yes, or no) for each production. This is called an auditory lexical decision task. If she only accepts SPOON as correct we would have a good idea that she has an accurate representation of the word. If she answers yes for additional incorrect items, it is likely that she has a fuzzy representation of the word. We would use the same procedure for all errors words. If Anna has experienced no difficulties in auditory discrimination tasks, we would be confident that she is hearing the test items accurately. However, if difficulties were found in the auditory discrimination task we would need to bear this in mind in the auditory lexical decision task as she may not be hearing the test stimuli clearly. Lexical decision tasks in which the examiner does not name pictures but requires the child to access their own representation and silently sort pictures into sound categories is one way of overcoming this difficulty.

KEY TO ACTIVITY 5.3

Task description Write a general description of the task	Therapist and child are looking at minimal pair pictures together. The child is required to name her favourite picture, which she then gets to keep if she produces the target correctly. The aim is for the child to produce an accurate /st/ cluster in word-initial position.
Materials Note the materials used	Minimal pair picture stimuli. The stimuli involve contrasts between words with an initial /st/ cluster and words with initial /t/, e.g. STABLE and TABLE. The written words are included along with the picture stimuli.
Procedures Outline what took place	Two minimal pair pictures are presented each time. The child is asked to name her favourite picture. The stimuli have been selected based on the child's errors, with some more desirable and exciting items containing target /st/ clusters. The child points to or picks up the one she wants, but often names the other picture. This gives the therapist opportunity to show confusion and talk about the difference between the two words.
Feedback What feedback was given to the child?	The therapist does not give the child the picture or move on to the next turn until the child has attempted correct production of her favoured item. The therapist models an exaggerated 'sssssss' sound and cues the child by talking about written forms and previously learnt names for sounds, e.g. snakey sound for /s/.
Techniques Were any supporting techniques used?	Explicit use of written forms.

Chapter 6
Working on Consonant Clusters in Single Words

This chapter describes the intervention that took place with Joshua, a boy aged 6;10 at the start of intervention. Joshua's case study illustrates some of the points made in the previous chapter about the use of consonant clusters in intervention and how psycholinguistic and phonological perspectives can be combined in intervention. However, these two perspectives should always be employed with awareness of the child's individual needs and broader social, emotional and family needs. Adopting this third perspective was particularly important in Joshua's case.

Case study: Joshua aged 6;10

Joshua was generally delayed in his development, and evidenced associated delays in his speech and language. He had been diagnosed as mildly autistic, and having deficits of attention, motor control and perception (DAMP)[1] which combines elements of Asperger's syndrome and Attention Deficit Hyperactivity Disorder (ADHD). He presented with challenging behaviours in addition to speech, language and academic delays. He attended a mainstream school and required individual support in order to cope with the demands of this environment. Joshua was first referred for speech and language therapy at CA 1;3 as he had failed to attain normal communicative milestones by this age and was not yet using single words. He had received regular intervention from this time and had made slow progress in his use and understanding of language. His speech still had many immaturities, but he was understood by most listeners. Joshua's social skills and behaviour were a great concern for his teachers and family.

In the following sections we present Joshua's assessment findings. The assessment results are presented in two sections: macro-assessment and micro assessment. The first section on macro-assessment looks at Joshua's speech processing profile, while the micro assessment section that follows focuses on his phonology.

Macro Assessment

The speech processing profile of Stackhouse and Wells (1997) was used as a framework for organizing the data from this part of the assessment. At each level of the profile at least one assessment was carried out.[2] In some cases results obtained from the standardized tests were incorporated into the profile, and in other cases unpublished, non-standardized tests or subtests from standardized materials were used. The ticks and crosses on the profile indicate Joshua's performance in relation to children of his chronological age, with one tick indicating age-appropriate skills, and the number of crosses showing the number of standard deviations above or below the mean. The completed profile is presented in Figure 6.1.

ACTIVITY 6.1

Study Joshua's speech processing profile presented in Figure 6.1 and answer the following questions.

(a) Does Joshua have difficulties with input or output?
(b) Outline two areas of relative strength.
(c) Outline Joshua's main areas of difficulty.
(d) What further information or assessments would you find valuable?

Check your answers with the Key to Activity 6.1 at the end of this chapter, then read on for further information on Joshua's speech processing profile in the sections that follow.

Overview of Psycholinguistic Speech Processing Profile

Generally, Joshua had more difficulties with output than with input. However, within each of the different levels, Joshua performed variably; his difficulties were often item-specific or test-specific rather than being a general problem with a particular level of processing.

Strengths

In terms of input, Joshua had strengths towards the lower part of the profile: he was able to discriminate between speech and non-speech sounds with ease. At a higher level his phonological representations were found to be generally accurate – a relative strength – although for some of the longer, less familiar words they were less clear. He had knowledge of the internal structure of phonological representations of CVC and CCVC words, as tested by sorting tasks and rhyme pictures.

√ = age appropriate performance
X = 1 standard deviation below the expected mean for his age
XX = 2 standard deviations below the expected mean for his age

INPUT

F Is the child aware of the internal structure of phonological representations?
√ – Picture rhyme detection (Vance *et al.*, 1994)
X– Picture onset detection (PhAB picture alliteration subtest, Frederikson *et al.*, 1997)

E Are the child's phonological representations accurate?
X – Auditory detection of speech errors (Constable *et al.*, 1997)

D Can the child discriminate between real words?
√ – Minimal pair auditory discrimination of clusters (Bridgeman and Snowling, 1988)
√ – Aston Index discrimination subtest (Newton and Thompson, 1982)
√ – PhAB alliteration subtest (Frederikson et al., 1997)
√ – Auditory discrimination test (Wepman and Reynolds, 1987)

C Does the child have language specific representations of word structures?

Not tested

B Can the child discriminate speech sounds without reference to lexical representations?
√ – Minimal pair auditory discrimination of clusters in non-words (Bridgeman and Snowling, 1988)

A Does the child have adequate auditory perception?
√ – audiometry

OUTPUT

G Can the child access accurate motor programmes?
X – Single word naming test (Constable *et al.*, 1997)
X – Word-finding vocabulary test (Renfrew, 1995)
X – Edinburgh Articulation Test (Anthony *et al.*, 1971)
XX – The Bus Story (Renfrew, 1969)

H Can the child manipulate phonological units?
√ – PhAB spoonerism subtest (Frederikson *et al.*, 1997)
√ – PAT rhyme fluency subtest (Muter *et al.*, 1997)

I Can the child articulate real words accurately?
X – Real word repetition subtest (Constable *et al.*, 1997)
√ – Aston Index blending subtest – real words (Newton and Thompson, 1982)

J Can the child articulate speech without reference to lexical representations?
X – Aston Index blending subtest – non-words (Newton and Thompson, 1982)
X – Non-word repetition subtest (Constable *et al.*, 1997)

K Does the child have adequate sound production skills?
√ – Stimulable for all sounds
√ – Oro-motor assessment (Nuffield Centre Dyspraxia Programme, Williams and Stephens, 2004)

L Does the child reject his own erroneous forms?
Informal observation – no.

Figure 6.1: Joshua's speech processing profile at age 7;2. (Reproduced by kind permission of Whurr Publishers from Stackhouse and Wells, 1997.)

He performed less well on the alliteration picture subtest of the *Phonological Assessment Battery* (PhAB) (Frederikson *et al.*, 1997) suggesting that he had more difficulties at the segmental level (in contrast to rime) and was not aided by the visual information contained in the pictures.

Weaknesses

Joshua had widespread difficulties on the output side of the profile. These were weighted to the top of the profile with Joshua having adequate sound production skills, although he lateralized /s/ on occasion. He produced consistent speech errors in his repetition and naming. Joshua's speech errors were generally like those of a younger child rather than being unusual or symptomatic of atypical development. His speech delay was in line with his language levels and cognitive skills. As one would expect, longer words that Joshua found hard to recognize on an auditory lexical decision task (see Constable *et al.*, 1997) were also harder for Joshua to produce in an accurate way. Joshua performed poorly on the naming and repetition tasks suggesting difficulties with his stored motor programs and also his online motor programming.

Micro Assessment

The *Phonological Assessment of Child Speech* (PACS) (Grunwell, 1985) was used to provide information on Joshua's speech production. Severity indices were introduced in Chapter 4 and are useful measures that can encapsulate the degree of difficulty a child experiences with his or her speech in a single number. Most typically used are indices such as percentage of consonants correct (PCC), or percentage of vowels correct (PVC). Joshua's PCC score falls in the mild-moderate range. A summary of the findings is presented in Table 6.1.

The most noticeable process in Joshua's speech was cluster reduction, frequently observed for clusters in word initial position, e.g. SPOON → [bun], SCHOOL → [kul]; GRANDDAD → ['gændæd]. Joshua reduced clusters in 43 of a possible 49 instances (87.7%). On some occasions elements of the [s] cluster were used in a reversed order in the word-final position (e.g. WASP → [wɒps]). Joshua's productive phonological knowledge (PPK) varied from cluster to cluster. Further examples of Joshua's cluster realizations and PPK classification for clusters as outlined by Gierut and Dinnsen (1987, and described in Chapter 3) are presented in Table 6.2. The clusters in Table 6.2 are presented in a developmental sequence based on early acquired to later acquired clusters.

Nineteen of the 27 word-initial consonant clusters were Type 6: sounds about which the child has no productive phonological knowledge and is thus never able to use correctly. Two of the clusters, /sk, st/, were consid-

Table 6.1: Summary of Joshua's speech data at CA 7;2

Assessment	Comments	
Severity indices	Percentage of consonants correct (PCC): 78% Percentage of vowels correct (PVC): 100% Percentage of phonemes correct (PPC): 86.7%	
Phonetic inventory	Word-initial position: [m, n, p, b, t, d, k, g, f, v, s, z, ʃ, ʧ, ʤ, j, l, w] Word-medial position: [m, n, ŋ, p, b, t, d, k, g, f, v, s, z, ʃ, ʒ, ʧ, ʤ, j, l, w] Word-final position: [m, n, ŋ, p, b, t, d, k, g, f, v, s, z, ʃ, ʒ, ʧ, ʤ, j, l, w]	
Stimulability	Able to produce all segments in isolation	
Phonological processes analysis (% use)	Developmental processes: cluster reduction (87.7%); consonant harmony (9%)	
Single-word speech sample	JACOB → ['ʤeɪpɪb]	SPOON → [bun]
	YELLOW → ['lɛləʊ]	SCHOOL → [kul]
	CATERPILLAR → ['tætikɪlə]	GRANDDAD → ['gændæd]
	HOSPITAL → ['hɒsbɪkɪl]	WASP → [wɒps]
	HOSPITAL → ['ɒʔəʔbɪl]	DESK → [dɛsk]
	BROTHER → ['bʊvə]	VEST → [vɛst]
	SCARF → [kɑf]	CLASS → [klæs]
	SCOOTER → ['kʊtə]	CLOCK → [kɒk]
Connected speech sample	SHE GOT A BLACK ONE → [ʃiʔ gɒʔ ə 'bæk wʊn]	
	THE THREE LITTLE PIGS → [dəʔ fwi 'lɪtə pɪg]	
	I'M THE BIG BAD WOLF → ['ɑɪm və bɪg bæd wʊf]	
	NOW THE TWO (ARE) LEFT → ['nɑʊ dəʔ tʊ lɛf]	
	FINGER PUPPET → ['fɪŋgə 'pʊʔpɛ]	

ered to be Type 4 'positional constraint' clusters since Joshua was able to use these correctly in the word-final position but not word-initially, e.g. he accurately produced the targets DESK and VEST. The remaining 6 clusters, /kl, kw, kr, br, gl, tw/, were Type 3 clusters, about which Joshua had the most phonological knowledge. He was able to accurately produce these clusters in the word-initial position in some words (e.g. CLASS) but seemed to have frozen forms for other lexical items (e.g. CLOCK → [kɒk]). Joshua also had immature or frozen forms of non-cluster words that he produced like a younger child, e.g. JACOB → ['ʤeɪpɪb], and YELLOW → ['lɛləʊ]. His production of these words alternated with accurate productions. Joshua found it hard to produce longer, multi-syllabic words. Sequencing errors (e.g. CATERPILLAR → ['tætikɪlə]) and other sound confusions (e.g. HOSPITAL → ['hɒsbɪkɪl]) were frequently noted in words with 3 or more syllables.

Turning our attention to Joshua's written representations of clusters, we found that many of his spoken errors on clusters were mirrored in his spellings. Joshua found it hard to write words with consonant clusters. He was reluctant to write words such as SPOON and SPOT at the initial assess-

Table 6.2: Summary of Joshua's productive phonological knowledge (PPK) for all consonant clusters

Consonant cluster	Examples	Productive phonological knowledge (PPK)* 1 = maximum PPK; 6 = no PPK
[tw]	[tælv] TWELVE; ['twɛnty] TWENTY	3
[kw]	[kin] [kwin] QUEEN	3
[sp]	[bun] SPOON	6
[st]	[dɑ] STAR; [vɛst] VEST	4
[sk]	[kɑf] SCARF; [dɛsk] DESK	4
[sm]	[məʊk] SMOKE	6
[sn]	[nəɪk] SNAKE, [nɔ] SNORE	6
[sw]	[sɒp] SWOP	6
[sl]	[sip] SLEEP	6
[pl]	[piz] PLEASE	6
[bl]	[bæk] BLACK	6
[kl]	[klæs] CLASS; [kɒk] CLOCK	3
[gl]	[glaɪd] GLIDE; [gʊv] GLOVE	3
[fl]	['faʊwə] FLOWER	6
[pr]	[pæm] PRAM	6
[br]	[breɪk] BREAK; ['bʊvə] BROTHER	3
[tr]	[ʧeɪn] TRAIN; [twi] TREE	6
[dr]	[daɪv] DRIVE	6
[kr]	[kwɒs] CROSS; ['kɒkədaɪl] CROCODILE	3
[gr]	['gændæd] GRANDDAD	6
[fr]	[fʊt] FRUIT	6
[θr]	[fwi] THREE	6
[skw]	[gɛə] SQUARE	6
[spl]	[pæʧ] SPLASH	6
[spr]	[pɪŋg] SPRING	6
[str]	[tɪŋg], [ʧɪŋg] STRING	6
[skr]	[kæʤ] SCRATCH	6

* From Gierut *et al.* (1987) and Gierut and Dinnsen (1987), see Table 2.1.
PPK type 3: can produce on occasion but has fossilized forms for some words.
PPK type 4: positional constraints – uses in final position only.
PPK type 6: no knowledge – never uses.

ment, and said that he could not do it. When asked to say how he thought he might write them he said you should write [bə] [u:] [nə] for SPOON. The fact that Joshua used the initial voiced, de-aspirated [bə] and not [pə] or [sə] indicated that he has processed the cluster as a whole and must have some awareness of his speech output and the influence of the neighbouring cluster components. These findings suggest that his online motor programming may not yet have the template for words with initial consonant clusters. The fact that the clusters do not appear in either speech or spelling suggests an under-specified phonological representation common to both these modalities. Ben, the child presented in Chapter 10 contrasts with Joshua. He was an older child whose spelling skills were relatively good but who had difficulties with articulating specific sounds.

In the following sections we present details of Joshua's intervention planning. As for the assessment sections, intervention planning is divided into two sections: macro intervention planning and micro intervention planning. Macro intervention planning focuses broadly on the psycholinguistic, phonological and psychosocial motivation for the intervention. Micro intervention planning focuses more specifically on the details of the intervention such as the design and selection of the stimuli as well as the tasks used.

Macro Intervention Planning

Intervention planning focused on three main areas with each one serving as a rationale for the work carried out. These included the following.

- A psycholinguistic rationale that aimed to answer the question: 'What aspects of the speech processing system should be worked on?'
- A phonological rationale that aimed to answer the question: 'Which aspects of the sound system should be targeted?'
- A psychosocial rationale which aimed to answer the question: 'What other aspects important to the child should be taken into account?'

Each of these is discussed in the sections that follow.

Psycholinguistic rationale: What aspects of the speech processing profile should be worked on?

In order to answer this question carry out Activity 6.2.

ACTIVITY 6.2

Turn to Figure 6.1, Joshua's speech processing profile at CA 7;2. Using the data presented in that profile, circle Joshua's main areas of difficulty on the speech processing model presented below. This speech processing model was described in Chapter 2. After you have circled Joshua's main areas of difficulty turn to the Key to Activity 6.2 at the end of the chapter, and then read on below.

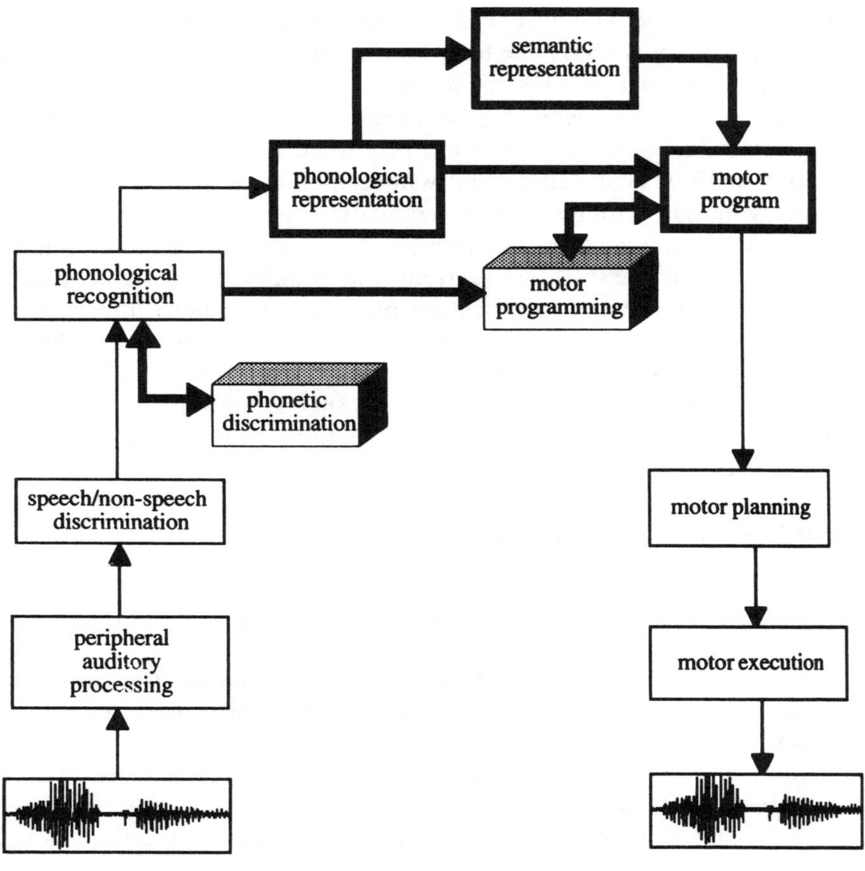

Joshua's main deficits were mapped from the speech processing profile onto the Stackhouse and Wells's (1997) speech processing model. Joshua's difficulties centred on the mapping of his phonological representations onto motor programs: creating and accessing motor programs was difficult for Joshua. Although his input phonological representations were generally accurate, motor programs were often inaccurate. Both motor programming (the online process) and stored motor programs were affected since he had difficulties with non-word repetition tasks as well as with picture naming. Since his semantic skills were weak he had limited top-down support in retrieving motor programs. In spontaneous speech he used some familiar words in an immature way and he repeated unfamiliar/new words in the same, immature way. Bryan and Howard (1992) describe a child whose non-word repetition was more accurate than spontaneous naming. The child in their study had 'frozen phonology' and had failed to update stored motor programs while his online motorprogramming skill *had* improved. Joshua is more similar to the child described by Waters (2001) whose stored motor programs were inadequate because of current limitations of online motor programming. Joshua's motor programming problems might be conceptualized as resulting from an immature template that acts to simplify words produced whether in naming or repetition. Joshua was highly consistent in his use of cluster reduction and seemed to not yet have the appropriate template for phonotactic structures which incorporate clusters (e.g. see Ingram and Ingram, 2001). Intervention needed to (a) update stored motor programs into more adult-like forms, and (b) get the online motor programming device to consistently compile accurate programs for storage by using an accurate template that incorporates the CCVC shape. Where Joshua had extra motor programs, the aim was to get him to abandon the immature motor program and retain the mature one.

In order to plan therapy that is tailor made for Joshua, we needed to answer the following questions. Each question is followed by an indication of where to look on Joshua's speech processing profile to answer the question.

(a) Can Joshua perceive consonant clusters?
 - Input
(b) Can Joshua produce clusters?
 - Output, lower right hand side of the speech processing profile
(c) Can Joshua repeat clusters in words/non-words?
 - Output, mid-right hand side of the speech processing profile
(d) Can Joshua produce clusters when naming words?
 - Output, top right hand side of the speech processing profile

Let us now consider each of these questions in turn.

(a) Can Joshua perceive consonant clusters?

Input skills were a relative strength for Joshua. In his speech processing profile shown in Figure 6.1 he did show some difficulties with input processing, but in general there were many ticks noted on the input side of the profile. His relative strengths with input were used in intervention to help build up the weaker areas on the output side. Joshua was encouraged to perceive fine phonological differences between words. Joshua had another strength in his ability to utilize phoneme–grapheme (sound to letter) conversion for spelling from dictation, and to use grapheme–phoneme conversion in reading tasks. The intervention programme drew on these skills to focus on the development of more accurate motor templates.

(b) Can Joshua produce clusters?

Yes, considering the information presented in Figure 6.1 and Table 6.1 Joshua was stimulable for all sounds and could repeat all clusters in isolation.

(c) Can Joshua repeat clusters in words/non-words?
Joshua had difficulty in repeating both real and non-words, although his difficulties were greater in the non-word repetition tasks. His difficulties with non-word repetition suggested that he has problems using online motor programming to devise new motor programs. Practitioners working with children with speech difficulties often select stimuli words that are familiar to the child, i.e. they aim to update the child's stored but 'frozen' forms. Working on online processing using new words as stimuli might lead not only to more efficient online motor programming and accurate storage of these new words, but also updating of any 'frozen forms' already stored. Novel words may help to break up habitual patterns as the child can use current skills to produce them (e.g. see MacWhinney, 1985; Gierut, 1999). This was our first hypothesis about Joshua's speech processing difficulties and how we might address these in intervention. However, Joshua had difficulties with language processing: standardized tests of language had revealed that his receptive vocabulary was delayed and sentence processing was a challenge. We were aware that it would be difficult for him to learn the meanings of new words, but considered that it could help to expand his vocabulary as well as helping to shake up existing inaccurate motor programs. It might also provide him with an opportunity to reflect on his own speech production and to improve his self-monitoring skills (see Figure 6.1, Level L). Teaching unfamiliar words with emphasis on phonological input, meaning and speech output may result in long lasting and more widespread change in online motor programming and in the way in which motor programs are stored.

(d) Can Joshua produce clusters when naming words?
Joshua's ability to name words from pictures was a weakness recorded on his speech processing profile. He consistently reduced clusters in such tasks. It was hypothesized that Joshua had established inaccurate motor programs for familiar words, and it was likely to be difficult to modify these habitual patterns immediately. He had (at least) two forms of many words in his output lexicon – an immature form and a more adult-like representation that he used inconsistently, e.g. HOSPITAL produced as both [ˈɒʔəʔbɪl] and [ˈhɒsbɪkɪl]. It was considered that introducing Joshua to new words might help him avoid this competition between new and old forms. Joshua could be introduced to new words in both the spoken and written form. It was hypothesized that he would be able to tackle the unfamiliar word using his good grapheme–phoneme conversion skills, and this might help establish the item in his input representations and his stored motor programs.

Phonological rationale: Which aspects of the sound system should be targeted?

Speech analysis carried out at the start of the study (see Tables 6.1 and 6.2), revealed that Joshua had a good phonetic repertoire, and was able to make most contrasts at a segmental level. However, at a syllable structure level, he consistently reduced clusters. All clusters were affected word-initially as well as some in word-final position. Joshua had difficulties with all clusters although to varying degrees. Because of the unclear picture of cluster development and intervention (see the literature review in Chapter 5), all clusters were targeted to allow for observation of the entire set of clusters in English, and their relationship with each other. Words were selected to represent each of the 27 clusters occurring word-initially in English. The intervention aimed to investigate the pattern of change that occurs when all clusters are treated in the same therapy programme.

Psychosocial rationale: What other aspects important to the child should be taken into account?

At the time of our involvement with Joshua, there was concern regarding Joshua's behaviour and social relationships. Joshua was unhappy at school, frequently involved in fights and aggressive outbursts. An educational psychologist noted that Joshua might benefit from social stories. These are short stories written according to a formula, and used to describe social situations that the child on the autistic spectrum finds difficult (see Gray, 1994; Rowe, 1999). They are tailor made for an individual child based on specific scenarios with which the child has difficulty. In order for Joshua's speech and language programme to have maximum relevance to his behaviour, cluster words targeted in intervention were addressed within a social stories context. Intervention focused on Joshua's speech using the social stories as a tool for bringing about more general behavioural change.

Micro Intervention Planning

Joshua received a total of 24 hours of intervention over a four month period. Therapy sessions lasted for approximately one hour each time and were carried out twice a week in Joshua's school. Sessions were missed in some weeks when Joshua was ill, or there were school holidays or outings.

The intervention used a multiple baseline design. A multiple baseline design involves staggering two or more baselines. In a single baseline design, often called an ABA design, pre-intervention assessment is carried out (A); this is followed by the intervention phase (B); and then post-intervention assessment (A). In a multiple baseline design, baseline measures are established and then treatment is introduced at different times. There are three variations of a multiple baseline design. Multiple baseline across

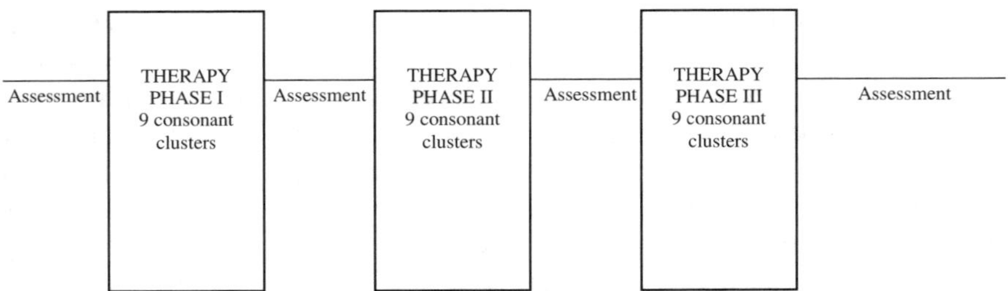

Figure 6.2: The outline design of Joshua's intervention programme.

behaviours (different behaviours are observed), across participants (different participants are observed), or across settings (different settings are used). In Joshua's intervention different clusters were assigned to each one of the three phases to be treated at different times. Each therapy phase addressed nine clusters (i.e. all 27 consonant clusters were addressed over the course of the programme) and was followed by a reassessment of all items. An outline design of Joshua's intervention is shown in Figure 6.2.

Three lists of stimuli were devised with one treatment list (list A) and two control lists (lists B and C). Each list consisted of 27 monosyllabic CCVC English words and met the following criteria.

(a) All 27 word-initial consonant clusters in English were included in each list.
(b) The treatment list (list A) consisted of real words, which were unfamiliar to Joshua as determined by picture naming and discussion. Words that could be used readily in social stories were preferred. Novel words were selected so that Joshua was explicitly given the opportunity to devise and store new motor programs. These were the words that formed the focus of therapy.
(c) List B consisted of untreated real words familiar to Joshua as determined by picture naming and spontaneous speech. These words were not used in therapy but would allow us to see if existing motor programs had been updated.
(d) List C consisted of untreated non-word items made by randomly joining the initial consonant clusters with a range of medial vowels and coda segments (see Chapter 3 for further information about designing matched non-word control stimuli). These words were not used in therapy but would allow us to determine whether Joshua was generalizing the online motor programming skills addressed in therapy to new words not directly targeted.

The three stimuli lists are presented in Table 6.3, together with the average age of acquisition (from McLeod *et al.*, 2001) and the PPK rating (from Gierut *et al.*, 1987) for each cluster.

Table 6.3: Joshua's stimuli lists

Consonant cluster	Age of acquisition*	Productive phonological knowledge** 1 = maximum 6 = no PPK	List A: treated words (novel)	List B: untreated control words (familiar)	List C: untreated control words (non-words)
[tw]	3;6	3	TWIT	TWELVE	[twɛm]
[kw]	3;6	3	QUIT	QUEEN	[kwɛp]
[sp]	5;0-6;0	6	SPITE	SPOON	[spɪb]
[st]	5;0-6;0	4	STATE	START	[stæd]
[sk]	5;0-6;0	4	SCOFF	SCARF	[skɑn]
[sm]	5;0-7;0	6	SMIRK	SMOKE	[smɒf]
[sn]	5;0-7;0	6	SNEER	SNAKE	[snuθ]
[sw]	6;0	6	SWIPE	SWING	[swɔk]
[sl]	7;0	6	SLY	SLEEP	[slɜv]
[pl]	4;0-5;6	6	PLAN	PLATE	[plus]
[bl]	4;0-5;6	6	BLAME	BLACK	[bləʊʃ]
[kl]	4;0-5;6	3	CLASH	CLASS	[klɑt]
[gl]	4;0-5;6	3	GLUM	GLOVE	[gleɪθ]
[fl]	4;0-5;6	6	FLED	FLAG	[flaɪm]
[pr]	5;0-6;0	6	PRAISE	PRAM	[præd]
[br]	5;0-6;0	3	BRAVE	BRIDGE	[braʊp]
[tr]	5;0-6;0	6	TRAIT	TRAIN	[træz]
[dr]	5;0-6;0	6	DREAD	DRESS	[drɛn]
[kr]	5;0-6;0	3	CRUEL	CRASH	[krutʃ]
[gr]	5;0-6;0	6	GREET	GRASS	[grɒdʒ]
[fr]	5;0-6;0	6	FROWN	FROG	[frʌb]
[θr]	7;0	6	THRIVE	THREE	[θrɑɪŋ]
[skw]	7;0	6	SQUIRM	SQUARE	[skwif]
[spl]	7;0	6	SPLIT	SPLASH	[splaʊt]
[spr]	8;0	6	SPRINT	SPRING	[sprɛk]
[str]	8;0	6	STRESS	STRING	[strug]
[skr]	8;0	6	SCREECH	SCREAM	[skreɪt]

* From McLeod *et al.* (2001). ** From Gierut *et al.* (1987).

The words in list A were addressed in therapy, using a task hierarchy which allowed Joshua to move from easier tasks tapping his strengths, to more challenging tasks. The ultimate aim of the programme was for Joshua to devise new and accurate motor programs for a range of new words containing word-initial consonant clusters, and to then lodge these as stored motor programs. In giving Joshua many listening opportunities and the chance to contrast his phonological input representations with his motor programs on the output side, it was hypothesized that he would be able to update motor programs for all clusters, realizing the mismatch that exists. The task hierarchy is outlined below:

(a) **TASK 1: Introduce targets**: Joshua was introduced to the new target words with emphasis on the meaning of the word in the context of a story. The social story was presented to him as a short booklet with illustrations. No production was required at this stage. This task tapped Joshua's auditory input skills, his visual input skills and orthographic knowledge, and his semantic knowledge.

(b) **TASK 2: Listen and judge**: A more specific listening task was carried out that moved beyond the normal developmental process of new word acquisition. Joshua was confronted with each new word as well as closely related foils for each one. Using a yes/no question format, he was asked to consider the exact phonological representation, e.g. SPITE – is the new word SPITE (yes/no) or SPRITE? (yes/no). Again, he was not required to produce the new word himself. This task more specifically tapped Joshua's phonological representations.

(c) **TASK 3: Build up links**: Joshua was explicitly helped to build up the motor programs by focusing on the written forms of words in the stories and talking about 'how we should say them' and how not to say them. The aim here was to use the newly-acquired semantic, phonological and orthographic knowledge from the first two sessions, to map out new motor programs. Joshua was encouraged to say the words and to experiment with and reflect on different ways of saying them. This task tapped phonological representations, semantic knowledge and orthographic knowledge and linked these representations with motor programming.

(d) **TASK 4: Produce**: In the final phase, Joshua read the story using the new words in context in connected speech. He was encouraged to think carefully about how to say the new words. This most challenging task tapped motor programming and motor programs, as well as Joshua's self-monitoring skills.

The 27 words from list A (Table 6.3) were incorporated into social stories. These were written based on guidelines from Gray (1994) and Rowe (1999). Each story begins with a description of a particular scenario. Stories include desired responses to the situation and are used to prepare children to cope with that scenario, as well as other new situations. The following procedure was adopted in preparing the stories and ensuring that all stimuli words from list A were included.

1. Six social stories were written.
2. Four or five of the stimuli words from list A were selected for inclusion in each story so that all 27 words were included at some point in the programme.
3. Each word appeared at least three times, and not more than five times, in a story.

4. Each story was worked through over four consecutive sessions using the task hierarchy outlined above. Thus, each session comprised one of the tasks from the task hierarchy.

Figure 6.3 provides an example of one of the social stories written for Joshua to introduce new words containing consonant clusters.

Figure 6.4 shows the design of the intervention in further detail.

1.

A Story About
Lining Up

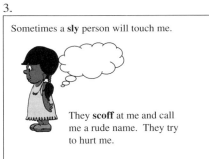

2.

When I hear the bell, it's time to line up.

All the children in my class stand in a line.

Sometimes we stand quietly.
Nobody touches me. Nobody annoys me.
My teacher **praises** me.

3.

Sometimes a **sly** person will touch me.

They **scoff** at me and call me a rude name. They try to hurt me.

4.

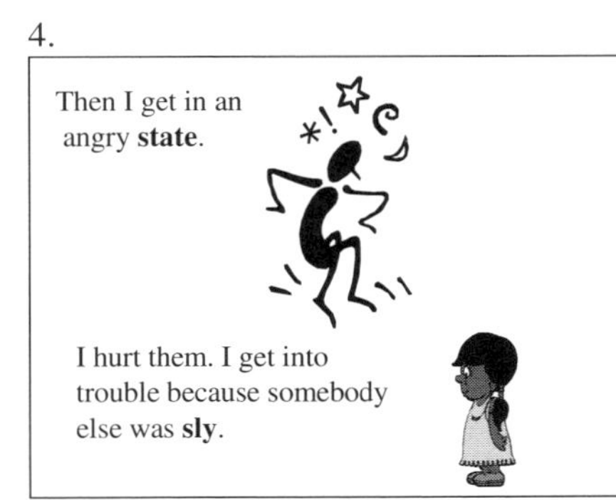

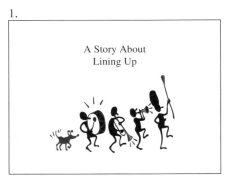

Then I get in an
angry **state**.
I hurt them. I get into
trouble because somebody
else was **sly**.

5.

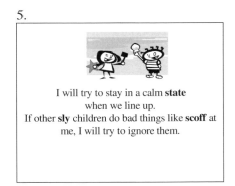

I will try to stay in a calm **state**
when we line up.
If other **sly** children do bad things like **scoff** at
me, I will try to ignore them.

6.

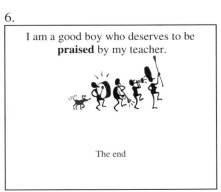

I am a good boy who deserves to be
praised by my teacher.
The end

Figure 6.3: Example of a social story used as context for introducing Joshua's new words: PRAISE; SLY, SCOFF, STATE.

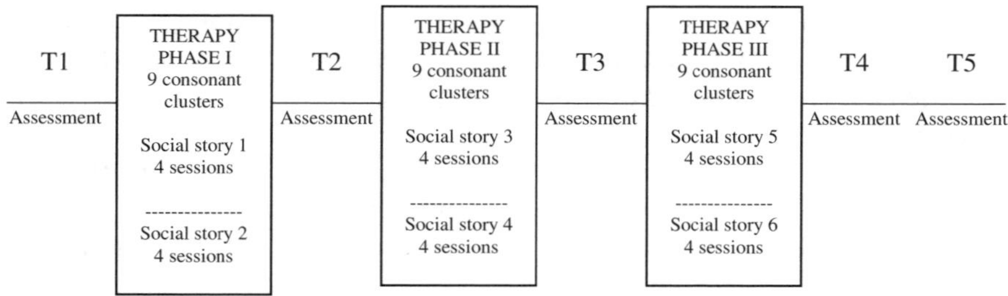

Figure 6.4: The design of Joshua's intervention programme.

Joshua received three phases of therapy with each phase focusing on nine randomly selected consonant clusters. Two social stories were used in each phase to introduce and contextualize the new words. Assessment of Joshua's ability to produce the new words took place at five points throughout the intervention programme (T1–T5) in order to monitor any progress made. Baseline evaluation took place prior to the intervention at T1, and then following each of the three phases of intervention, as is typical for a multiple baseline design. Each phase comprised eight sessions, i.e. working through the four tasks of the task hierarchy twice, for two social stories and the associated nine clusters. On completion of the programme (T4), re-assessment took place, and at T5 long-term follow-up evaluation took place, 7 months after intervention has ceased. The assessment involved obtaining single word productions for each of the items in each of the lists as well as obtaining Joshua's written spelling attempts for all words.

Table 6.4 outlines what took place in each phase of therapy, together with excerpts from the therapist's case notes from each session.

ACTIVITY 6.3

Consider the intervention plans outlined in this section. Comment on the following aspects of the programme design.

(a) What are the strengths of the design that will enable us to determine if any changes observed in Joshua's speech are due to the intervention?
(b) Can you foresee any difficulties with the design, and suggest ways of improving it?
(c) What questions would you pose about the intervention outcomes?

Turn to the Key to Activity 6.3 at the end of this chapter, and then read on to see the specific questions that we posed about Joshua's intervention.

Table 6.4: Example of recorded comments on Joshua's intervention sessions

Phase I

Consonant clusters: [pr], [sl], [sk], [st] [gl], [fr], [str], [skr], [tr]

Story 1: A story about lining up

Stimuli words: PRAISE; SLY, SCOFF, STATE		Comments
Session 1	Task 1: Introduce	Joshua listened attentively and said that he liked the story.
Session 2	Task 2: Listen and judge	Joshua missed two sessions due to illness. We went over the story again and I reminded him about the new words: he had forgotten them all. We played the phonological representations game in which he had to judge if similar-sounding words were correct or not (80% correct).
Session 3	Task 3: Build up links	We wrote and practised saying the words today. PRAISE is hardest for him – he typically says 'plays' or 'lays'.
Session 4	Task 4: Produce	Joshua read the story very well and made good attempts at all the target words. He was producing [s] clusters although still needs to leave a little break between [s] and stop. Joshua was very excited to take the story home.

Story 2: A story about talking and reading

Stimuli words: GLUM, FROWN, STRESS, SCREECH, TRAIT		Comments
Session 5	Task 1: Introduce	Introduced new story today. Joshua read it together with me and started colouring in some of the pictures.
Session 6	Task 2: Listen and judge	Went over new words today – Joshua had remembered some of them (50%). Enjoyed phonological representations games – scored 100% correct. He has appropriate phonological representations of the target words, which is quite surprising because it seems like he is not listening when I say or talk about them.
Session 7	Task 3: Build up links	Joshua told me how to spell the words and we talked about how to say them (70% accuracy). I had to remind him to put the [s] in front of the [s] cluster words but otherwise he did well.
Session 8	Task 4: Produce	Joshua did well today: TRAIT and GLUM were correctly produced on all attempts (100% accuracy). Others were harder for him but some attempts. Noticed that he said GREEN correctly in spontaneous speech during game.

Table 6.4: *Continued*

Phase II

Consonant clusters: [θr] [pl] [br] [kw] [fl] [sm] [spr] [tw] [kl]

Story 3: A story about working on my own

Stimuli words: THRIVE, PLAN, BRAVE, QUIT		Comments
Session 9	Task 1: Introduce	Joshua grabbed the story and started reading aloud before I could! Noted some accurate clusters in the story, but not using spontaneously.
Session 10	Task 2: Listen and judge	Re-read the story and spoke about new words. Joshua had remembered some parts of the story. He enjoyed the phonological representations game, scoring 80% correct.
Session 11	Task 3: Build up links	He did well despite the fact that some are confusing to write (e.g. <quit>). He is trying to say all parts of the cluster now and knows when he forgets!
Session 12	Task 4: Produce	We returned to the story today and Joshua read it very well. All his clusters were fine. I gave him a lot of praise and he seemed very proud.

Story 4: A story about walking away from fights

Stimuli words: FLED, SMIRK, SPRINT, TWIT, CLASH		Comments
Session 13	Task 1: Introduce	Joshua liked the new story about fighting. He was concerned about some of the details in the story and the pictures so we spent some time talking about who was represented in the pictures.
Session 14	Task 2: Listen and judge	Joshua was still concerned about the pictures today, and whether he was the boy depicted in them. He read the story well and showed some understanding of the words. When I tried to explain what some of the words meant, he interrupted or started to hum. He scored 90% correct on the representations game. He said that 'print' was wrong for SPRINT but then carried on reading and saying 'print' still indicating a mismatch between input and output.
Session 15	Task 3: Build up links	Joshua was able to help me write the new words and say them. He could say them all when he spoke slowly (100%).
Session 16	Task 4: Produce	Completed this story today. Joshua said some accurate cluster words although at times he forgot but could correct himself. He seemed very inconsistent today and unmotivated.

Table 6.4: *Continued*

Phase III

Consonant clusters: [bl] [dr] [kr] [gr] [sp] [sn] [sw] [skw] [spl]

Story 5: A story about doing something different

Stimuli words: BLAME, DREAD, CRUEL, GREET		Comments
Session 17	Task 1: Introduce	Joshua insisted on reading the story to me first, rather than letting me read it to him. There was a mistake in the story and Joshua did not notice.
Session 18	Task 2: Listen and judge	Re-read the story and went over new words and phonological representations. He did well with this (80% correct).
Session 19	Task 3: Build up links	Very good spelling today (70% clusters correct). Noticed that Joshua was inserting schwa between two initial clusters in his speech, e.g. BLAME → [bəleɪm]. This might be because of how they've been emphasized, or maybe a phase required before getting them correct. He reflects this in his spelling too, on occasion, e.g. <belame>.
Session 20	Task 4: Produce	Good reading and good cluster production (70% correct).

Story 6: A story about being kind and helpful

Stimuli words: SPITE, SNEER, SWIPE, SQUIRM, SPLIT		Comments
Session 21	Task 1: Introduce	Joshua was introduced to the new story today. We both had a chance to read it.
Session 22	Task 2: Listen and judge	Joshua scored 100% on the phonological representations task
Session 23	Task 3: Build up links	Joshua did well with the spelling and was able to say most of the words correctly when pointing to the letters. SPLIT is hard for him though: he could either say 'spit' or 'plit' but not all three consonants together. He was getting frustrated about this.
Session 24	Task 4: Produce	Re-read the story today. Joshua did well but needed some reminding about initial [s] sounds. SPLIT remains challenging for him.

The Questions We Asked

We asked the following questions about Joshua's intervention.

(a) Is the intervention effective? If so, there will be improvements in Joshua's speech production of treated items (list A) beyond chance level.

(b) Does generalization occur? If so, there will be improvements in Joshua's production of matched untreated control words (lists B and C). Improvement in Joshua's production of familiar words with word-initial clusters (list B words) would suggest that the stored motor programs have been effectively updated. Improvement in Joshua's production of non-words with word initial clusters (list C words) would suggest that the online motor programming mechanism had improved.

(c) Is there a relationship between pre-intervention PPK and intervention success? For each of the consonant clusters, Joshua had varying degrees of productive phonological knowledge (PPK).

(d) Does the pattern of change observed over intervention follow a developmental trend as outlined in the literature (e.g. by McLeod *et al.*, 2001)?

(e) Will targeting a small set of consonant clusters (as in the first phase of intervention) have an effect on the remainder of the consonant clusters?

(f) How does the intervention affect Joshua's written representations of words? The intervention relies heavily on exposure to written forms with both reading and writing of treated items. Does the spelling of the treated words improve through this exposure? If so, will this generalize to the untreated words? This would suggest that orthographic representations have been updated in the case of the familiar words, and that accurate phoneme to grapheme conversion is taking place for the non-words.

Intervention Outcomes: Our Questions Answered

In this section we attempt to answers the questions posed about Joshua's intervention:

(a) Is the intervention effective?

Yes, Joshua made significant improvements in his ability to accurately realise the clusters in the treated words in list A. A statistically significant difference was found in his spoken production of clusters when comparing pre- (T1) and post-intervention (T4) performance. We used the statistical procedures ANOVA (analysis of variance) and t-test to provide the statistical evidence of change. Pring (2005) describes the use of these tests with specific reference to intervention cases and communication disorders. Before the intervention Joshua produced the target PRAISE as [peɪz], and FROWN as [faʊn]. After intervention he was able to produce these words more accurately, e.g. [pweɪz] and [fraʊn]. If we had scored these items on a right or wrong basis we might not have detected all the change that had occurred, e.g. from [peɪz] to [pweɪz] is a positive change although he is still gliding the liquid /r/ and has yet to produce the adult target PRAISE.

(b) Did generalization occur?
There were statistically significant improvements in Joshua's production of the clusters in the matched untreated control words (lists B and C). Joshua's production of untreated, but familiar control words (e.g. SCARF and PRAM) changed over the course of intervention from [gaf] to [skaf], and [pæm] to [præm]. The improvement in Joshua's production of familiar words with word-initial clusters (list B words) suggests that his stored motor programs have been effectively updated. Improvement in Joshua's production of non-words with word-initial clusters (list C words) suggests that the online motor programming mechanism has been altered.

Looking beyond the stimuli specifically designed to evaluate the intervention, we carried out more general speech sampling. A post-intervention PACS (Grunwell, 1985) was carried out at CA 8;8 to provide information on Joshua's phonological system (Table 6.5).

The speech samples obtained at CA 8;8 were compared with the summary of findings at the initial assessment. Many of the findings were the same as for the initial assessment: Joshua's severity indices had not changed (see Chapter 11 on intelligibility). However, it was noted that Joshua's word-initial cluster reduction had decreased significantly from 88% to 66%. There was no evidence of cluster reversal (e.g. WASP → [wɒps]) at this second assessment. In addition to using more clusters in the word-initial position, Joshua was also using more clusters word-finally, although this was not yet consistent and did not constitute a significant difference from T1. Joshua still found it hard to produce longer, multi-syllabic words (e.g. HOSPITAL → ['hɒsbɪkɪl]; TOMATO → [mə'tɑtəʊ]). He also still had many immature 'frozen' forms of words which he produced like a younger child, e.g. YELLOW → [lɛləʊ]. No generalization was noted to unrelated speech difficulties which suggests that intervention hit the targeted aspects directly and brought about specific changes in clusters, the targeted area of Joshua's speech. Joshua's cluster reduction remained a dominant aspect of his speech and one which required further intervention. Joshua was no longer lateralizing /s/: his front teeth had now appeared and it was easier for him to produce a correct /s/. Joshua's teachers and parent continued to express concern about his speech difficulties on completion of the intervention. Although intervention outcomes were positive, Joshua required further support for his speech, language and literacy needs.

(c) Is there a relationship between pre-intervention PPK and intervention success?

Table 6.5: Comparison of Joshua's speech data at CA 7;2 (pre-intervention) with CA 8;8 (post-intervention)

Assessment	Pre-intervention CA 7;2	Post-intervention CA 8;8
Severity indices	PCC 78% PVC 100% PPC 86.7%	PCC 76% PVC 100% PPC 85.5%
Phonetic inventory	Word initial: [m, n, p, b, t, d, k, g, f, v, s, z, ʃ, ʧ, ʤ, j, l, w] Word medial: [m, n, ŋ, p, b, t, d, k, g, f, v, s, z, ʃ, ʒ, ʤ, j, l, w] Word final: [m, n, ŋ, p, b, t, d, k, g, f, v, s, z, ʃ, ʒ, ʧ, ʤ, j, l, w]	Word initial: [m, n, p, b, t, d, k, g, f, v, s, z, ʃ, ʧ, ʤ, j, l, w] Word medial: [m, n, ŋ, p, b, t, d, k, g, f, v, s, z, ʃ, ʒ, ʧ, ʤ, j, l, w] Word final: [m, n, ŋ, p, b, t, d, k, g, f, v, s, z, ʃ, ʒ, ʧ, ʤ, j, l, w]
Stimulability	All segments	All segments
Phonological processes analysis (% use)	Developmental processes: cluster reduction (87.7%); consonant harmony (9%)	Developmental processes: cluster reduction (66.6%); consonant harmony (7%)
Single word speech sample	JACOB → [ˈʤeɪpɪb] YELLOW → [ˈlɛləʊ] CATERPILLAR → [ˈtætikɪlə] HOSPITAL → [ˈhɒsbɪkɪl] HOSPITAL → [ˈɒʔəʔbɪl] BROTHER → [ˈbʊvə] SCARF → [kɑf] SCOOTER → [ˈkʊtə]	JACOB → [ˈʤeɪpɪb] YELLOW → [ˈlɛləʊ] CATERPILLAR → [ˈtætikɪlə] HOSPITAL → [ˈhɒsbɪkɪl] BROTHER → [ˈbrʊvə] SCARF → [skɑf] SCOOTER → [ˈskʊtə]
Connected speech sample	SHE GOT A BLACK ONE → [ʃiʔ gɒʔ ə bæk wʊn] THE THREE LITTLE PIGS → [də fwi ˈlɪʔtə pɪg] I'M THE BIG BAD WOLF → [ɑɪm və bɪg bæd wʊf]	AND I GOT A TRACKSUIT → [æn ɑɪ gɒtə ˈtwæksut] I'M NOT ALLOWED TO OPEN IT ON FRIDAY → [ɑɪm nɒt ə ˈlaʊd tuʔ əʊpɪn ɪt ɒn ˈfrɑɪdeɪ]

For each of the consonant clusters, Joshua had varying degrees of productive phonological knowledge (PPK). Gierut *et al.* (1987) suggest that clusters about which the least is known (Type 6) are the most efficient ones to address. In Joshua's case, the majority of consonant clusters were in the Type 6 category, sounds about which Joshua had no phonological knowledge and never used correctly. Two of the clusters, /sk, st/, were considered to be Type 4 clusters since Joshua was able to use these correctly in the word final position but not word-initially. The remaining six clusters, /kl, kw, kr, br, gl, tw/, were clusters from Type 3, about which Joshua had the most phonological knowledge. He was able to produce these correctly on occasion but seemed to have frozen forms for some specific words. Table 6.6 shows the PPK classification of clusters together with a summary of outcomes for each cluster.

Table 6.6: Joshua's stimuli lists showing clusters for which intervention was deemed a success*

Consonant cluster Shaded clusters = clusters successfully addressed	Age of acquisition from McLeod *et al.* (2001)	Productive phonological knowledge (PPK)** 1 = maximum PPK; 6 = no PPK
[tw]	3;6	3
[kw]	3;6	3
[kl]	4;0-5;6	3
[gl]	4;0-5;6	3
[br]	5;0-6;0	3
[kr]	5;0-6;0	3
[st]	5;0-6;0	4
[st]	5;0-6;0	4
[sk]	5;0-6;0	4
[sm]	5;0-7;0	4
[sn]	5;0-7;0	6
[sw]	6;0	6
[sl]	7;0	6
[pl]	4;0-5;6	6
[bl]	4;0-5;6	6
[fl]	4;0-5;6	6
[pr]	5;0-6;0	6
[tr]	5;0-6;0	6
[dr]	5;0-6;0	6
[sp]	5;0-6;0	6
[gr]	5;0-6;0	6
[fr]	5;0-6;0	6
[θr]	7;0	6
[skw]	7;0	6
[spl]	7;0	6
[spr]	8;0	6
[str]	8;0	6
[skr]	8;0	6

* Based on scoring in the post-intervention assessments.
** From Gierut *et al.* (1987).

The Type 6 clusters varied widely in the pattern of changes observed: some were efficiently modified (e.g. /tr/) while others showed no change (e.g. /sp/). Each of the three-part clusters (e.g., /spl, spr/) made very limited change. The two clusters classed as Type 4 also made very limited change, suggesting that although Joshua initially had more phonological knowledge of these sounds, this did not aid the remediation process. Many of the /s/ clusters were problematic for Joshua to acquire and this is something that has been noted in the literature (e.g. Barlow, 2001) and was discussed in Chapter 5. Six clusters were classed as Type 3 clusters – sounds about which Joshua knew the most. No /s/ clusters were included in this set. Joshua made progress with each of these clusters suggesting that having some knowledge is a good prognostic factor for intervention.

(d) Does the pattern of change observed over intervention follow the developmental trend as outlined in the literature?

Pre-intervention baselines showed that Joshua was following a normal developmental sequence in his consonant cluster development. Table 6.3 shows the range of word-initial consonant clusters together with norms for age of acquisition (from McLeod *et al.*, 2001). It can be seen that Joshua's clusters classified as having a PPK of 3 are the ones expected to develop earliest. Scores were awarded for post-intervention productions. The successful clusters are highlighted in Table 6.6, which shows that all the Type 3 clusters were considered a success, with the exception of [kl], which fell short of the criterion for success. Second, it is striking that the /s/ clusters were not so successfully treated – with the exception of /sw/. In general, Joshua followed developmental trends as, by the end of intervention, he had acquired all of the earliest acquired clusters, e.g. those usually mastered by 3;6 (/tw, kw/) and those that children typically begin to acquire at 4;0 (e.g. /pl, bl/) and 5;0 (e.g. /tr, dr/). The /s/ clusters, including the three-element clusters, remain challenging for Joshua. Three-element clusters are typically some of the last elements of children's speech sound acquisition. In general, it seems that intervention was able to expedite normal phonological development, although the /s/ clusters seemed not to fit in with this pattern, functioning as a separate group and somewhat resistant to change. These findings are in line with previously published literature outlined in Chapter 5.

(e) Did targeting a small set of consonant clusters (as in the first phase of intervention) have an effect on the remainder of the consonant clusters?

Yes, Joshua made some improvements on untreated clusters prior to their intervention. The clusters addressed in phase II improved slightly between T1 and T2 (prior to intervention) for speech, but these gains did not reach significance. The phase III clusters showed some significant gains prior to their intervention for two of the lists for speech (between T2 and T3), and one of the lists for spelling (between T1 and T2). Joshua's awareness of the concept of a cluster at a general level may have increased in the first phase of intervention, thus bringing about spontaneous change in clusters not yet targeted. This may provide evidence for the fact that for some children clusters can be taught as a concept, and that a limited number of exemplars are sufficient to bring about change to all clusters, although /s/ clusters may not fit with this pattern.

(f) How does the intervention affect Joshua's written representations of words?

The intervention relied heavily on exposure to written forms with both reading and writing of treated items. A significant improvement was noted in Joshua's spelling of consonant clusters when comparing pre- and post-intervention results. More specifically, Joshua made significant spelling improvement over the course of intervention for both the treated wordlist (A) and the familiar controls (list B). For these two lists, Joshua's written representations improved hand-in-hand with his spoken representations. For example, for the treated words Joshua's spellings changed as follows.

Target	Pre-intervention Spelling	Post-intervention Spelling
STATE	<s>	<steb>
SCOFF	<s>	<scoff>
PRAISE	<biss>	<plasie>

No significant change was noted for spelling the non-words (list C), showing a mismatch with his greatly improved spoken production of list C words.

What Did We Learn from Joshua's Intervention?

Including all clusters in Joshua's treatment programme allowed for the adoption of a holistic perspective on cluster development. Joshua seemed to follow broad developmental trends (as outlined by McCleod *et al.*, 2001) in his acquisition of clusters, but different patterns of change were noted for different words and different clusters. In general, it was found that Joshua's pattern of response depended more on his lexical knowledge than on a particular cluster, i.e. non-words changed in a similar way as a group, rather than all /sk/ words acting as a group. Non-words seemed to respond differently to real words. In terms of phonology it was noted that the /s/ clusters seemed to respond differently to other clusters. This finding is supported by the literature and /s/ clusters are frequently described as adjuncts, consonants adjoined more loosely to a word than a true cluster (Barlow, 2001; Velleman, 2002). The special status of /s/ clusters has been supported by intervention studies, which have found that treatment of these adjuncts does not result in generalization to other clusters (Gierut, 1999). Furthermore, it has been noted that the adjuncts as a group may be acquired before other clusters, or after – but essentially that they can be clearly distinguished as a group from the other clusters. /s/ clusters certainly seemed most challenging for Joshua, but this may be because he had some difficulties in articulating [s] at the start of the intervention.

A multiple baseline design was used with different clusters being treated at different phases of intervention. In the early phases of intervention there was a clear effect of intervention on the particular clusters targeted in that phase, but by the third phase of intervention this pattern was not clear, with clusters from that set improving prior to the specific treatment targeted at them. This finding is not entirely surprising (Seron, 1997), and suggests that the concept of a cluster might have been the most important aspect of intervention. A small set of exemplars might have been sufficient in bringing about change rather than attempting to include all clusters. The questions of 'how many exemplars to use?' and 'which exemplars to use?' are important ones (see Chapter 3). While some authors have suggested that the answer to the first question is just one feature contrast (Blache, Parsons and Humphreys, 1981) or one segment (Gierut *et al.*, 1987), others such as Edwards (1983) and Hodson and Paden (1991) have suggested multiple exemplars are preferable. A phonotactic approach to therapy (e.g. as advocated by Velleman, 2002) fits well with this point of view. Velleman suggests that focusing on the concept of a new word shape (e.g. CCVC) may well result in generalization beyond the treated sounds. As noted in Chapter 3, the answer to these questions of 'how many' and 'which' stimuli to use is most likely, 'it depends on the children and their individual profiles of strengths and weaknesses'.

Unfamiliar words were used as the main stimuli for intervention, and this was based on a specific rationale used with some success in previous studies (e.g. MacWhinney, 1985; Gierut, 1999). In the present study, these words did seem to have the overall effect of bringing about improvement in Joshua's speech processing, but it has been questioned whether other stimuli might have had a similar, or even more desirable effect. On the one hand, real and familiar words might have been more motivating for Joshua who tended to forget the new words. Children have a finite set of cognitive skills brought to the learning process. Learning non-familiar words was taxing for Joshua and using familiar words might have freed up more cognitive resources for learning. Alternatively, using non-words might have been another effective strategy that would have reduced the semantic load placed on Joshua.

Joshua's intervention gave us a window into the consonant cluster development of a child with PSDs. Intervention was shown to be effective in promoting acquisition of clusters following a normal, developmental sequence. It was suggested that working on a small set of clusters brought about widespread change in all clusters. Much of this discussion has emphasized the importance of stimuli selection, a theme introduced in Chapter 3 but of importance to all intervention. Joshua's intervention addressed a specific aspect of his phonological processing, adding to clinical and theoretical knowledge of word-initial consonant clusters, while contextualizing this linguistic work within social stories in order to have wide-ranging relevance to the child in question and his behavioural difficulties. Although we did not evaluate Joshua's behaviour in any formal way, comments from his parents and school staff suggested that the social stories had had a positive effect on his behaviour in the specific situations addressed.

Joshua needed a great deal of direct and intensive work to bring about significant changes in his production of consonant clusters. Still there remained a need for further work on perfecting his clusters - and his speech more generally. Providing this level of therapy is expensive and raises a number of service delivery challenges which are discussed in greater detail in Chapter 13. Positively, Joshua's intervention showed how a targeted programme of intervention can bring about changes not only in speech, but also in spelling and social behaviours.

Summary

This chapter has described the intervention that took place with Joshua aged 6;10 in order to address his consonant clusters. The key points are as follows.

- The speech processing profile was used as a starting point in organizing Joshua's assessment results, followed by more detailed phonological analysis.
- Intervention planning was motivated by the three key strands of psycholinguistics, phonology and the child's psychosocial needs.
- The psycholinguistic strand emphasized the need for therapy tasks to be targeted at appropriate parts of the speech processing system with a carefully ordered task hierarchy.
- The phonological strand emphasized the need for therapy stimuli to be carefully selected and controlled for in the light of Joshua's speech data.
- The psychosocial rationale emphasized the need for therapy to be relevant to Joshua's behavioural difficulties and his family's most urgent concerns.
- Developmental norms of consonant cluster acquisition and productive phonological knowledge were used to inform intervention planning and in making sense of intervention outcomes.
- Non-words can be used effectively to tap a child's online motor programming, although the use of such stimuli can place high demands on children with language and memory difficulties.
- Intervention outcomes were positive as Joshua's word-initial cluster reduction decreased significantly from 88% to 66%.

- Joshua's spelling of words with consonant clusters, and his behaviour in specific social situations improved following intervention.
- Joshua's cluster reduction remains a dominant aspect of his speech and one which requires further intervention.
- The intervention with Joshua showed him to be following a developmental hierarchy of acquisition, but responding slowly with his /s/ clusters which behaved in a different way to the other clusters.
- Generalization occurred to other clusters following the first phase of intervention with a subset of clusters, suggesting that Joshua was using his increasing knowledge of the concept of a cluster to generalize to untreated clusters.
- Joshua's intervention raises issues for service delivery which are returned to in Chapter 13.

KEY TO ACTIVITY 6.1

(a) Does Joshua have difficulties with input or output?
He has difficulties with both input and output, but has more problems on the output side.

(b) Outline two areas of relative strength.
Joshua has relative strengths at levels D and H of the profile. At level D he showed age-appropriate auditory discrimination of real words on a range of tests. At level H he showed age-appropriate phonological awareness skills. He also has strengths at levels A, B and K.

(c) Outline Joshua's main areas of difficulty.
Joshua has difficulties with the output side of the profile, most notably at level G (Can the child access accurate motor programs?) and with repeating more complex real and non-words (Levels I and J).

(d) What further information or assessments would you find valuable?
We wanted to know what is causing his difficulties at Level G, e.g. is there a relationship between

- auditory lexical decision and naming (Levels E and G)?
- non-word and real word repetition and naming (Levels I, J and G)?
- speech and spelling?

Additional assessments we wanted to carry out included:

- an evaluation of Joshua's new word learning;
- further evaluation of his naming skills following Constable *et al.* (1997);
- asking Joshua to speak and spell the same words (see Chapter 10).

KEY TO ACTIVITY 6.2

Speech processing model showing Joshua's main areas of difficulty at CA 7;2. Reproduced by kind permission of Whurr Publishing, from Stackhouse and Wells, 1997.

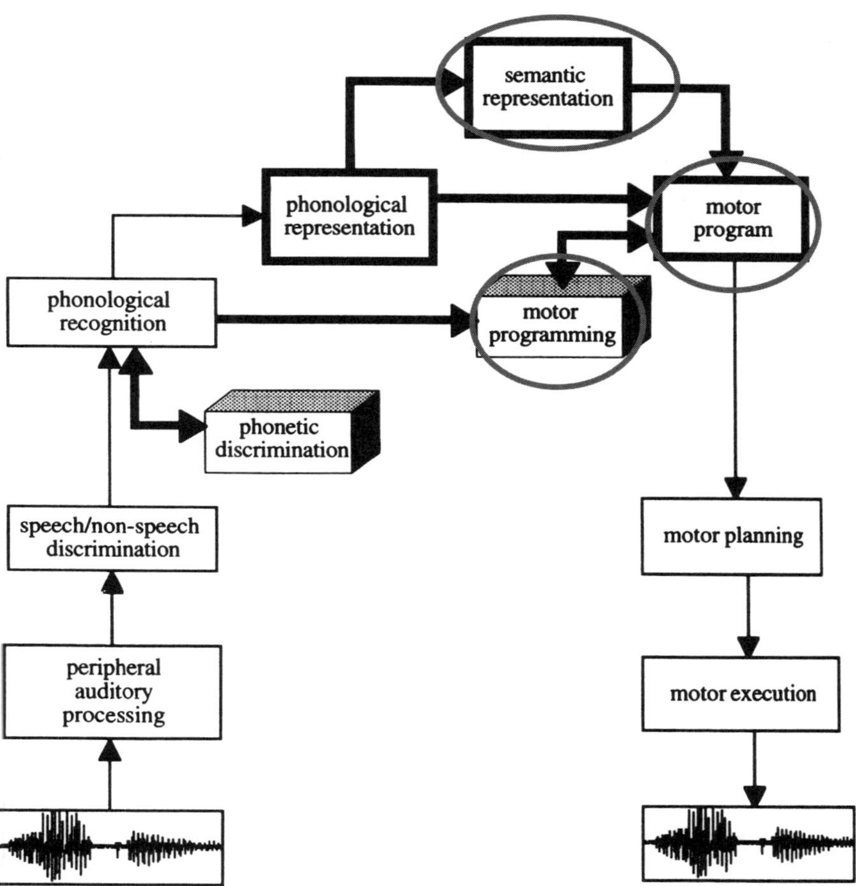

KEY TO ACTIVITY 6.3

(a) What are the strengths of the design that will enable us to determine if any changes observed in Joshua's speech are due to the intervention?

The multiple baseline design will give us a window into any changes occurring in Joshua's phonological system. Specific clusters are addressed in specific phases of intervention. We may therefore expect to see a corresponding improvement in only the treated clusters for each phase. The intervention focuses very specifically on consonant clusters. We might therefore expect to see an improvement in Joshua's production of clusters but not in other aspects of his speech, or more general language development. Choosing sets of control words that are closely matched to the treated words ensures that the specific effects of therapy can be monitored and the extent of any generalization observed.

(b) Can you foresee any difficulties with the design and suggest ways of improving it?

A stable baseline was not demonstrated prior to the start of the intervention. He may have been making improvements in his production of clusters already, even before the intervention started. It may be that working on a small subset of clusters results in generalization to other untreated clusters so that the effects of the multiple baseline design are not clear. However good a research design, children can be variable in their behaviour and responses.

(c) What questions would you pose about the intervention outcomes?

Examples of questions you may have posed include the following.

- Does the intervention bring about changes in Joshua's production of consonant clusters?
- Does generalization occur?
- Is there a relationship between pre-intervention productive phonological knowledge (PPK) and intervention outcomes?
- Is the pattern of change in Joshua's consonant clusters predicted by developmental norms?
- Will targeting a small set of consonant clusters, e.g. as in the first phase of intervention, have an effect on the remainder of the consonant clusters?
- How does the intervention affect Joshua's written representations of words?
- Do the social stories have any impact on his behaviour/social awareness?

These questions are discussed in greater detail in the text.

Notes

1. While DAMP is seldom given as a diagnosis in the United Kingdom, the term is one that originated in Scandinavia some 20 years ago and is widely used in parts of Northern Europe. Gillberg (2003) suggests that about 1.5% of the general population of school-age children in Sweden are affected by the condition. Gillberg (2003) provides a review of the condition and notes that the diagnosis is typically made by psychiatrists or paediatricians.
2. With the exception of Level C which is not routinely assessed in monolingual children (Stackhouse and Wells, 1997).

Chapter 7
Stimuli Design: Connected Speech

Traditionally speech and language therapists focus on children's production of specific, individual speech sounds and their use of these sounds in the production of single words (e.g. Forrest, Elbert and Dinnsen, 2000; Williams, 2000a, b; Barlow and Gierut, 2002). Therapy often involves single-word naming tasks, reading of single words, guessing games and word games involving single words or pictures of single objects. In Chapters 3–6 we have focused on stimuli design at the level of segments and clusters in single words. The implicit rationale behind single word approaches to therapy is that single word production is easier for children, and this is the first step towards positive outcomes: if children can produce the target sound or word accurately at this level, then they have a good foundation for going on to produce the sound or word in their connected and spontaneous speech. This may well be an appropriate approach for many children, however there is increasing evidence, coming from intervention studies (e.g. Stiegler and Hoffman, 2001), linguistic studies of children with speech difficulties (e.g. Wells, 1994) and intelligibility literature (e.g. Chin, Tsai and Gao, 2003, and see Chapter 11) of the need for speech therapy that explicitly addresses connected speech. Phonological difficulties in connected speech are often more numerous and qualitatively different to those in single words (e.g. Andrews and Fey, 1986; Morrison and Shriberg, 1992). You may well be able to think of children who are able to produce single words with relative accuracy, but whose intelligibility dramatically decreases when they use everyday, spontaneous speech.

This chapter focuses on stimuli design at the level of connected speech. We start by considering what is meant by the term 'connected speech', and when and why working on connected speech could be useful. Connected speech is contextualized within a psycholinguistic framework, again emphasizing the importance of combining psycholinguistic and phonological approaches to intervention for the school-age child with PSDs. Chapter 8 presents a case study of Katy, aged 6;5 at the start of the intervention, a child whose intervention involved both single word and connected speech therapy phases.

What is Connected Speech?

Children and adults rarely speak in single words. When we talk we usually produce a continuous and connected stream of sounds. Although adults might use longer sentences and speak more rapidly than young children, connected speech is the norm for our communication. This can sometimes come as a surprise when reading some textbooks! Phonetics and phonology often focus heavily at a single word and segmental level, leading us to think of speech as a sequence of individual consonants and vowels. However, connected speech is more than just a string of individual segments joined together in an independent way. Each segment has a strong influence on the segments that surround it - as you will find out in the following activity (from Stackhouse and Wells, 1997 p. 226).

ACTIVITY 7.1

Say the following phrases in a normal, natural way as you might in everyday speech:

(a) GREAT ELEPHANT
(b) GREAT TIGER
(c) GREAT CAT
(d) GREAT BEAR

For each phrase write down how you think you have produced the final /t/ in GREA<u>T</u>. Are there differences in the realization of that sound for each phrase and how might you account for them? Turn to the Key to Activity 7.1 at the end of the chapter, and then read the following.

In most accents of English, the final consonant of GREAT, in the context of GREAT ELEPHANT, is an audibly released alveolar plosive. However, this changes in the subsequent phrases. In GREAT TIGER, the final consonant of GREAT is realized as a closure of the larynx and a silent period of contact between the tongue tip (or blade) and the teeth ridge, preceding the [t] of the following word. In GREAT CAT, it is realized differently again. Now the period of silent contact is between the back of the tongue and the soft-palate, anticipating the [k] of CAT. For GREAT BEAR, the period of contact does not involve the tongue at all: instead there is a closure of the lips, anticipating the [b] of BEAR. These are examples of the way in which sound segments are affected by neighbouring sounds. In the activity above, the examples all illustrate assimilation, an important connected speech process at the segmental level, and one that is discussed in greater detail in the sections that follow.

Typical speech in conversation consists of utterances of varying lengths, characterized by a flow of words connected together by specific phonetic and phonological features arising from the particular sequences of sounds that occur at word junctions. Stackhouse and Wells (2001) refer to phonetic and phonological glue that binds words together in ordinary, everyday speech. This glue is, very broadly, of two kinds: segmental and prosodic. In this section we briefly review some of the most important segmental and prosodic connected speech processes.

Segmental Processes in Connected Speech

Junction or juncture refers broadly to the way in which words or syllables are joined together with each other across word boundaries. Stackhouse and Wells (1997, p. 226) describe junction as 'subtle phonological features, occurring particularly around word boundaries, which are found in the speech of fluent adults and which serve to glue the utterance together into a cohesive entity'. Authors such as Wells (1994) and Newton and Wells (2002) make a broad distinction between open and close junctures. When a speaker of English produces two words in sequence, there may be features which serve to keep the words distinct. These are termed open junctures and are typically associated with a formal style of speech and/or emphatic utterances such as repair or reading aloud (Wells, 1994), e.g. THAT SIDE → [ðæt saɪd]. Close junctures are associated with non-emphatic utterances in colloquial speech, e.g. THAT SIDE → [ðæs: aɪd]. Describing syllable juncture using this two-term system has not been widely employed in studies of child phonology. However, this close/open dichotomy is a useful one in bringing together these processes. Studies by Newton (1999) and Newton and Wells (2002) suggest that children as young as 2–3 years of age show examples of close juncture (e.g. assimilation) and that this develops prior to open juncture. These authors studied a normally-developing boy called Christopher, aged between 2;4 and 3;4. From the very onset of multi-word production he was noted to attempt to glue adjacent words together, even though he could not yet do so in an adult way. For example at CA 2;4, Christopher realized the phrase LOST BERTIE as [lɒʔbɜti], an example of close juncture. As the year progressed and Christopher developed his language, some open junctures appeared but close junctures (e.g. assimilation) were always in the majority. The authors concluded that children do not start out by learning words and how to combine these, but rather produce chunks of speech that they initially treat as whole units, only later being able to break them down into words and syllables. This has important implications for intervention since working on words in isolation and building up towards phrases is not following a normal developmental pattern, contrary to what has often been presumed.

Howard (2004) carried out an investigation of the connected speech of five school-aged children (aged 9–16 years) with persisting speech difficulties using electropalatographic (EPG) and perceptual techniques. Findings revealed that all children were making use of some connected speech processes characteristic of typically developing children, but that in addition they all also exhibited a range of more unusual connected speech processes - often at word junctures. The children varied considerably in their connected speech patterns, but in general findings supported the notion that the traditional focus on single-word production in the assessment and treatment of speech disorders needs to be modified to allow for a more extensive consideration of spontaneous speech production.

Many accounts of connected speech and children's connected speech development prefer to describe juncture phenomena in terms of processes such as assimilation, elision and liaison. We define and discuss these terms in the sections that follow.

Assimilation

Assimilation is the process by which a segment is influenced and modified by its neighbouring segments. Some phonetic research favours the term co-articulation, which can be broadly defined as the way in which speech segments overlap in time and in space to such an extent that it is often difficult to determine where one segment begins and another segment ends (Hardcastle and Hewlett, 1999). We use the term assimilation here, although see Hardcastle and Hewlett (1999) for further discussion of this issue and the variable use of the terms co-articulation and assimilation.

Assimilation may occur in many different directions. Some sounds are influenced by the segments which follow them as demonstrated in the different productions of /t/ in GREAT in Activity 7.1. Other sounds vary because of what precedes them, e.g. during the production of [s] in the word SUE, the lips are rounded, but are spread when saying SEE in anticipation of the following vowel; the lip-rounding of the vowel has infiltrated the temporal domain of the consonant. Another example is to consider /p/ in English which often has a less explosive (i.e. deaspirated) sound when it is preceded by /s/. Say the word SPOT, now say it again but without the /s/. Then compare the /p/ in what you just said with the quality of the sound in the word POT. The /p/ in POT has a lot of aspiration (puff of air) but the /p/ in SPOT does not and sounds more like a /b/. Assimilation is helpful for speakers, as it allows us to produce components of more than one speech sound at a time, thereby speeding up the speech process and making it less effortful for our articulators. However, we cannot be too casual as speakers, or our listeners would not understand, and therefore we need to balance our assimilation against the listeners' decoding skills giving them enough cues so that they can process what we are saying.

Assimilations are traditionally classified into three main types based on the changes that can affect the sounds:

1. **Voice assimilation**. Assimilation of English plural forms is a good example of this, e.g. The /s/ in the suffix is devoiced when it follows a voiceless consonant (e.g. BOOKS → /bʊks/), but becomes voiced when it follows a voiced consonant (e.g. BUGS → /bʌgz/).
2. **Place assimilation**. This refers to changes in the place of articulation of a segment (usually a consonant). **IMP**OSSIBLE and **INT**ANGIBLE are examples of how prefixes are adapted in light of the following consonants. This is an example of where assimilation in speech has become part of spelling conventions.
3. **Manner assimilation**. Here one sound changes the manner of its articulation to become similar in manner to a neighbouring sound. Examples of this process are harder to find in English, and assimilation of manner is found only in very fast speech. In general, speakers change sounds so that they obstruct the airflow less and therefore require less energy. An example of manner assimilation would be in a phrase like THAT SIDE where it is typical not to release the [t] sound, produced rapidly as [ðæs: aɪd].

Elision

Elision is the process by which sounds that would be pronounced in slow, careful speech seem to disappear in everyday speech. It is the way in which sounds are omitted in the rapid flowing of speech. An extreme example of elision in English would be the contracted use of 'gonna' for GOING TO, and slightly less extreme, LOTS OF THEM produced as [lɒts ə ɛm]. As for assimilation, languages differ in the extent and nature of elisions permitted, but all languages show some tendency towards this process. From the point of view of co-articulation studies, elision is not a separate process from assimilation, but rather an extreme result of co-articulation whereby two sounds are articulated so closely in time to each other that a sound or sounds between them are completely obscured.

Chapters 5 and 6 focused on consonant clusters and there it was emphasized that many children, both those with normally-developing speech and those with difficulties, will find the production of consonant sequences a challenge, e.g. in words like STRENGTH. Consonant clusters occur more frequently in connected speech as they arise both when morphemes are added to a root word, e.g. STRENGTHS, and when a word which ends with a cluster is followed by a word beginning with a cluster, e.g. PINK SKIRT → [pɪŋkskɜt] which contains four consonants in succession. Kelly and Local (1989) describe a girl aged 5;2 who experienced speech difficulties. In order to cope with complex consonant sequences in connected speech, she made use of other strategies, namely consonant lengthening (or gemination) and glottal closure, and in so doing retained the rhythmic structure of the target adult forms (see Stackhouse and Wells, 1997, pp. 227–8 for further details of this child's speech).

Liaison

This term refers to the phonological adjustments made when a word ends with a vowel and the next word begins with a vowel. In such cases, depending on the final vowel of the first word, a glide (i.e. [w, j]) can be heard between the two words, e.g. compare your own production of TWO EGGS, THREE EGGS, FOUR EGGS. Wells (1994) describes Zoë, aged 5;11 who typically produced staccato forms in her connected speech, e.g. GO OVER → [gəʊʔhəʊfə], rather than what might typically be expected in normally developing children or adults: [gəʊwəʊvə].

Prosodic Processes in Connected Speech

Prosody is the term applied to patterns of intonation and rhythm in human speech. It is considered in this chapter since phonological knowledge and in particular the ability to process and use prosody, is needed in order to 'weld together a prosodic arrangement of familiar word forms and a relation observed between the referents of those word forms' (Chiat, 2001, p. 122).

Prosody can be categorized as either lexical (word stress) or supralexical, moving beyond single words. The focus of this chapter is on connected speech and therefore we do not consider word stress in any detail here but rather give a brief overview of supralexical prosody. First, focus on the role of intonation, which serves to group words into cohesive utterances, and this is an ability that emerges with the onset of two-word utterances (Corrin, Tarplee and Wells, 2001) and continues to be refined up to and beyond the age of 8 years (Dankovicová, Pigott, Wells and Peppé, 2004).

In Chapter 2 (Figure 2.4) we introduced the developmental phase model from Stackhouse and Wells. The assembly phase was described as the phase of speech development that involves bringing it all together so that difficulties at this level might result in stammering, prosodic difficulties or speech that is perceived as 'mumbley.' Stackhouse and Wells note:

> As the child's utterances become longer and more complex, there is a requirement to get to grips with the intonational systems of the language, since these have an important function in, for example, signalling the ends of a speaker's turn in conversation, and in highlighting the key word or words of an utterance. Thus, in English speakers routinely draw attention to important or new information by emphasizing it, and the means of emphasis is pitch prominence, with extra loudness and lengthening. This is often referred to as the system of tonic or nuclear prominence, and the child has to learn how to use it.
>
> (Stackhouse and Wells, 1997, p. 222)

The development of children's use of the intonational system has not been widely researched but there is some evidence to suggest that in normally-developing children it becomes established during the fourth year (Fletcher, 1985; Wells and Local, 1993). Stackhouse and Wells (1997, pp. 223–5) present connected speech data from David, a boy aged 5;4, who showed an atypical intonation system. The pervasive prosodic pattern in this boy's speech was to give the final syllable of each utterance greatest emphasis. This resulted in the disruption of normal stress patterns in words such as POSTMAN, e.g. [pəʊst'mæn] instead of more typical ['pəʊstmæn] when these occurred at the ends of David's utterances. Turning to rhythm or stress, the way in which stress is distributed over an utterance enables listeners to predict upcoming information and thus makes for efficient listening. David produced the phrase I ALREADY SAID THAT with the emphasis falling on the final word THAT. In the normal production of this phrase SAID would normally be emphasized. The use of an intonational system also helps us to predict when we can have our conversational turn. In David's case his consistent emphasis of the final syllable did give clear signals to his conversational partners about when he had completed his conversational turn.

ACTIVITY 7.2

Consider the data presented below from Simon CA 10;11.

Single-word data from naming task

Target	Simon's single-word production
STOP	[tɒp]
KICK	[kɪk]
MICHELLE	[mi'ʃæ]
SWIMMING	['wɪmi]
SPOON	[spun]

Connected speech data: Simon was asked to make a sentence using the target words.

Target word	Simon's sentence production
STOP	[dɒ də ka:] stop the car
KICK	[i ki mi] he kicked me
MICHELLE	[jɔ nəɪm ɪ mi'dæ] your name is Michelle
SWIMMING	[lɛ gəʊ 'wɪmə] let's go swimming
SPOON	[dæ maɪ bun] that's my spoon

Now answer the following questions about Simon's speech.

(a) What are your general observations about Simon's single-word speech and his connected speech?
(b) Compare Simon's production of each target word in isolation with his production in the sentence.
(c) Based on what you know about normal connected speech processes, give an example of one instance when you might expect assimilation or elision to occur in connected speech. This knowledge is important because it would not be appropriate to penalize Simon for errors in scoring for accuracy given that assimilation is a normal process.
(d) What are some of the factors that may have affected Simon's performance on the second task?

Now turn to the Key to Activity 7.2 at the end of this chapter for our thoughts on Simon's speech.

Why and When? Motivating for the Use of Connected Speech Stimuli

It is widely acknowledged that children with developmental speech difficulties are harder to understand in connected speech than in single-word production. Grunwell (1987, p. 54) notes that 'it is quite common to find that a person may perform satisfactorily on an articulation test, where utterances are restricted to single words, but will continue to use disordered and inadequate patterns in his everyday speech'.

Studies of children with childhood apraxia of speech (CAS) have suggested that it is connected speech, rather than single words or repetition tasks when most difficulties arise. For example, Stackhouse and Snowling (1992) investigated the speech of two children diagnosed with CAS and found a greater proportion of segmental errors in connected speech as opposed to in single-word naming tasks. For normally-developing controls there was no significant difference between the tasks. There are many children referred for speech and language therapy who present with age-appropriate speech at a segmental or single-word level. However, connected speech proves specifically challenging for these children, and intelligibility of spontaneous speech is markedly lower than their single-word production (e.g. see Stackhouse and Wells, 1991, 1997; Stackhouse and Snowling, 1992; Wells, 1994; Camarata, 1998; Newton, 1999). Practitioners are often at a loss as to how such difficulties can be explained or should be addressed, because our theoretical knowledge of the relationship between connected and single-word speech is limited.

Camarata (1998) emphasizes the importance of connected speech within an intervention context, in his argument about a speech–language overlap. He suggests that single-word speech assessments are likely to represent children's highest level of speech competence, and that children's speech should routinely be investigated in syntactic contexts and 'running speech'. From a clinical perspective, this is by no means a new suggestion. However, what is new is the suggestion made by Camarata and others (e.g. Stackhouse and Wells, 2001; Howard, 2004), and re-emphasised here, that intervention planning should explicitly consider connected speech. Camarata (1998) questions whether 'the conventional wisdom regarding treating speech disorders is in fact true', i.e. the 'traditional' hierarchies for speech intervention which move from single sounds to single words and finally to connected speech may be inappropriate for intervention planning. A search of the literature reveals few intervention papers which focus on improving children's speech at a connected speech level. Intervention papers emphasizing connected speech are typically concerned with client groups such as children with dysfluent speech (Ingham, Kilgo, Ingham *et al.*, 2001), hearing impairment (Allen, Nikolopoulos, Dyar and O'Donoghue, 2001) and Down syndrome (Stoel-Gammon, 2001) rather than children with persisting speech problems alone. Ingham *et al.* (2001) evaluated the use of a fluency-inducing strategy with young adults. The training programme described, like many other dysfluency interventions for both children and adults, focused on the level of connected speech since this clearly has the greatest relevance for the client. Allen *et al.* (2001) investigated the intelligibility of children who have had cochlear implants. Intelligibility is the focus of Chapter 11, but the functional concerns associated with investigations of speech intelligibility are relevant to investigations and interventions addressing connected speech. Stoel-Gammon's (2001) work with children with Down syndrome also addresses these concerns rather than focusing specifically at a segmental level. A paper by Fazio (1997) focused on intervention with low-income children with and without specific language impairment. The children were required to learn a poem, and evaluated in terms of their ability to remember and produce the poem. Although the main theoretical concerns of the paper are with phonological awareness and memory, the paper does also provide interesting insights into the challenges of connected speech production especially for children with speech and language difficulties.

Turning to assessment now, it is also not surprising that current assessment procedures are concerned primarily with single words, focusing on the child's ability to produce individual segments and contrasts. The majority of phonology assessments commonly used by practitioners comprise single-word naming tasks. Objectives for phonological therapy focusing on single words are typically identified on the basis of phonological analysis of the contrasts present in or absent from the child's system, and analysis of the child's phonotactic structures (Grunwell and Yavas, 1988; Howell and Dean, 1994). For some children this is likely to be sufficient, but for others they may make gains in their single-word production which do not generalize to their connected speech. Indeed working with school-age children whose speech difficulties are persisting may already ring warning bells about limited generalization and slow progress.

There are, however, some assessments which do provide information about connected speech. *The Diagnostic Evaluation of Articulation and Phonology* (DEAP) (Dodd *et al.*, 2002) includes some evaluation of connected speech with comparisons made between single-word production and production in connected speech. Stackhouse *et al.* (forthcoming) include assessments of connected speech in their compendium of psycholinguistic tests for children. These include the following.

- Connected Speech Process (CSP) Repetition Test (Newton, 1999). The test aims to assess a child's use of the connected speech processes of assimilation, elision and liaison. A set of sentences is presented to the child, either read live by the tester or using a pre-recorded tape. The child's repetition of each sentence is recorded for later analysis.
- Final Consonant Juncture Repetition Test (from Pascoe, Stackhouse and Wells, 2005). The test aims to assess the child's use of final (coda) consonants in a connected speech environment; and to compare that to the child's use of final consonants in words produced in isolation. The child is required to repeat a list of short, phonologically controlled phrases such as THE X IN THE PICTURE, where X represents the different target words; and to repeat the same list of words in isolation.

Intervention studies have also provided evidence of young children's ability to generalize from single words treated in therapy to connected speech. Elbert, Dinnsen, Swartzlander and Chin (1990) investigated changes in the speech of 10 children (aged between 3 and 4 years) with phonological difficulties following intervention. Changes in both single words and conversational speech were analysed, both before and after intervention, and three months later. Conversational analysis results suggested that for most of the children, there were system changes both in single words and in conversational speech. The authors concluded that many children with phonological disorders are able to extend their correct production to conversation without direct treatment on spontaneous speech. This is a point discussed in greater detail in Chapter 9 on generalization. For now, the important point to note is that not all children – especially older ones whose problems have persisted – will generalize spontaneously into connected speech following intervention with single-word stimuli. The children in the study by Elbert *et al.* were young children, probably very different to children with PSDs. Children with PSDs may need to have their connected speech specifically and skilfully addressed in order for them to make gains in intelligibility at a functional level. Some children may only become ready for connected speech work following single-word work. For some, connected speech work may never be needed, and for others targeting connected speech straight away may be the most efficient course of action. Until we have more intervention research focusing on the relationship between single words and connected speech, the evidence base will not be able to offer clear answers to these questions. However, adopting a psycholinguistic approach and using it in conjunction with a phonological approach may suggest the most effective course of therapy for a given child. In the following section we turn our attention to understanding connected speech within the psycholinguistic framework, and describe an assessment battery, the *PEPS-C* (Wells and Peppé, 2001, 2003) used for evaluating children's prosodic abilities within a psycholinguistic framework. Before moving on to this section of the chapter, carry out the reflective learning task in Activity 7.3.

ACTIVITY 7.3

In the first book of this series, Stackhouse and Wells (1997) encouraged readers to consider 'What do tests really test?' This is always a helpful question to ask about assessments. Consider what assessments – standardized, published or your own – you routinely use that would provide helpful information about connected speech. Make a list of the assessments and the type of information they provide. How could this information be used in intervention planning?

Connected Speech and the Psycholinguistic Framework

Most psycholinguistic models do not account for all the aspects involved in speech and language processing, and choose to focus on specific parts of the process. Stackhouse and Wells's (1997) model focuses mainly on speech processing, with the authors noting:

> Although [the model] attempts to handle the processing of connected speech and the influence of phonetic context, it does not deal in any detail with sentence processing and grammatical development. Within this limitation, it attempts to be reasonably comprehensive.
>
> (Stackhouse and Wells, 1997, p. 146)

One way of conceptualizing connected speech in the psycholinguistic model is by considering that at each level of the model, single word or connected speech tasks can take place. For example, consider Levels B and D of the speech processing profile (Figure 2.1 in Chapter 2) which ask: Can the child discriminate between non-words/real words? Auditory discrimination tasks could be carried out at a single-word level, e.g. can the child discriminate between single words CAT/CAP. Alternatively, the processing demands of the task could be increased to involve processing of connected speech. For example, the child might be asked whether the following sentences are the same or different: I LIKE YOUR CAT/I LIKE YOUR CAP. In an alternative version of the task they might be shown pictures representing the sentences, and asked to point to the picture they think best represents what they have heard (see Cassidy, 1994, and Stackhouse *et al.*, forthcoming, for further details of tasks such as this). Repetition tasks on the output side of the profile can also be carried out at a single-word level (e.g. asking the child to repeat UMBRELLA), or with the child repeating sentences (e.g. asking the child to repeat HIS UMBRELLA IS YELLOW, see Vance, Stackhouse and Wells, 1995, and Stackhouse *et al.*, forthcoming, for further details of sentence repetition tasks). The speech processing routes and the levels of the speech processing model that are tapped are the same for the single word or connected speech task, but connected speech tasks add a level of complexity or an extra load at each level.

Stackhouse and Wells's psycholinguistic framework emphasizes speech processing rather than expressive language. The lexical representation (see Stackhouse and Wells, 1997, Chapter 6) includes a grammatical component which specifies knowledge of, for example, how a word is used in sentences or changed into a plural form. The model does not, however, attempt to account for where grammatical encoding takes place if one is moving beyond a single-word utterance. Stackhouse and Wells suggest that it is at the level of motor planning (see Figure 2.3 in Chapter 2) that connected speech is explicitly brought into play. Here motor programs for individual words are assembled into one overall plan for speech production with individual segments influencing their neighbouring sounds. However, they note that input processing and phonological representations may also be involved in connected speech. Loucas and Marslen-Wilson (2000) have shown age-related changes in children's connected speech processing so that different levels may have different roles in connected speech processing at different times during development.

Chiat (2000, 2001) explicitly incorporates grammar into her model of children's speech and language processing. Verbs and their associated argument structure lie at the heart of her model of grammatical processing while integrating with other aspects of speech and language processing, making it a fairly comprehensive developmental model in terms of the speech/language interface. Research has been carried out to investigate the relationship between phonology and syntax. It is known that syntactic complexity frequently results in reduced phonological accuracy (Panagos and Prelock, 1982; Paul and Shriberg, 1982). This is thought to occur because of limited processing resources so that increased syntactic processing demands result in decreased resources available for phonological processing.

Profiling Elements of Prosodic Systems - Children (PEPS-C) (Wells and Peppé, 2001) is a prosodic assessment battery devised within the psycholinguistic framework. The battery was designed to assess linguistic intonational abilities in school-age children with the ultimate aim of providing an assessment of prosodic abilities in children with speech and language difficulties. The battery examines four areas in which the role of intonation is well established.

- Chunking: Prosodic delimitation of an utterance into two or three meaning units.
- Affect: Strong liking versus reservation, expressed through contrasting pitch movements.
- Interaction: Confirming an understanding versus checking an understanding, also expressed through contrasting pitch movements.
- Focus: Indicating which item is most important in an utterance, expressed through accent placement.

The child's ability to express and understand each of the above, using prosodic resources, is examined. The ability to perceive and produce prosodic contrasts without reference to meaning is also examined. This permits comparison of input with output skills. Group studies of normally-developing children and those with speech/language difficulties have been carried out using this battery (e.g. Wells and Peppé, 2003; Wells, Peppé and Goulandris, 2004). A computerized version of the test has been developed by Peppé and McCann (2003) with further information available from http://sls.qmuc.ac.uk/RESEARCH/Autism/PEPS-C.htm.

There is a great need for further research addressing the development of connected speech and its processes. Research findings to date already have important implications for intervention with children with PSDs. The following section draws together some suggestions for best practice when assessing and addressing connected speech. Some of the ideas have been evaluated systematically through research, and where this is the case, a reference is supplied. Other suggestions have yet to be tested, but are presented here for further development in practice and research.

Connected Speech: Suggestions for Assessment and Intervention

Assessment

- Attempt to include connected speech assessment in addition to assessment at the single-word level (e.g. see Howard, 2004).
- Some published tests of connected speech include the *PEPS-C, DEAP* and procedures included in a *Compendium of Psycholinguistic Assessments for Children* (Stackhouse and Wells, forthcoming).
- Any favourite tests can be adapted to assess connected speech, and tests listed in Appendix 2 include, or can be modified to include, connected speech.
- When carrying out connected speech assessment attempt to take into account any language processing demands since we know that increased language demands may mean reduced capacities available for phonology (Panagos and Prelock, 1982).
- Make comparisons between stimuli words produced as single words, and in sentences (as for Activity 7.2, although it can be better to give the child sentences to repeat rather than having them create their own).
- Consider processes of normal connected speech at a segmental and a prosodic level.
- When analysing assessment results take into account the normal processes of connected speech, e.g. elision or assimilation across word boundaries.
- Consider how children may be compensating for segmental difficulties in their use of connected speech processes (e.g. Kelly and Local, 1989) and what the functional outcomes of difficulties with connected speech production may be.

Intervention

- When designing and selecting stimuli for intervention, consider that you may wish to include stimuli at the connected speech level.
- Children with PSDs may benefit most from intervention that is targeted at their connected speech since this is likely to have most functional relevance to them (cf. stammering intervention literature, e.g. Ingham *et al.*, 2001).
- Many children with PSDs will not be able to automatically generalize single-word skills to a connected speech level and will require

specific intervention for this (Pascoe, Stackhouse and Wells, 2005 and see case study presented in Chapter 8).

- Individual differences should always be taken into account since children will vary in their responses to intervention, and there may be issues of readiness regarding when it is appropriate to work on connected speech.
- Working on single words initially, and building up to phrases is not following a normal developmental pattern (Wells, 1994; Newton and Wells, 2002) and thus may not always be the best approach to adopt in intervention.
- When carrying out connected speech activities in intervention, take into account the language processing demands of tasks, e.g. getting children to make up their own sentences promotes sentence building and connected speech skills, but may need to be used in later stages of intervention when they can spare the extra processing resources needed for the language processing demands.
- Take into account the normal processes of connected speech, e.g. assimilation and elision. It would not be appropriate to work on final /t/ in a phrase such as THAT SIDE since in normal speech the /t/ is often elided.

In the following chapter we describe the intervention that took place with Katy, a girl aged 6;5 (from Pascoe, Stackhouse and Wells, 2005) illustrating in some detail the way in which connected speech stimuli were designed and used in intervention with a child with PSDs.

Summary

The key points are as follows.

- Connected speech stimuli are an important part of intervention for school-age children with persisting speech problems.
- Difficulties in connected speech can prove intractable for some children, but need to be addressed in order for intervention to have functional benefits for these children.
- Connected speech is more than a string of individual segments joined together. Each segment has influences over surrounding segments.
- Connected speech processes can be divided into segmental and prosodic processes.
- At a segmental level, we use the term junction to refer broadly to the way in which words are joined with each other across syllable boundaries.
- Open juncture occurs in formal, emphatic speech where all individual segments are precisely realized.

- Close juncture is also referred to as assimilation and refers to the way in which sounds are influenced by the neighbouring sounds.
- Close juncture develops before open juncture, which provides evidence of children's early holistic speech processing and has implications for intervention.
- Elision is the complete omission of sounds in the rapid flow of speech.
- Liaison refers to the phonological adjustments made when a glide is inserted between adjacent vowels across a word boundary.
- At a prosodic level, intonation and rhythm of speech are considered to emerge along with two-word utterances and to be refined beyond the age of 8 years.
- Connected speech can be contextualized in the psycholinguistic framework where it can mean a greater processing load at each level of the speech processing profile than for single words.
- Further research is needed into the development of connected speech processes and the use of connected speech stimuli in intervention for children with PSDs.

KEY TO ACTIVITY 7.1

(a) GREAT ELEPHANT
The final consonant of GREAT is an audibly released alveolar plosive.

(b) GREAT TIGER
The final consonant is realized as a closure of the larynx and a silent period of contact between the tongue tip (or blade) and the teeth ridge, preceding the [t] of the following word.

(c) GREAT CAT
The period of silent contact is between the back of the tongue and the soft-palate, anticipating the [k] of CAT.

(d) GREAT BEAR
The contact does not involve the tongue at all: instead there is a closure of the lips, anticipating the [b] of BEAR.

KEY TO ACTIVITY 7.2

(a) What are your general observations about Simon's single word speech and his connected speech?

His single-word productions are more accurate than his productions of the same words in connected speech.

(b) Compare Simon's production of each target word in isolation with his production in the sentence.

STOP: [tɒp]; [dɒ də kɑː]

- Simon is unable to produce the /st/ cluster in STOP at the single word level. In his sentence, production of STOP moves further away from the adult target with prevocalic voicing [t] → [d], and final consonant deletion.

KICK: [kɪk]; [i ki mi]

- Simon is able to produce the target word accurately in the single word naming task. In his sentence he omits the final [k] as well as any morphological markers, e.g. kicks, kicked.

MICHELLE: [miˈʃæ]; [jɔ nəɪm ɪ miˈdæ]

- Simon deleted the final [l] in both attempts. He produces an accurate [ʃ] at the single word level. This was a sound that had recently been worked on in intervention, and he was careful about remembering to use it! In connected speech however he reverts to his immature substitution of [ʃ] → [d].

SWIMMING: [ˈwɪmi]; [lɛ gəʊ ˈwɪmə]

- Simon's productions are similar for this target with little difference noted between single word and connected speech context.

SPOON: [spun]; [dæ maɪ bun]

- Simon produces an accurate realization of SPOON in the single word task. In connected speech he reverts to his immature production [bun] evidencing cluster reduction and prevocalic voicing.

(c) Based on what you know about normal connected speech processes, give an example of one instance when you might expect elision or assimilation to occur in connected speech.

When Simon produces [dɒ] for stop he moves further away from the adult target with prevocalic voicing [t] → [d]. He also shows final consonant deletion as the [p] is not realised. However, if you say STOP THE CAR very fast (and very loudly with an American accent, as Simon did!) then you may not in fact realise the [p].

(d) What are some of the factors that may have affected Simon's performance on the second task?

Creating sentences to incorporate given words is a task with high language demands. Simon is likely to have been focusing his cognitive resources on formulating the sentences, so that he did not remember many of the sounds that he had worked on in therapy and had in fact mastered at a single-word level.

Chapter 8 Working on Connected Speech

In this chapter we describe the intervention that took place with Katy, a girl aged 6;5 with severe and persisting speech difficulties (Pascoe, Stackhouse and Wells, 2005). Katy's speech difficulties meant that despite several years of intervention her intelligibility to unfamiliar listeners was low. Psycholinguistic and phonological assessments suggested particular levels of speech processing, and phonological forms that were problematic for Katy. These were then used as the basis of our intervention which focused both on single words and connected speech in a structured way. The selection of the single word stimuli was based on principles outlined in Chapters 3 and 4 on using segments in single words. The selection of the connected speech stimuli was based on ideas introduced in Chapter 7, e.g. connected speech is more than just a string of individual segments joined together in an independent way; each segment has a strong influence on the segments that surround it. Through this case study we aim to show one way in which connected speech stimuli have been used in intervention for a child with PSDs.

Case Study: Katy Aged 6;5

Katy was a child with severe and persisting speech difficulties. She had been diagnosed with ataxic cerebral palsy and had associated delays in all aspects of her motor development including speech. There were no other significant medical or social factors to report. Katy lives with both her parents and an older brother.

Academically Katy was coping in a mainstream classroom but required additional one-to-one support from assistants. Her speech and language difficulties were numerous and severe, affecting all aspects of her academic work. These included unintelligible speech, receptive language delay and literacy difficulties. Katy had received speech and language therapy from the age of 2;3. She required ongoing classroom support, and speech and language therapy. When we first met Katy, her speech remained the primary area of concern as at age 6;5 it was still very hard for unfamiliar listeners to understand her. Katy's case has been published elsewhere in greater detail (see Pascoe, Stackhouse and Wells, 2005), but here it is discussed with particular attention to stimuli design and the way in which single words and connected speech intervention was implemented.

Macro Assessment

The speech processing profile from Stackhouse and Wells (1997) was used to collate the data from this part of the assessment. At each level of the profile, with the exception of level C,[1] at least one assessment was carried out. In some cases these were standardized measures, and in other cases consisted of unpublished and non-standardized materials. The ticks and crosses used on the profile indicate Katy's performance in relation to other children of her chronological age: with one tick indicating age-appropriate skills, and crosses showing the number of standard deviations below the mean for her age-matched peers. The completed profile is presented in Figure 8.1 with a discussion of these results following.

ACTIVITY 8.1

Study Katy's speech processing profile presented in Figure 8.1 and answer the following questions.

(a) Does Katy have difficulties with input or output?
(b) Outline two areas of relative strength.
(c) Outline Katy's main areas of difficulty.
(d) What further information would you find valuable?

Check your answers with the Key to Activity 8.1 at the end of this chapter, then read on for further information on Katy's speech processing profile in the sections that follow.

Overview of Speech Processing Profile

Katy had weaknesses throughout her speech processing profile, on both the input and output sides. The entire output side, from Levels G to K, was affected. The input side showed some more specific difficulties with discrimination of both real words (Level D) and non-words (Level B).

√ = age appropriate performance
X = 1 standard deviation below the expected mean for her age
XX = 2 standard deviations below the expected mean for her age

INPUT

F Is the child aware of the internal structure of phonological representations?

√ – Picture onset detection (PhAB picture alliteration subtest, Frederikson *et al.*, 1997).

E Are the child's phonological representations accurate?

√ – Auditory detection of speech errors (Constable, 1993).

D Can the child discriminate between real words?

X – Minimal pair auditory discrimination of clusters (Bridgeman and Snowling, 1988)
X – Aston Index discrimination subtest (Newton and Thompson, 1982)

C Does the child have language specific representations of word structures?

Not tested

B Can the child discriminate speech sounds without reference to lexical representations?

XX – Minimal pair auditory discrimination of clusters in non-words (Bridgeman and Snowling, 1988)

A Does the child have adequate auditory perception?

√ – audiometry

OUTPUT

G Can the child access accurate motor programmes?

X – Word-finding vocabulary test (Renfrew, 1995)
X – Edinburgh Articulation Test (Anthony *et al.*, 1971)
X – The Bus Story (Renfrew, 1969)

H Can the child manipulate phonological units?

X – PhAB Spoonerism subtest (Frederikson *et al.*, 1997)
X – PAT rhyme fluency subtest (Muter *et al.*, 1997)

I Can the child articulate real words accurately?

X – Aston Index blending subtest – real Words (Newton and Thompson, 1982)

J Can the child articulate speech without reference to lexical representations?

XX – Aston Index blending subtest – non-words (Newton and Thompson, 1982)

K Does the child have adequate sound production skills?

? Some difficulties. Nuffield motor assessment; oral examination and DDK

L Does the child reject her own erroneous forms?

Informal observation – no.

Figure 8.1: Katy's speech processing profile at age 6;5 (based on Pascoe *et al.*, 2005).

Non-word discrimination was relatively harder for Katy than real word discrimination.

Strengths

Katy had built up relatively good stores of phonological and semantic knowledge. Her knowledge in these areas was not age-appropriate or in keeping with her peers, but in terms of her own profile they were relative strengths. Building up such representations may have taken her longer than for normally-developing children, because of difficulties in speech production and obtaining kinaesthetic feedback. Katy had some age-appropriate phonological awareness skills (e.g. rhyme and alliteration identification from pictures, Level F). Her strengths lay on the input side of the profile with phonological and semantic knowledge that had been built up over time.

Weaknesses

On the input side of the profile, Katy had difficulties with auditory discrimination tasks – with both real and non-words – and made errors when discriminating between closely related consonant sequences, e.g. [ts] and [st] in VO*ST* ~ VO*TS*, and individual segments, e.g. [s] and [t] in VOS ~ VOT. In terms of output she had widespread weaknesses in her accessing of motor programs, as well as her repetition of real and non-words, and her manipulation of phonological units. Non-words were, again, particularly challenging for Katy who found these harder to process and produce than real words. Her difficulties with phonological manipulation on the output side were not surprising given that Katy had had little opportunity to experiment with sound production in the way that typically developing children do. Katy's output constraints may well have resulted in limited feedback to the rest of the system, and created widespread problems throughout the rest of the system.

Micro Assessment

Phonological Assessment of Child Speech (PACS) (Grunwell, 1985) was used to provide information on Katy's speech production. Severity indices have been introduced in previous chapters. These are useful measures which can encapsulate the degree of difficulty children experience with their speech in a single number. Most typically used are indices such as percentage of consonants correct (PCC), or percentage of vowels correct (PVC). Katy's PCC score falls in the severe range. A summary of the findings is presented in Table 8.1.

Table 8.1: Summary of Katy's speech data at CA 6;5

Assessment	Comments	
Severity indices	Percentage of consonants correct (PCC): 22% Percentage of vowels correct (PVC): 74,1% Percentage of phonemes correct (PPC): 41,9%	
Phonetic inventory	Word-initial position: [m, n, p, b, d, t, k, g, f, w, j, r, ʤ] Word-medial position: [m, b, d, t, k, g, w] Word-final position: none	
Stimulability	All segments except [v, ð, ʃ, ʒ, ʧ]	
Phonological processes analysis (% use)	Developmental processes: cluster reduction (100%); final consonant deletion (96%); prevocalic voicing (40%); stopping of fricatives and affricates (21%); gliding (21%) Non-developmental processes: vowel distortion (25%)	
Single word speech sample	BAG → [bæ]	APPLE → [ˈæbə]
	WEB → [wɛ]	GARAGE → [gæˈwɪ]
	FISH → [vɪ]	VEGETABLES → [vɛˈbɛ]
	CHRISTMAS → [gɪˈmɛ]	SINK → [dɪ]
	PRAM → [bæ]	LIGHT → [jɑɪ]
	EGG → [ɛ]	QUEEN → [ki]
	BEES → [bɪ]	CLASS → [gæ]
Connected speech sample	THE LITTLE GIRL IS MICHELLE → [jɪ ˈlɪtə gɜ ɪ mɪ ˈdæ]	
	THE THREE LITTLE PIGS → [də fi lɪʔə bɪ]	
	I'M (THE) BIG BAD WOLF → [ɑɪ bɪ bæ wʊ]	
	THE CHILDREN ARE NAUGHTY → [jəˈtʊdɛ ɑˈnɔdɪ]	
	FINGER PUPPET → [ˈfɪŋgə ˈpʊpɛ]	

Based on Pascoe, Stackhouse and Wells, 2005.

ACTIVITY 8.2

Consider Katy's speech data presented in Table 8.1. Now answer the following questions about the data.

(a) Which segments or processes would you wish to address in therapy?
(b) Why did you choose these particular targets?
(c) How would you attempt to combine the phonological information with the psycholinguistic information presented previously, in Figure 8.1?

Now turn to the Key to Activity 8.2 at the end of this chapter to see how we answered these questions. Then read the following sections.

Katy's speech was delayed for her age with some deviant substitutions also noted, e.g she distorted vowels in words such as CHILDREN producing instead [ˈtædə] or [ˈtʊdə]. Her syllable structure was typically open: she did not use final consonants. Her speech was laboured and staccato. Katy's speech production at a connected level had a similar degree of accuracy to her single word speech. Many of the words in her connected speech were produced as single words with primary stress and many pauses between items that would normally be elided or assimilated in the connected speech of normally-developing children (Newton and Wells, 2002). Her speech sounds were not glued together in a normal way.

In terms of speech sound realizations, Katy was able to realize several segments in the word initial position. She was able to indicate contrasts between plosives /p, b, t, d, k, g/, nasal /m/ and approximants /w, j/. Within words she was able to mark some of these contrasts although with less regularity ([b, d, g, m]) in targets such as BA<u>B</u>Y, CHIL<u>D</u>REN, ME<u>G</u>AN AND CHRIST<u>M</u>AS. In word-final position, Katy realized few consonants. The PACS analysis sheet for this section showed that for the vast majority of instances no consonants were produced, e.g. BAG → [bæ]; WEB → [wɛ]; FISH → [vɪ]. The PACS requires detailed analysis of a single word and connected speech sample. In order to calculate the prevalence of particular simplifying processes a count is made of all potential instances in the speech sample when a process might have been used. A second count is then made of the actual instances in which the process was used, and the two figures used to calculate a percentage to indicate how frequently the process was used. Katy's scores from the PACS suggest that 70 of 75 realizations involved final consonant deletion. This is based on her single word data, although comparisons with her connected speech data suggested that there was no significant difference between the scores obtained for the two. Katy was also not able to produce any of the consonant clusters in an adult-like way. In word-initial position, she attempted these but reduced them in the manner of a much younger child, e.g. PRAM → [bæ]. In all other word positions neither element of a cluster was realized. At a phonotactic level, it was noted that Katy typically had open syllable structure favouring V and CV syllable structure for monosyllables, e.g. EGG → [ɛ], WEB → [wɛ], and VCV and CVCV structure for disyllables, e.g. APPLE → [æbə]; GARAGE → [gæˈwɪ].

A phonological process analysis revealed a range of processes which included the following.

- Final consonant deletion: consistently carried out on all consonants (95.3%) in this position (e.g. BEES → [bɪ]).
- Cluster reduction: consistently carried out in all word-initial clusters (100%), (e.g. PRAM → [bæ]).
- Weak syllable deletion: carried out in 15% of possible instances, (e.g. VEGETABLES → [vɛˈbɛ]).

- Stopping: carried out in 21% of possible instances, (e.g. SINK → [dɪ]).
- Gliding: carried out in 21% of possible instances (e.g. LIGHT → [jɑɪ]).
- Voicing: carried out in 45% of possible instances word-initially, e.g. FISH [vɪ], and 37.5% within words, e.g. APPLE → ['æbə].

All these processes acted together to reduce Katy's speech intelligibility.

Intervention Planning

Intervention planning focused on three main areas; each one giving direction to the work carried out. These included the following.

- Psycholinguistic perspective: We aimed to answer the question: 'What aspects of Katy's speech processing system should be worked on?'
- Phonological perspective: We aimed to answer the question: 'Which aspects of the sound system should be targeted?'
- Psychosocial perspective: As for the other children described we aimed to consider Katy and her own likes and dislikes, learning styles and previous therapy experiences.

We decided to focus on Katy's output, updating her motor programs and giving her practice in motor planning by putting the new programs into context. We decided to address the most dominant process in Katy's speech: her final consonant deletion. It was hypothesized that Katy had an incomplete phonotactic frame or template for words in her online motor programmer, and a set of stored motor programs that also reflected the incorrect, immature, simplified frame, typically with open syllable structure such as CVCV or CV. The intervention aimed to use Katy's stronger phonological and semantic representations as well as her orthographic knowledge to highlight the difference between her simplified productions and the correct adult targets. Intervention involved activities that gave Katy explicit opportunities to use her strengths. These activities included:

- reading - using her orthographic decoding skills;
- meaningful minimal pair work (following Weiner, 1981) - drawing on her semantic knowledge;
- tasks involving picture naming which give Katy the opportunity to access her own (accurate) phonological representation and relate it to the (inaccurate) stored motor program, giving her the opportunity to revise the latter.

Katy's speech processing profile also revealed difficulties with motor planning. Motor planning is considered to involve phonetic aspects of speech production, moving beyond the abstract linguistic knowledge of motor programming/motor programs. It is at the motor planning stage that connected speech processes such as assimilation come into play. While motor programming is perceived as being a single word phase, motor planning involves the connection of words into strings of speech. Once motor programs have been revised, motor planning may need to be more specifically addressed so that Katy is able to use the new words with their coda segments in connected speech. Katy's intervention aimed to alter her habitual open syllable structure, and get her producing any segment in the syllable-final, word-final (SFWF) position. Katy's intervention programme concentrated on a range of consonants typically occurring in SFWF position and aimed to increase her awareness of the fact that consonants are needed here to make important meaning contrasts.

Katy received a total of 30 hours of intervention. This was subdivided into three phases, as follows with each phase involving a different treatment:

- Phase I: therapy on a specific set of single words;
- Phase II: therapy on a wider range of single words;
- Phase III: therapy on connected speech.

Phase I aimed to increase Katy's awareness of final consonants and encourage her to produce CVC stimuli items from a small set of targeted words. Phase II aimed to encourage generalization of CVC production to a broader range of single words. Intervention in this phase was guided by broad themes (e.g. animals, numbers, household objects). Sessions gave Katy the opportunity to produce CVC words in a wider and more natural range of contexts. Written forms of the words were used to remind Katy about her final consonant production in some instances, together with silent posting tasks and meaningful minimal pair activities (following Weiner, 1981). Phase III aimed to facilitate production of CVC targeted words from Phase I, putting these in sentences graded in terms of phonetic difficulty. Intervention in this phase involved literacy skills as Katy was required to read the stimuli sentences written below illustrations of the items, and match sentences with appropriate pictures. Katy was assessed at five points over the course of the intervention:

- T1: Pre-intervention baseline assessment
- T2: Assessment after Intervention Phase I
- T3: Assessment after Intervention Phase II
- T4: Assessment after Intervention Phase III
- T5: Follow-up assessment carried out 7 months after intervention had stopped.

The design of Katy's intervention is shown in Figure 8.2.

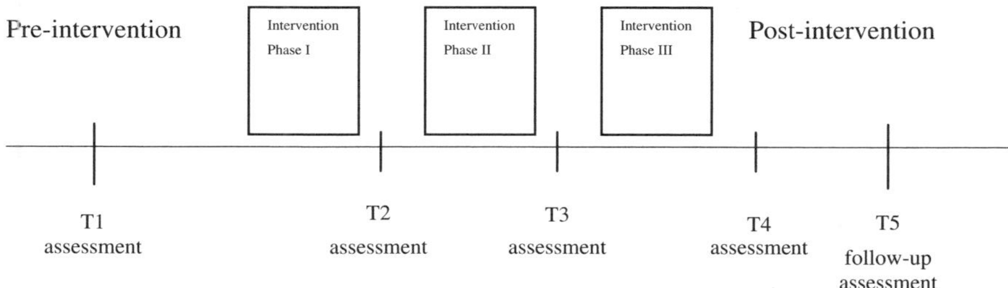

Figure 8.2: Katy's intervention design.

Stimuli Selection: Single Words

Now let us consider how we set about designing and selecting the single word stimuli for Katy. These single words were used in Phase I of the intervention programme where we aimed to update Katy's stored motor programs to include the CVC word shape. We aimed to compile two matched wordlists: List A that would consist of words to be addressed in intervention, and List B that would consist of matched control words that would not be included in intervention. We used the following criteria to help us create the two lists:

1. Each list consisted of 16 monosyllabic words.
2. CVC words were favoured, although in some instances CCVC words had to be used since all requirements for matched items could not be met. Where CCVC words were selected they were matched across the lists.
3. Items were matched by rime across the lists, e.g. N*OTE*, G*OAT*. Where rime could not be matched, items were matched by coda segment, e.g. LEA*F*, HOO*F*.
4. Irregular orthographic forms were balanced across the lists.
5. Items were chosen to highlight the functional importance of final consonants and, thus were words that, with the final consonant removed, made another real-word minimal pair (e.g. NOTE/NO). The vowel nucleus was therefore either a long vowel or a diphthong.
6. Items were matched across the lists for children's average age of acquisition and estimated spoken language frequency using the MRC psycholinguistic database (http://www.psy.uwa.edu.au/mrcdatabase).

ACTIVITY 8.3

Using the list of criteria 1–5 above, create two matched lists of single words which might have been suitable for Katy. List A should consist of words to be addressed in intervention, and List B should consist of matched control words that would not be included in intervention. Each list should contain six words.

Remember, the idea behind the careful creation of these lists, is that the two lists are as similar in as many ways as possible so that any differences in Katy's post-intervention performance on the two wordlists can be attributed to the different treatments (i.e. intervention and no intervention) rather than because of some inherent property of the lists (i.e. one list was actually easier than the other).

Now turn to the Key to Activity 8.3 at the end of this chapter, then read the following.

Two lists of stimuli were devised, and are presented in Table 8.2. List A consists of the words that were worked on in intervention. List B consists of the control words that were never worked on.

Table 8.2: Katy's matched stimuli lists

Item no.	List A treated words worked on in intervention	List B untreated control words
1	NOTE	GOAT
2	PLANE	TRAIN
3	HEART	PART
4	NAIL	HAIL
5	CAGE	PAGE
6	SLIDE	LIED
7	WHEEL	KNEEL
8	RAKE	STEAK
9	STORK	WALK
10	LEAF	HOOF
11	SAUCE	PURSE
12	ICE	DICE
13	ROPE	GRAPE
14	PIPE	SHEEP
15	BARN	LINE
16	ROAD	TOAD

Stimuli Selection: Connected Speech

Stimuli for the connected speech phase of treatment (Phase III) were also chosen according to phonological criteria. A graded hierarchy of sentences was devised around each of the target single words shown in Table 8.2 as follows:

- facilitatory sentence
- neutral sentence
- challenging sentence.

For example, in the case of treatment item number 13 (see Table 8.2), the target word ROPE, the facilitatory sentence used as a starting point was:

THIS **ROPE** PULLED THE CAR

where the onset consonant of the following word PULLED is the same as the coda consonant of the target word ROPE. Given Katy's phonological abilities at the beginning of the study, it was thought that she would be able to produce the initial [p] in PULLED even if she omitted the final [p] in ROPE. In order to achieve an acceptable realization of this final consonant, she would merely have to lengthen the closure phase for the (single) consonant articulation.

At the next level of the neutral sentence, Katy would be required to produce a sentence where the target would be followed by a vowel (i.e. a more neutral context) such as ROPE in:

THERE'S **ROPE** ON THE ROAD

The third and most challenging condition would be where Katy was required to change her place of articulation (and voicing) between the final segment in the target, e.g. [p] in ROPE and the onset of the next word in the sentence, e.g. [g] in a sentence such as:

THIS **ROPE** GOT FRAYED

It should be noted however that hetero-organic adjacent consonants such as those selected for the most challenging sentences are not necessarily the articulatory challenge one might suppose, since assimilation occurs across word boundaries. Assimilation refers to the way in which neighbouring segments affect each other in connected speech (see Chapter 7). Thus, for example, in a sentence such as: THIS NOTE COST £2 it would be inappropriate to encourage Katy to produce the final [t] in NOTE since this segment would typically be absent in normal English speech. Nevertheless, we wanted to observe the assimilation occurring spontaneously in Katy's connected speech. The most challenging sentences of the hierarchy were therefore split into two subgroups:

- sentences where no assimilation was expected, and thus were challenging for Katy to produce as in THIS ROPE GOT FRAYED above; and
- sentences where assimilation was expected as in THIS NOTE *COST* £2 above.

These sentences were monitored in the pre- and post-intervention assessments, but not directly worked on.

ACTIVITY 8.4

Based on the ROPE example given above, create connected speech stimuli that would be appropriate to use in Katy's intervention programme. Select three words from List A in Table 8.2. Each word should then be incorporated into three short phrases or sentences in which

- sentence 1 is facilitatory, giving Katy maximal support in terms of word glue;
- sentence 2 is neutral where the target is followed by a vowel;
- sentence 3 is challenging involving adjacent consonants with different places of articulation. For each 'sentence 3' consider whether assimilation would be expected in typical speech and indicate this with an asterisk. You may wish to use the following table to order your sentences.

Word	Sentences
e.g. ROPE	1. THIS ROPE PULLED THE CAR 2. THERE'S ROPE ON THE ROAD 3. THIS ROPE GOT FRAYED
a.	1. 2. 3.
b.	1. 2. 3.
c.	1. 2. 3.

Now turn to Key to Activity 8.4 at the end of this chapter to see the complete list of connected speech stimuli we used with Katy. Then read the following.

Devising connected speech stimuli for Katy took time, however it is suggested that the time spent on this type of stimuli design is time well spent. Another challenge in creating such stimuli is that phonological demands sometimes mean creating semantically improbable sentences. Semantic oddity is something that children usually enjoy and so can be used to your advantage in creating funny pictures and scenarios.

Outcomes: Single Words

In the single word phases of intervention Katy was involved in meaningful minimal pair therapy games with the aim of updating her immature motor programs to include the CVC word shape. Single word assessment was carried out at five points in the intervention programme to evaluate her progress with both the treated words that were being addressed in intervention, and the matched control words. At these assessments she was required to name single words from pictures such as NOTE and GOAT, and other stimuli words listed in Table 8.2. The focus of the assessment was on Katy's final segment production: she was awarded two points for final consonants that were accurately realized, one point for using an inaccurate final consonant, and no points for omission of a final consonant. Raw scores were converted to percentages. The following activity provides the opportunity to develop scoring skills.

ACTIVITY 8.5

The table below shows Katy's production of single words before intervention at T1, and after completion of intervention at long-term follow-up at T5. The words shown in the table are stimuli words from List A, the treated words that were worked on in intervention. Your task is to consider each of Katy's productions and give a score of 0, 1 or 2 as outlined above. Remember the focus of the assessment was on Katy's final segment production:

- 2 points for final consonants that were accurately realized;
- 1 point for using an inaccurate final consonant;
- 0 points for omission of a final consonant.

Stimulus	Katy's production at T1	T1 Score	Katy's production at T5	T5 Score	Difference between scores
NOTE	[nəʊ]		[nəʊt]		
PLANE	[peɪ]		[pleɪn]		
HEART	[ɑ]		[hɑt]		
NAIL	[neɪʔə]		[neɪʔjə]		
CAGE	[keɪ]		[keɪk]		
SLIDE	[daɪ]		[daɪd]		
WHEEL	[wiʔə]		[wiʔjə]		
RAKE	[reɪ]		[weɪ]		
STORK	[dɔʔgə]		[dɔk]		
LEAF	[jif]		[ji]		
SAUCE	[dɔ]		[dɔ]		
ICE	[aɪ]		[aɪt]		
ROPE	[wɔ]		[wəʊp]		
PIPE	[paɪ]		[paɪp]		
BARN	[bɑ]		[bɑn]		
ROAD	[wɔ]		[wəʊd]		
		T1 Total score:		T5 Total score:	Total difference between scores:

Once you have completed the scoring exercise, answer the questions that follow.

(a) Did Katy improve in her final consonant production?
(b) The scoring of speech results is not always clear cut. Outline any difficulties you experienced.
(c) How would you resolve this difficulty?

Now turn to the Key to Activity 8.5 at the end of this chapter, and then read the following section.

Overall, a statistically significant main effect for intervention was found using two-way mixed ANOVA ($F(2, 44) = 38.310$, $p < 0.001$) (see Pring, 2005, for further details of how ANOVA might be used). This means that over the course of the intervention programme, Katy made significant improvements in her use of final consonants. After the first phase of intervention that focused specifically on single words, Katy's use of final consonants in single words increased significantly. This change was noted not only for the treatment words from List A (as shown in Activity 8.5), but also for the untreated, matched control set of words from List B. This suggests that generalized change had been brought about, rather than being limited to the specific items that she had met in the intervention.

After the second phase of intervention on a wider range of single words, further significant gains were made in single word speech production. Again, this change was not limited to the treatment lists but also for the untreated, matched control set of single words suggesting that generalized change had been brought about. However, there was no carryover spontaneously to target words in connected speech after Phases I and II of intervention.

In the third phase of intervention we focused specifically on connected speech using the carefully graded sentence stimuli. The outcome of this is discussed in the next section, but here we focus on what happened to Katy's single word production after this phase. The results for Katy's single word speech production over the three phases of therapy and at each of the assessment points are presented in Figure 8.3. This shows a decrease in the accuracy of Katy's production of CVC stimuli in single word naming tasks, i.e. compare the lines on the graph at T3 and T4. This decrease may be attributable to the focus of the intervention in each of the phases: Phases I and II focused on single word production and had an effect at this level for the matched stimuli lists. Phase III involved work on connected speech only; no work was done directly on single word production. The single word task may have been perceived by Katy as less important than tasks involving connected speech. On the other hand, a recency effect may have been acting so that at each post-intervention assessment Katy performed well on whatever had been addressed most recently in the preceding intervention, but these gains were not maintained in the longer term. However, data from T5 (long-term

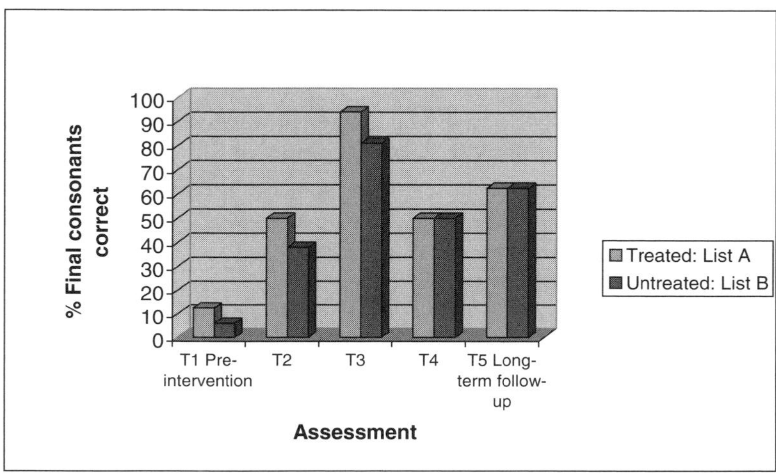

Figure 8.3: Katy's CVC production in single words.

follow-up) suggests that a recency effect was not operating. Gains in connected speech were maintained after intervention ceased, and the decline in her single word speech production did not continue, a slight increase in performance being noted at T5.

Outcomes: Connected Speech

Katy's ability to produce CVC words in connected speech was assessed by asking her to repeat each stimuli item in a short carrier phrase. Katy had to produce words like NOTE and GOAT in a short 'neutral' phrase, i.e. where the target word was followed by a vowel, e.g. THE NOTE IN THE PICTURE, or THE GOAT IN THE PICTURE. As for the single word speech assessment, the focus was on Katy's final segment production of the stimuli words: she was awarded two points for final consonants that were accurately realized, one point for using an inaccurate final consonant, and no points for omission of a final consonant. Raw scores were converted to percentages.

As for single words, a two-way mixed ANOVA showed that there was a statistically significant main effect for intervention. At the early assessments, Katy found the production of the neutral sentences very challenging. She did not use any final consonants in connected speech at the T1 pre-intervention assessment, or T2 or T3 assessments. Remember that connected speech was not being addressed in the early phase of the intervention programme, and there was no carryover from work on single words in Phases I and II to connected speech. However, following Phase III which specifically targeted connected speech there was a significant change on both stimuli lists, i.e. the words in both Lists A and B.

Katy greatly enjoyed intervention Phase III with its focus on connected speech and reading sentences. It seemed to have more relevance to her beyond the therapy room, and she said that she thought the single word games had been 'babyish'. In terms of the speech processing model (Figure 2.3 in Chapter 2), the first two phases of intervention focused on motor programs, while the third phase was targeting motor planning. For Katy, and possibly for other children, generalization of single words into connected speech may be dependent on the specific targeting of motor planning. The intervention in Phase III was very successful in getting her to use the CVC stimuli in sentences, something that she had been completely unable to achieve before. It is likely that Katy's attention had shifted to the production of larger units of speech which involve motor planning, rather than being focused at the single word level. We were able to manipulate the word glue that links words in such a way as to gently support Katy in her production of final consonants.

Katy's improvement in connected speech was not limited to the treatment list but also extended to the untreated, matched control list suggesting that generalized change had been brought about. Although we had

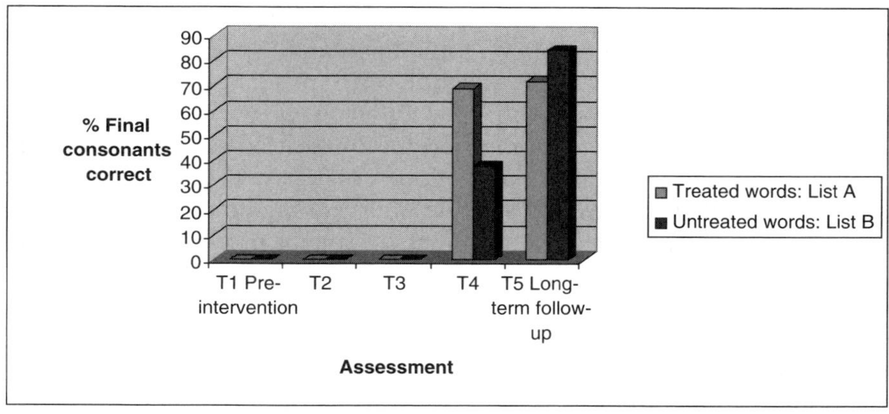

Figure 8.4: Katy's CVC production in connected speech.

not worked specifically on her production of words such as GOAT and TRAIN (i.e. the List B words) in sentences, she showed improvement in her production of these words in sentences. This improvement was only noted following the phase of intervention that focused on connected speech. Gains made with connected speech were maintained in the long term, after a period of no intervention for 7 months, when T4 and T5 performances were compared. An important message arising from this work is that improvement in connected speech was only brought about by specifically addressing connected speech in a carefully structured way. Figure 8.4 shows the changes which occurred in Katy's connected speech production.

An important question to consider in future research is whether the single word intervention phases were a necessary prerequisite prior to the connected speech phase, or whether intervention might have started with the connected speech work straight away. Considerations such as this one are discussed in greater detail in the following section.

What Did We Learn from Katy's Intervention?

Many children are able to apply what they have learnt at a segmental or whole-word level to conversational speech, and some studies have explicitly measured this type of generalization (e.g. Wright, Shelton and Arndt, 1969; Elbert *et al.*, 1990; Almost and Rosenbaum, 1998). However, this is not always the case, and many children with persisting speech difficulties find it difficult to apply what they have learnt at a single word level into spontaneous speech in the real world. Indeed, therapists may discharge children at this point hoping that generalization will occur into spontaneous speech without intervention (Joffe, Penn and Doyle, 1996).

There is little research addressing the relationship between connected speech and single word speech production in intervention despite the fact that connected speech has important implications from a functional point of view and in terms of intervention efficiency. The work with Katy suggested (1) that she needed specific intervention aimed at motor planning in order for generalization of final consonant production to extend into her connected speech, and (2) that intervention might have been more efficient if this level had been addressed first. For children with motor programming difficulties it may be developmentally more appropriate to start by addressing larger chunks of speech, rather than following the traditional hierarchy of single sounds at the most basic level of motor programming (see Chapter 7).

It would be valuable to be able to distinguish between children who (a) will be able to generalize spontaneously what they learn in therapy at a single word level into connected speech, and (b) are not going to be able to generalize in this way, and whose therapy should thus target the level of connected speech specifically. The intervention with Katy allows for generation of some hypotheses about making this distinction. It may be that children with very severe speech difficulties are not able to automatically generalize into connected speech, or that children beyond the critical age of CA 5;6 (see Chapter 1) are not able to generalize single word changes into connected speech. Other factors may include the underlying nature of the speech processing system or the particular phonological processes involved. These hypotheses will need to be tested out through other case studies. One child, Zoë, described by Stackhouse and Wells (1993) had severe speech difficulties but was able to generalize from single words to connected speech. This child did not have final consonant deletion, and it may be that this process makes children vulnerable in terms of limited generalization.

Katy's intervention was effective in improving her speech production at the single word and connected speech level by reducing the frequency of final consonant deletion and increasing her percentage of consonants correct. However, there are two important caveats to note. The intervention took place with just one child so results cannot be generalized to other children. The findings from this study need to be viewed in conjunction with related case-study interventions such as those carried out by Stackhouse and Wells (1993) – and see also the intervention studies of Bryan and Howard (1992) and Ebbels (2000).

Katy was highly motivated by the connected speech intervention, and this is something that may have important implications for many older children with persisting difficulties. Using connected speech may have more immediate and functional relevance to them, and if we can motivate them in this way, then half the battle is won. Connected speech is a more natural phenomenon than communicating in single words: Katy seemed to enjoy the connected speech activities more than the intervention targeting single words. Children's motivation may increase when communicative relevance seems greater. Furthermore, in connected speech, processes such as assimilation provide natural support, for example, for children such as Katy attempting to realize final sounds. The careful selection of hierarchically graded connected speech stimuli for this part of the intervention was useful in building on Katy's strengths and gently leading her to more challenging steps. Intervention approaches that use connected speech stimuli in this way are seldom used, yet are potentially valuable for many children with severe difficulties. Examples of facilitative phonetic contexts can be found in the speech therapy literature (e.g. see Kent, 1982; Grundy, 1989; Grunwell, 1992), but often these facilitative contexts do not extend across word boundaries.

There is a great deal more work needed in finding out about connected speech and how to incorporate it into intervention. Practitioners can contribute to this by considering children's connected speech and the extent to which they can address this effectively through careful selection of stimuli to scaffold change in connected speech. In this chapter we have given an example of how we employed connected speech stimuli (as well as single word stimuli) in intervention. The connected speech intervention was particularly effective in bringing about changes in Katy's motor planning for connected speech but only when it was worked on directly.

Summary

This chapter described the assessment and intervention that took place with Katy, a girl aged 6;5 with severe speech difficulties. The key points are as follows.

- Intervention planning involved consideration of psycholinguistic, phonological and psychosocial data.
- Katy's strengths in her psycholinguistic profile (e.g. phonological representations) were used to support her weaknesses (e.g. motor programs and motor planning) in the intervention.
- Children's relative strengths, i.e. in terms of their own speech processing profile, should not be confused with age-appropriate skills when they are compared to other children of the same age.
- Katy's intervention involved successive phases tapping firstly her stored motor programs, and then her motor planning for connected speech.
- Connected speech stimuli were specifically designed to support her use of final consonants.
- Katy made significant gains in both her single word and connected speech production.

- The improvements in her connected speech required direct and carefully focused work to bring about the change. No spontaneous generalization from single words to connected speech was noted prior to this.
- Generalization occurred to matched untreated words.
- Katy's motivation to be involved in connected speech activities was greater than for single words.
- The use of a naturally occurring speech phenomenon such as word junction was effectively used to support changes in Katy's speech.

KEY TO ACTIVITY 8.1

(a) Does Katy have difficulties with input or output?
Katy has difficulty with both speech input and output, although output is more affected.

(b) Outline two areas of relative strength.
Katy has relatively good phonological representations (Level E) and some good phonological awareness skills (Level F). Alliteration stands out as a strength as she was successful at both Levels D and F.

(c) Outline Katy's main areas of difficulty.
The entire output side (Levels G to K) is affected. Level B (discrimination of non-words) and Level D (discrimination of real words) are affected on the input side.

(d) What further information would you find valuable?
Further speech data would be valuable. We specifically asked: What is the relationship between:

- Katy's poor auditory discrimination at Levels B and D, and her output skills?
- Katy's Level G performance and the lower levels on the output side, such as Level I and J?
- Katy's speech output and her spelling?
- Katy's input and output phonological awareness skills?
- Katy's single word speech production and connected speech and intelligibility?

KEY TO ACTIVITY 8.2

(a) Which segments or processes would you wish to address in therapy?

Katy was able to indicate contrasts between word-initial and within-word consonants. However, she was not using final consonants at all. We decided to address her final consonant production first.

(b) Why did you choose these particular targets?
We considered that her inability to indicate final consonants was having a major impact on her intelligibility.

(c) How would you attempt to combine the phonological information with the psycholinguistic information presented previously, in Figure 8.1?
Katy had difficulties with her stored motor programs. These seemed to contain immature or inaccurate word templates: e.g. all CVC words were a CV (or in some cases V) shape. Our intervention aimed to make Katy aware of the shortcomings of her CV templates for CVCs by drawing her attention to the contrasts in meaning between CV and CVC words. Motor planning also presented problems for Katy. We considered that intervention should give Katy the opportunity to use her new and accurate CVC templates in connected speech which would tap the level of motor planning and improve her intelligibility.

KEY TO ACTIVITY 8.3

Examples of words for matched stimuli lists for Katy

Item No.	List A Treated words worked on in intervenion	List B Untreated control words
1	NOTE	GOAT
2	PLANE	TRAIN
3	HEART	PART
4	NAIL	HAIL
5	CAGE	PAGE
6	SLIDE	LIED
7	WHEEL	KNEEL
8	RAKE	STEAK
9	STORK	WALK
10	LEAF	HOOF
11	SAUCE	PURSE
12	ICE	DICE
13	ROPE	GRAPE
14	PIPE	SHEEP
15	BARN	LINE
16	ROAD	TOAD

KEY TO ACTIVITY 8.4

Examples of sentence stimuli for Katy

LIST A

1 = Facilitatory sentences
2 = Neutral sentences
3i = Most challenging sentences (hetero-organic adjacent consonants without assimilation)
3ii = Sentences not directly addressed (assimilation of final consonants in stimulus words)

No.	Stimulus word	Sentences
1	NOTE	1: This NOTE teaches Father Xmas 2: There's a NOTE under the table (3ii: This NOTE can't be read)
2	PLANE	1: The PLANE knocked it 2: There's a PLANE in the sky (3ii: This PLANE must be loaded)
3	HEART	1: This HEART tastes nice 2: There's a HEART on my jumper (3ii: This HEART can break)
4	NAIL	1: This NAIL looks pretty 2: There's a NAIL in the wood 3i: This NAIL got painted twice
5	CAGE	1: The CAGE joined my class 2: There's a CAGE on the bed 3i: The CAGE got stolen
6	SLIDE	1: This SLIDE dumped me 2: The SLIDE in the park is nice 3i: The SLIDE bounces him
7	WHEEL	1: The WHEEL looks broken 2: There's a WHEEL on the bike 3i: This WHEEL got fixed
8	RAKE	1: This RAKE cost £10 2: There's a RAKE on the ground 3i: This RAKE takes a bath
9	STORK	1: The STORK carries a baby 2: There's a STORK on the log 3i: This STORK teaches swinging
10	LEAF	1: The LEAF feels wet 2: The LEAF is in the air 3i: This LEAF got torn
11	SAUCE	1: The SAUCE seems nice 2: There's SAUCE in the jar (3ii: The SAUCE shouldn't burn)
12	ICE	1: This ICE seems cold 2: The ICE is in the bucket (3ii: This ICE should melt)

No.	Stimulus word	Sentences
13	ROPE	1: This ROPE pulled the car 2: There's ROPE on the road 3i: This ROPE got frayed
14	PIPE	1: The PIPE pushes through the roof 2: There's a PIPE on the wall 3i: This PIPE curls round the floor
15	BARN	1: The BARN needs painting 2: There's a BARN on the farm (3ii: The BARN must be cleaned)
16	ROAD	1: The ROAD divides the hill 2: There's a ROAD over the river (3ii: This ROAD brings us home)

KEY TO ACTIVITY 8.5

Stimulus	T1	T1 Score	T5	T5 Score	Difference between scores
NOTE	[nəʊ]	0	[nəʊt]	2	+2
PLANE	[peɪ]	0	[pleɪn]	2	+2
HEART	[ɑ]	0	[hɑt]	2	+2
NAIL	[neɪʔə]	½	[neɪjə]	1	+½
CAGE	[keɪ]	0	[keɪk]	1	+1
SLIDE	[daɪ]	0	[daɪd]	2	+2
WHEEL	[wiʔə]	½	[wijə]	1	+½
RAKE	[reɪ]	0	[weɪ]	0	0
STORK	[dɔʔgə]	1	[dɔk]	2	+1
LEAF	[jif]	2	[ji]	0	–2
SAUCE	[dɔ]	0	[dɔ]	0	0
ICE	[aɪ]	0	[aɪt]	1	+1
ROPE	[wɔ]	0	[wəʊ]	0	0
PIPE	[paɪ]	0	[paɪp]	2	+2
BARN	[bɑ]	0	[bɑn]	2	+2
ROAD	[wɔ]	0	[wəʊd]	2	+2
		T1 Total score:		T5 Total score:	Total difference between scores:
		4		20	+16

(a) Did Katy improve in her final consonant production?

Yes. Without carrying out statistical analysis, these results show a general trend of improvement from T1 to T5.

(b) The scoring of speech results is not always clear cut. Outline any difficulties you experienced.

Items such as NAIL and STORK posed a challenge. At T1 Katy produced [neɪʔə] and at T5 she said [neɪjə]. At T1 she produced [dɔgə], and at T5 she said [dɔk]. The difficulty lies in whether Katy should be given any credit for introducing this additional final syllable as it may be an attempt to mark the final consonant.

(c) How would you resolve this difficulty?

We chose to award ½ a point when Katy emphasized the coda with insertion of a glottal stop and schwa, e.g. [neɪʔə]. When she inserted schwa following a perceptible English consonant we awarded 1 point, e.g. [neɪjə] and [dɔgə]. [dɔk] was awarded 2 points since the final consonant was present and accurate. Incorporating these rules into our scoring system meant Katy's progress could be more sensitively measured.

Note

1. This is not routinely assessed in monolingual children.

Chapter 9
Generalization

Implicit in every intervention is the hope that children will generalize what they have learnt in therapy to segments, clusters or words not directly addressed. Teaching every speech sound, every word or particular language structure would be time consuming and demotivating for child and therapist. Therapists normally rely on the fact that once they have worked together with a child on some exemplars of speech or language, this will be sufficient for the client to generalize the knowledge of wider aspects of speech and/or language. An efficient approach to intervention is one which results in widespread change throughout a child's system. Bunning (2004) notes that, 'Generalization of therapeutic gains is not something that happens as a natural consequence of therapy . . . It requires deliberate planning' (p. 9). In this chapter we aim to make this process more explicit since generalization is key to a successful therapy outcome. We introduce Rachel, a girl aged 7;1 whose intervention illustrates some of the points made in previous chapters about working with children with PSDs, and more specifically illustrates how generalization arising from a specific speech intervention can be evaluated and interpreted.

The design and selection of targets to be addressed in therapy is an important decision facing practitioners as they plan intervention. In Chapters 3–8 we focused on some specific aspects of stimuli design and selection. These issues are important since the ultimate aim of intervention is to encourage generalization throughout the speech processing system, and careful selection of targets may maximize the generalization achieved, and thus ultimately the efficiency of intervention. However, there are a great many unanswered questions regarding generalization, and it is challenging to predict how widely a particular child will generalize new skills learnt in therapy. Joffe and Serry's (2004) review of the phonological therapy evidence base reveals that intervention studies have considered generalization to varying degrees and that evidence for generalization varies considerably.

This chapter starts by exploring what is meant by generalization, what we know about generalization and how evaluation of generalization can inform our knowledge of both therapy and theory. Intervention studies which have added to our knowledge of generalization are reviewed, as well as some of our own intervention cases that have a contribution to make to the area. We aim to show how widely patterns of generalization can differ, but also indicate some trends based on a small number of children we have studied in depth and our review of the literature.

What is Generalization?

Generalization can be defined as the extent to which a targeted area addressed in intervention results in changes beyond the specific aspect addressed. Some texts also use the term 'carryover' to refer to generalization. In this chapter we use the term generalization throughout. Generalization can be considered at two broad levels.

- *Across-item generalization*: generalization from treated items (e.g. words directly targeted in therapy) to untreated items. The degree to which the untreated control items resemble the treated items is an important variable, i.e. these may range from very closely matched single words, to words with a different phonotactic structure, or sentences.
- *Across-task generalization*: generalization from a treated task (e.g. naming of CVC words) to another task (e.g. spelling of the same CVC words to dictation, or auditory discrimination of the same and closely related CVC words). To evaluate across-task generalization a constant wordlist is needed since it enables comparison of task performance between tasks and levels of processing, without confounding the issue by introducing stimulus variability (Stackhouse and Wells, 1997, 2001).

The descriptions of across-item and across-task generalization both mention untreated items or tasks needed to evaluate generalization. These may also be called controls. If we only observe the effects of intervention on treated items then we will not be able to evaluate the extent of generalization that may be happening to untreated items or task. The design and selection of untreated control items is discussed in further detail in later sections of this chapter, but for now let us turn our attention to more general issues about generalization and intervention design.

Generalization and Intervention Design

As practitioners we strive for generalization, but as researchers we need to demonstrate that what we do has specific, carefully delineated effects. How can we reconcile the two? Therapists aim to bring about generalization within the speech and language system since we could not hope to teach every language structure that a child needs to know. When addressing /s/ clusters in intervention with a child, we would be delighted to note not only improvement in the child's production of words containing /s/ clusters but also gains in intelligibility, listening and attention, and ability to construct sentences. After all we want children to improve in as many areas and as quickly as possible. However, when systematically evaluating the effect of the specific /s/ cluster intervention, a reasonable assumption may be that the child was improving anyhow, e.g. because of classroom-based language teaching rather than because of the specific /s/ cluster intervention itself. The /s/ cluster intervention may not have been the specific cause of these widespread changes in the child's abilities. If we wanted to evaluate the effect of the /s/ cluster intervention in a systematic way we might make the following hypotheses based on our theoretical knowledge of the speech processing system:

- /s/ clusters will improve in the treated words that are worked on in intervention;
- /s/ clusters will improve in untreated, control words matched to the treated items;
- the increased accuracy of /s/ clusters will improve intelligibility.

Changes in other unrelated language areas such as sentence construction ability were not predicted based on our theoretical understanding of the speech processing system. Thus, changes in such general language skills may suggest that there are other factors, e.g. maturation or classroom language work affecting the child's performance. Obviously, this is not a bad thing, but the clear demonstration of the specific effects of our /s/ cluster intervention has now been confounded by the intrusion of other variables. Although it may not be possible to ever completely rule out factors such as maturation and classroom input, we need to control for these as best we can when attempting to demonstrate the value of our interventions.

A study by Howell and Dean (1994) provides a good example of dealing with this issue. They aimed to determine whether their Metaphon therapy programme specifically affected the processes targeted in therapy or whether it affected the speech and language system more generally. The Metaphon program is a good example of a structured metaphonological approach to therapy for speech difficulties. The program aims to provide children with explicit information about the sound system of their language and to enable them to bring about changes in their speech output. Therapist and child share a vocabulary (a meta-language) about speech sounds that is built up during the course of therapy (e.g. 'long' to talk about fricative sounds: 'ffffffff', and 'short' for plosive sounds: /p/). Metaphon has two phases: Phase I consists of games and activities which focus on the sound system, and Phase II gives opportunities for children to use their newly acquired knowledge in communicative settings. In the intervention study, Howell and Dean (1994) hypothesized that there would be significant changes in the treated areas of phonology, phoneme segmentation and communicative awareness. However, they predicted that there would be no corresponding change in scores on a vocabulary assessment, sentence segmentation and sentence structure tasks. The rationale behind such research is that practitioners need to carry out therapy that is specific in targeting its goals.

The Metaphon intervention took place with 13 pre-school children (aged 4–5 years) who had been admitted to speech and language therapy and had phonological difficulties. The study was designed as a series of single-case studies in which children acted as their own control. The design allowed for the consideration of individual responses to remediation and comparison across the group as a whole. The intervention involved phases of assessment, treatment, and re-assessment. Dosage was a half hourly session of therapy given once weekly for approximately 22 weeks. The intervention aimed to test the following predictions.

1. There would be a significant change in scores on the phonological assessment.
2. There would be a significant change in scores on phoneme segmentation and communicative awareness tasks.
3. There would be no corresponding change in vocabulary, sentence segmentation and sentence structure tasks.

This study found that Metaphon therapy was effective as significant changes in the children's scores on phonological assessment were noted. However, it was also noted that a certain amount of Metaphon therapy is required for significant change to take place in phonological production. The effectiveness of Metaphon holds good regardless of the severity and nature of the child's phonological problems. Metaphon is also thought to be an economical treatment procedure for pre-school children: five hours of therapy was sufficient to bring about significant change for most children in the study (Dean *et al.*, 1995a, b). In general, children were found to have made significant gains in their phoneme segmentation and communicative awareness skills. As predicted, the study found no corresponding change in scores on the more general language tasks such as vocabulary, sentence segmentation and sentence structure. More global language improvement would have suggested that other variables such as maturation or classroom influences had brought about the change, and that this was not due to the specific therapy implemented (Hegde, 1985).

Generalization is an excellent example of a concept that has both practical and theoretical importance. Observing patterns of generalization that occur as a result of specific interventions can tell us about the nature of speech processing and how it develops in children. Our own predictions about the type and extent of generalization that occur will be based around our theoretical knowledge and beliefs. For example, if we believe that each lexical item has discrete, local representations then we would not expect to see across-item generalization. Whereas, if we assume that words are representations of interconnected micro-features shared by many different words (e.g. Coltheart and Byng, 1989; Patterson, 1994) then we would expect generalization to other untreated words. Furthermore, the pattern of generalization noted post-intervention would inform views about how the lexicon might be organized. In terms of across-task generalization, if our chosen theory assumes that, for example, there is a common output lexicon for both spoken and written forms then we would be expecting that intervention addressing speech production (or more specifically motor programs) would result in improved spelling skills on the same set of words. Predictions about reading and writing will depend on whether our theory assumes, for example, that the orthographic representations underlying word recognition in reading and word production in writing are the same ones. Evidence regarding this issue, from intervention studies with adults, is conflicting: Carlomagno and Parlato (1989) did find generalization from reading to writing, whereas Scott and Byng (1989) did not. We do, however, need to be cautious about applying results of studies of adults to our understanding of children. Adults with acquired difficulties suffer disruption to a fully developed system, whereas children in the process of developing speech, language and literacy may experience more complex knock-on effects due to difficulties in the interaction between each of these areas. Furthermore, there are likely to be differences between typical and atypical populations. Children with persisting speech difficulties may often show minimal generalization as a characteristic of their difficulties.

In carrying out routine intervention and research, we need to have a clear rationale for:

(a) the aspect of the speech processing system targeted;
(b) the nature of the change we aim to bring about;
(c) the extent of generalization that might feasibly occur;
(d) control measures that we would not expect to change as a result of intervention.

Working within an explicit psycholinguistic framework can help us in addressing these points.

What Do We Know about Generalization?

A survey of the intervention literature reveals the following patterns of generalization when working with children with speech difficulties.

- Treatment of a segment in one word position (e.g. word-initial position) can generalize to other word positions (e.g. word-final) (Elbert and McReynolds, 1975).
- Treatment of one representative aspect of a sound category can facilitate improvement across that category (within-class generalization). This has been documented for place, manner and voicing of production, e.g. treatment of fricatives /s/ and /θ/ enhanced changes in other untreated fricatives (Costello and Onstine, 1976). This type of generalization is thought to be influenced by the relationship that exists between segments. The fact that children seem to generalize across segments that have common features is an indication that these groupings have a psychological reality.
- Treating a phonological process with a few examples can extend to all segments involved in that process (Weiner, 1981; Crary and Hunt, 1982). Weiner (1981) worked on the error pattern of final consonant deletion and this facilitated improvements in a broad range of final consonants disrupted by the same pattern.
- Treatment of a segment using just 3–5 different exemplar words could result in widespread generalization to the treated segment in other words (Elbert, Powell and Swartzlander, 1991).
- Treatment of more marked clusters will cause generalization to less marked clusters even if the latter are not targeted in treatment (see Chapter 5). One child in such a study who initially produced no clusters was treated for the cluster /bl/ and generalized to nine other clusters (Gierut, 1999). In another study, treatment of specific three-element clusters (e.g. /spr/) did not generalize to other three element clusters, although some children generalized to untreated singletons (including affricates) and to untreated two-element clusters (Barlow, 2001).
- Working on maximally opposed words is more effective than minimal pair work, and results in greater generalization (Gierut, 1990). Contrasting one new segment with an unrelated known segment resulted in greater generalization than the more traditional target-substitute format. Similar positive results were obtained by systematically varying contrasts along the dimensions of place, manner and voicing (Gierut, 1989, and see Chapter 3 for further discussion of this issue).
- Treatment of words can generalize to connected speech in some cases (Wright, Shelton and Arndt, 1969; Elbert, Dinnsen, Swartzlander and Chin, 1990).

Generalization is, however, not as clear cut as it might seem from these statements. Many of these findings indicate the potential for generalization given the right therapy conditions and the right child or children. There is no guarantee that such widespread generalization will occur for all children as a result of all treatments. Children with persisting speech difficulties vary widely in their responses to intervention so that it is hard to predict which children will show widespread generalization and which children will generalize in more limited ways. Many of the research findings outlined above are based on work with young pre-school children, aged 3–5 years, who may well have a very different generalization response from that of school-age children with PSDs.

Generalization is a challenge to achieve, and even more of a challenge to understand. Focusing on individual studies and evaluating the nature of intervention and the extent of generalization that took place can be helpful in attempting to understand this complex phenomenon. In order to do this we return now to the intervention studies described in Chapter 2 (see Table 2.1 and the Appendix at the end of Chapter 2). These studies were all carried out with school-aged participants. The studies varied widely in their design and the way in which specificity was controlled for. Specificity is a term used to refer to the specific effects of intervention. Many of the studies included control measures so that the authors could state with relative confidence that the results seen were due to the specific effects of intervention. Typically such control measures included incorporation of an unrelated language processing task so that it could be demonstrated that general developmental improvements were not responsible for the outcomes observed. For example, in Crosbie and Dodd's (2001) auditory intervention with Amy, aged 7;0 they noted, 'An unrelated skill not targeted during therapy, reading, was measured before and after the period of therapy so that any change in Amy's ability to discriminate between words could be attributed to therapy and not other factors' (p. 186).

Demonstrating a stable baseline prior to the start of intervention is another way in which we can demonstrate the specific effects of a therapy: if spontaneous change was not occurring before intervention started then it seems unlikely that any effects of intervention will be because of maturation. Stable pre-intervention baselines were demonstrated in the papers by Broom and Doctor (1995a, b), Crosbie and Dodd (2001), Best (2005), and Pascoe *et al.* (2005). Another way of demonstrating that any changes observed are due to specific interventions is to withdraw intervention and monitor the changes that occur following a period with no intervention. One might expect to see some further generalization to related structures or tasks, but again no significant changes in unrelated and general skills. A significant decline in the particular area addressed will suggest a recency effect – a transitory change due to the recent work done but not of any lasting benefit to the child. Carrying out a longer term follow-up is both a control measure, i.e. it ensures that any other confounding variables such as maturation can be ruled out, and a way of providing functional data on generalization beyond the therapy setting. Gibbon and Wood (2003) noted that a year after their EPG therapy there was evidence of 'carryover from clinical settings to day-to-day environments, making it possible to discharge [the participant] from therapy. This demonstrated that the positive changes in articulatory patterns . . . were clinically significant and long lasting' (p. 369). In the study by Pantelemidou *et al.* (2003), the authors carried out their final assessment some five weeks after the completion of therapy, following a period with no intervention, in order to evaluate any generalization.

More specifically we evaluated generalization in each of the studies by noting:

- whether generalization occurred for untreated items, i.e. across-item generalization;
- whether it extended to related language processing tasks, i.e. across-task generalization.

Our survey of these papers revealed that across-task generalization (e.g. progress in auditory discrimination of closely related CVC words, having focused on production of these words) is more rarely achieved than across-item generalization (e.g. progress with untreated words containing /s/ clusters, having treated a set of words containing /s/ clusters). While all the studies showed positive outcomes, generalization varied widely between them. Some studies did not achieve - or could not demonstrate - any significant generalization (e.g. Broom and Doctor, 1995a, Norbury and Chiat, 2000) although there was significant improvement in targeted words or aspects of speech. Many of the studies were able to show across-item generalization, e.g. untreated wordlists improved in the studies of Broom and Doctor (1995b), Crosbie and Dodd (2001), Spooner (2002) and Stiegler and Hoffman (2001). The studies by Bryan and Howard (1992), Waters *et al.* (1998) and Pascoe *et al.* (2005) were able to demonstrate both across-item generalization as well as across-task generalization. Bryan and Howard showed improvement in the speech production of their participant, as well as in his auditory discrimination. Waters *et al.*'s child improved in terms of his speech production as well as his phonological awareness and literacy. Katy, described by Pascoe *et al.*, improved not only in her speech, but also in her auditory discrimination of closely related words and her spelling.

Stiegler and Hoffman (2001) carried out a single-case study looking at the effectiveness of a discourse-based treatment for word-finding problems in 9-year-old children. This novel approach involved picture-elicited narratives, story retelling and conversations on familiar topics, with the aim of reducing children's overt word-finding behaviours. The intervention was effective in achieving this goal, and in addition generalization was noted to spontaneous, conversational speech. These authors noted that therapy addressing 'specific language concepts in single-skill fashion' has shown a disconcerting lack of efficiency (e.g. see Damico, 1988; Fey, 1988; Norris and Hoffman, 1993). They caution that single-skill training may not be justified in terms of time and money spent, and advocate the use of more discourse-based treatments, as well as further studies of generalization so that efficiency can be optimized. However, we also know that broad-based language approaches are typically not effective in remediating specific aspects such as phonology (e.g. Fey, Cleave, Ravida *et al.*, 1994). It seems that there may be a threshold in terms of age and specificity of speech–language difficulties beyond which whole-language interventions are less appropriate. Table 2.3 (Chapter 2) summarizes the studies by design, controls and generalization observed.

The questions of 'how many exemplars to use?' and 'which exemplars to use?' are vitally important ones in phonological intervention. Carrying out a phonological analysis can inform our choice with regards to the latter question, but the first question remains a challenge. While some authors have suggested that just one feature contrast (Blache, Parsons and Humphreys, 1981) or one segment (Gierut *et al.*, 1987) is sufficient in bringing about generalization, others such as Edwards (1983) and Hodson and Paden (1991) have suggested multiple exemplars are preferable. A phonotactic approach to therapy (e.g. as advocated by Velleman, 2002) fits well with this point of view. Velleman suggests that focusing on the concept of a new word shape (e.g. CCVC – see Katy's case discussion in Chapter 8) may result in generalization beyond the treated sounds. Giving children many, wide ranging examples of a particular structure will facilitate their acquisition of it.

Elbert, Powell and Swartzlander (1991) investigated this issue more systematically in their study, entitled: 'Toward a technology of generalization: How many exemplars are sufficient?' They examined the number of minimal word-pair exemplars needed for 19 pre-school children with speech difficulties to meet a generalization criterion. They found that 59% of their child participants required just three exemplars to obtain the necessary level of generalization. Five exemplars were sufficient for 21% of the children, while it was necessary to teach 10 different exemplars to 14% of the participants. For 7% of the participants, generalization did not occur despite intervention focusing on 10 exemplars. They concluded that although generalization usually occurred following treatment with a small number of exemplars, there was great variability from child to child. There was no apparent relationship between specific sounds and the likelihood of generalization; however, the data from some children suggested that treatment of one sound enhances learning of subsequent sounds. It seems likely that the answer to the question of how many exemplars do we need, may depend on the child, the exact nature of the difficulties, age and motivation.

There is a great deal of work to be done in improving the efficacy of speech and language intervention and our understanding of generalization. The question of whether we can say that one intervention is better than another is important. Broom and Doctor (1995a, b) emphasize the wide diversity between children diagnosed with the same condition and suggest that it is unlikely that there is one treatment that will be successful with all children. However, what is needed is an improved understanding of the type of therapy that works best with an individual child or various sub-groups of children. In the following section, we introduce one child with persisting speech difficulties.

Case Study: Rachel aged 7;1

Rachel had a normal developmental history with no significant medical or social factors to report. She was in her second year of formal schooling in a mainstream school and making pleasing progress academically. Rachel had persisting difficulties with her speech production: she spoke slightly later than her older sibling had, and her speech was a cause of concern to her family, her teachers, the school nurse and now, increasingly, to herself. Her speech had been variously described as 'immature', 'unclear' and 'unintelligible to strangers'. Rachel had received speech therapy – approximately 12 hours of direct therapist contact over a four-year period. However, difficulties remained and there was concern that Rachel might be at risk for spelling and reading difficulties linked to her persistent speech problems.

Assessment

The speech processing profile was used as a framework for organizing the findings from the assessment. At each level of the profile, excluding Level C, which is not routinely assessed in monolingual children (Stackhouse and Wells, 1997), at least one assessment was carried out. In some cases these were standardized measures, and in other cases these were unpublished and non-standardized materials. The ticks and crosses on the profile indicate Rachel's performance in relation to children of her chronological age, with one tick indicating age-appropriate skills, and further ticks or crosses showing the number of standard deviations above or below the mean. The completed profile is presented in Figure 9.1.

√ = age appropriate performance
X = 1 standard deviation below the expected mean for her age
XX = 2 standard deviations below the expected mean for her age
XXX = 3 standard deviations below the expected mean for her age

INPUT

F Is the child aware of the internal structure of phonological representations?
√ – Picture rhyme detection (Vance *et al.*, 1994)
√ – Picture onset detection (PhAB picture alliteration subtest, Frederikson *et al.*, 1997)

E Are the child's phonological representations accurate?
√ – Auditory detection of speech errors (Constable *et al.*, 1997)
√ – Sorting tasks

D Can the child discriminate between real words?
X – Minimal pair auditory discrimination of clusters (Bridgeman and Snowling, 1988)
√ – Aston Index discrimination subtest (Newton and Thompson, 1982)
√ – PhAB alliteration subtest (Frederikson *et al.*, 1997)

C Does the child have language specific representations of word structures?

Not tested

B Can the child discriminate speech sounds without reference to lexical representations?
XXX – Minimal pair auditory discrimination of clusters in non-words (Bridgeman and Snowling, 1988)

A Does the child have adequate auditory perception?
√ – audiometry

OUTPUT

G Can the child access accurate motor programmes?
X – Single word naming test (Constable *et al.*, 1997)
√ – Word-finding vocabulary test (Renfrew, 1995)
X – Edinburgh Articulation Test (Anthony *et al.*, 1971)
X – The Bus Story (Renfrew, 1969)

H Can the child manipulate phonological units?
√ – PhAB Spoonerism subtest (Frederikson *et al.*, 1997)
√ – PAT rhyme fluency subtest (Muter *et al.*, 1997)

I Can the child articulate real words accurately?
X – Real word repetition subtest (Constable *et al.*, 1997)
√ – Aston Index blending subtest – real words (Newton and Thompson, 1982)

J Can the child articulate speech without reference to lexical representations?
√ – Aston Index blending subtest – non-words (Newton and Thompson, 1982)
X – Non-word repetition subtest (Constable *et al.*, 1997)

K Does the child have adequate sound production skills?
√ – Stimulable for all sounds
√ – Oro-motor assessment (Nuffield Dyspraxia Programme, Connery. 1992)

L Does the child reject her own erroneous forms?
Informal observation – No

Figure 9.1: Rachel's speech processing profile at CA 7;1.

ACTIVITY 9.1

Study Rachel's speech processing profile presented in Figure 9.1 then answer the following questions.

(a) Does Rachel experience any difficulties with input? Outline the levels of input processing at which any difficulties occur.
(b) Does Rachel have any difficulties with output? Compare her performance at various levels of speech production.
(c) Are there any links that you might be looking for between her input and output?

Now, turn to the Key to Activity 9.1 at the end of this chapter for our responses to these questions. Then read on to find out more about Rachel in the sections that follow.

Phonological Assessment of Child Speech (PACS) (Grunwell, 1985) was used to provide information on Rachel's speech production. Severity indices were introduced in Chapter 3 and are useful measures that can encapsulate the degree of difficulty a child experiences with his or her speech in a single number. PCC (percentage of consonants correct), PVC (percentage of vowels correct) and PPC (percentage of phonemes correct) were used. The severity of Rachel's speech difficulties was estimated at two points before the intervention separated by about 6 weeks. The difference between these scores at the two pre-intervention points was not a significant one indicating a stable pre-intervention baseline. This is an important aspect of the intervention design in showing that spontaneous change was not occurring prior to the intervention beginning. The severity indices suggest that Rachel's speech difficulties are very mild. These indices were calculated by using a speech sample of about 50 to 100 words. A count was made of all the possible consonants (or vowels) that would have been realized in an idealized adult production of the words. Because this count was based on single words it does not give an impression of Rachel's intelligibility in connected speech. Issues about the complex relationship between single words and connected speech were discussed more fully in Chapters 7 and 8.

Nevertheless, Rachel had some specific difficulties. She found it hard to produce longer, multi-syllabic words, e.g. sequencing errors such as CATERPILLAR → [tæ'tikɪlə], and other sound confusions such as HOSPITAL → ['hɒsbɪkɪl] were frequently noted in words with three or more syllables. Cluster reduction was observed on some occasions but limited only to simplification of /s/ clusters. This process occurred both word-initially (e.g. SPOON → [pun], SCHOOL → [kul]) and word-finally (e.g. ASK → [æs] or [æt]). Cluster reduction of /s/ clusters occurred for 72% of possible instances. In the word-final position, she was also frequently noted to include all elements of the /s/ cluster but in a reversed order (e.g. DESK → [dɛks]). This output difficulty with /s/ clusters mirrors the difficulties she experienced on the Bridgeman and Snowling task (Levels B and D, Figure 9.1) in discriminating between closely related word pairs like LOST and LOTS. Chapters 5 and 6 had consonant clusters as their focus. It was noted in these chapters that /s/ clusters often develop at different stages from other clusters, i.e. either earlier or later than the others, and often respond differently as a group to intervention.

Stopping of [s] was also a frequent feature of Rachel's speech (e.g. SCISSORS → [ˈdɪdəd]) and occurred in all word positions for approximately 78% of possible instances. Some inconsistent stopping of /θ, f, z/ was also noted on occasion (e.g. WITH → [wɪʔ]; LEAF → [lit], BOYS → [boɪd]). A summary of Rachel's speech data is presented in Table 9.1.

Rachel's difficulty with [s] production both in isolation and in clusters is the most striking aspect of the speech analysis, and one that affected her intelligibility. The question of whether to address [s] in isolation or in clusters is one that needed to be considered at this point: would greater generalization be likely to occur through addressing singleton [s] in words, or through addressing /s/ clusters? Now that you know more about Rachel's speech difficulties, carry out Activity 9.2 which focuses on intervention planning.

Table 9.1: Summary of Rachel's speech data at CA 7;2

Assessment	Comments	
Severity indices	Percentage of consonants correct (PCC): 96.1%	
	Percentage of vowels correct (PVC): 100%	
	Percentage of phonemes correct (PPC): 97.5%	
Phonetic inventory	Word-initial position: all segments present	
	Word-medial position: all segments present	
	Word-final position: all segments present	
Stimulability	Stimulable for all segments	
Phonological processes analysis (% use)	Developmental processes: stopping (78%), reduction of [s] clusters (72%)	
Single word speech sample	CATERPILLAR → [tæ ˈtikɪlə]	ASK → [æs]
	HOSPITAL → [ˈhɒsbɪkɪl]	ASK → [æt]
	SPOON → [pun]	WITH → [wɪʔ]
	SCHOOL → [kul]	LEAF → [lit]
	DESK → [dɛks]	BOYS → [boɪd]
	SCISSORS → [ˈdɪdəd]	
Connected speech sample	THE MAN WON'T BUY IT → [θə mæn wəʊnt baɪ ɪt]	
	THIS MAN IS SWIMMING → [ðɪs mæn ɪz ˈwɪmɪn]	
	IT WERE SCARY → [ɪt wɜ ˈgɛərɪ]	
	AT CHRISTMAS → [æt ˈkwɪtmɪt]	

ACTIVITY 9.2

Consider the speech data presented in Table 9.1, and the evidence presented from the literature in Chapters 5 and 6 about intervention and consonant clusters. Now answer the following questions.

(a) What aspect of Rachel's phonological system would you choose to target in intervention?
(b) Why would you select the target?

Now, turn to the Key to Activity 9.2 at the end of this chapter for our responses to these questions. Then read on to find out more about Rachel's intervention in the sections that follow.

Intervention Planning

Rachel had difficulties with both input and output: phonetic discrimination, stored motor programs and online motor programming and planning. Rachel's main deficits were mapped from the speech processing profile onto the Stackhouse and Wells (1997) speech processing model introduced in Chapter 2 (Figure 2.3). Figure 9.2 shows that phonological recognition is problematic for Rachel as measured by the discrimination tasks (Levels B and D in Figure 9.1). Her stored knowledge of phonological representations and semantics was relatively good. However, her stored motor programmes and online motor programming are circled as problematic since her scores on Levels G, I and J in the speech processing profile were lower than the scores of her age-matched peers in Figure 9.1. Because of the uncertain relationship between input and output, and the likelihood that these deficits have affected Rachel's speech processing in a circular way (i.e. input deficits result in problems with output; output deficits result in problems with input), both input and output were considered as targets, i.e. to work on the speech processing system as a whole (Waters, 2001). Rachel's intervention was required to carefully affect positive change in the areas of weakness, using the stronger areas to gently 'scaffold' the desired change.

Rachel's intervention programme had three parts.

- The first part specifically addressed her auditory discrimination skills. Using the strengths of her peripheral auditory processing and her literacy skills, Rachel was given the opportunity to reflect and discriminate between closely related word pairs.
- The second, parallel aim of the programme was for Rachel to produce words in a carefully supported way. It was hypothesized that Rachel had established inaccurate motor programs for familiar words, and

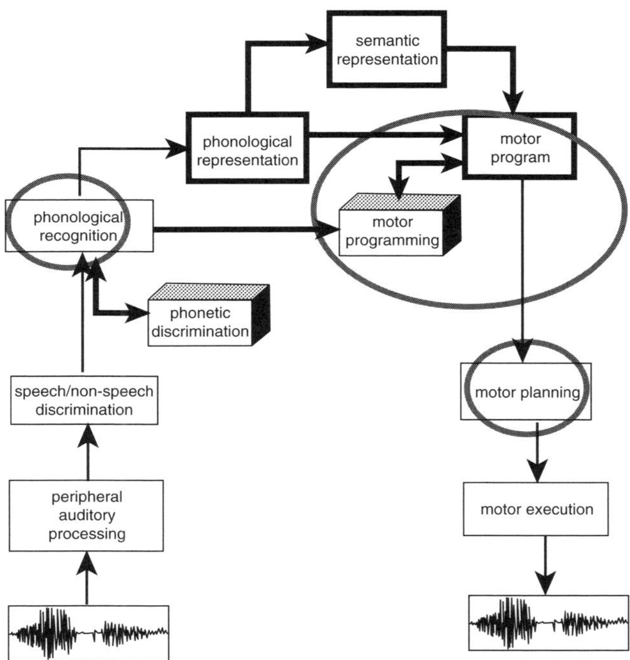

Figure 9.2: Speech processing model showing Rachel's main areas of difficulty at CA 7;1. (Reproduced by kind permission of Whurr Publishers from Stackhouse and Wells, 1997.)

it was likely to be difficult for her to modify these habitual patterns immediately. By teaching Rachel new words using a multi-faceted approach that tapped her strengths of semantic knowledge and literacy, new and accurate motor programs might be built up, and shake up the already existing inaccurate programs. This would also provide Rachel with an opportunity to reflect on her own speech production and to improve her self-monitoring skills (see Figure 9.1, Rachel's speech processing profile, Level L).

- The third aspect of the programme aimed to combine the input and output skills. Rachel was given opportunities to discriminate between closely related word pairs as well as encouraged to produce stimuli items. Again, many of these words would be unfamiliar to her. Drawing on Rachel's knowledge of written forms as well as her semantic knowledge would support the process of new word learning. The intervention tasks, together with the changes we were aiming to bring about in Rachel's speech processing system, are shown in Table 9.2.

Table 9.2: Rachel's intervention tasks and each one's psycholinguistic focus

Intervention	Example of tasks	Aspects of speech processing system targeted
Speech treatment	'Meaningful minimal pair therapy' (e.g. following Weiner, 1981)	Mainly targets: motor programming and stored motor programs. Also involves motor planning at connected speech level
Auditory discrimination treatment	Listening and posting games (e.g. see Waters, 2001)	Mainly targets: phonological recognition skills
Speech and auditory discrimination treatment	Combination of above tasks	Mainly targets: phonological recognition, motor programming and stored motor programs

Rachel received 10 hours of intervention which consisted of three different treatments:

- speech treatment
- auditory discrimination treatment
- combined speech and auditory discrimination work.

Evidence from intervention studies suggests that /s/ clusters appear to be different from other clusters in their response to intervention. In particular, treatment of /s/ + stop clusters (i.e. /st, sp, sk/) has been shown to result in little generalization to other clusters suggesting that they may not be a good starting point if one hopes to affect all clusters through intervention. However, Rachel has difficulties specific to /s/ clusters rather than affecting all clusters, and there is evidence from the literature that working on /s/ clusters may result in improvement in these sounds as well as improvements in singleton /s/ (Hodson, 1997). We targeted three different stimuli sets:

- words with word-final /sp/ clusters, e.g. WASP
- words with word-final /st/ clusters, e.g. FAST
- words with word-final /sk/ clusters, e.g. FLASK

The requirements for each of the three treatment lists were as follows.

(a) Each list consisted of 10 monosyllabic CVCC or CCVCC words. Although CVCC words were preferred, in some cases CCVCCs had to be used. Where this was the case these were balanced across the lists.

(b) Each list represented a different /s/ cluster: List A represented the cluster /sp/; list B contained the /st/ words and list C contained the /sk/ items. The words had these clusters in the word-final position.
(c) Words were matched across the lists in terms of the Kucera-Francis written frequency (MRC Psycholinguistic database)[1] and for spelling irregularities.
(d) Words familiar to Rachel were preferred, but where this was not possible due to phonetic constraints, familiarity of words was balanced across the three lists. Rachel's familiarity with the words was determined by picture-naming and discussion.
(e) Words which could have the final consonant clusters reversed to yield a real word (e.g. CLASP ~ CLAPS) were favoured, although this was not possible for all items.
(f) Each list of words was treated in a different way: List A was randomly selected as the speech-only treatment list; List B was randomly selected as the discrimination-only treatment list; and List C as the discrimination and speech treatment list.

The three stimuli lists are presented in Table 9.3.

The main aims of the intervention were to improve Rachel's speech processing so that she was able to discriminate closely related sounds more accurately, and to improve the accuracy of her speech production for consonant clusters. The intervention was designed to address these aims, and in addition to allow for comparison in the change brought about for each list. We had considered the aspects of the speech processing model that were being targeted by each part of the intervention. However, the

Table 9.3: Rachel's stimuli lists for treatment

List A: /sp/ Speech treatment	List B: /st/ Auditory discrimination treatment	List C: /sk/ Auditory discrimination and speech treatment
CLASP	HASTE	RISK
GASP	WEST	DESK
LISP	GUST	DISK
CRISP	BOAST	BRISK
CUSP	JEST	CASK
GRASP	VEST	TASK
RASP	FEAST	FLASK
WASP	ROOST	DUSK
WISP	CRUST	KIOSK
UNCLASP	RUST	TUSK

next question we asked ourselves was: What is the extent of the generalization that might feasibly occur, and how would we evaluate this? Issues related to this important question are discussed in the following section.

Untreated Control Items

In Chapter 3 we introduced the notion of using control stimuli to evaluate the wider effects of intervention. Control wordlists need to be designed to answer specific questions about intervention. The questions asked about intervention will tell us how the stimuli need to be designed. For example, if we want to know whether an intervention has been effective in bringing about changes in specific features of speech that were addressed in an intervention, e.g. word-final /k/, then we would need to design a wordlist which contains items matched to the therapy stimuli as closely as possible, but which were not addressed in intervention. If therapy involved working on words such as BOOK, PACK, SOCK, then our control wordlist might consist of matched words such as BACK, PECK, SICK. These words have been designed by keeping the consonants constant and altering vowels. The aim is to create wordlists which are as identical as possible so that if improvement is shown on one list we are able to make fair comparisons between the two lists without having to take into account semantic or phonological differences.

For another child we might want to evaluate intervention aimed at updating a child's motor programs to include CCVC words (e.g. FLAT) rather than immature attempts at FLAT such as 'fat'. In order to evaluate whether generalization had extended beyond updating of stored motor programs to the child's online motor programming ability we would need to devise novel words or non-words of the same CCVC structure. In Activity 3.3 in Chapter 3, we showed examples of 10 core vocabulary words used with a child with inconsistent speech. We also showed 10 non-words matched to these core words. These non-words were not worked on in intervention but were used to monitor the effects of intervention on other parts of the child's speech processing system. Our hypothesis was that by revising Ruth's stored motor programs for commonly used words we might shake up her online motor programming too. One way of testing this was to get her to repeat non-words, and make comparisons between her performance before and after intervention.

ACTIVITY 9.3

Imagine you have been planning Rachel's intervention. Answer the following questions about generalization.

(a) What questions would you want to ask about generalization arising from the intervention programme as planned above?
(b) For each question, give an example of the stimuli you would use to evaluate this.
(c) What additional control measures would you employ so that you can make claims for the effectiveness and specificity of your intervention, i.e. how will you prove that she was not just improving anyhow or through classroom work?

Now turn to the Key to Activity 9.3 at the end of this chapter. Then read the following.

In Rachel's case we posed a range of questions about the extent of generalization that might occur and used a fairly long list of control words to monitor the extent of this. The questions we asked were as follows.

(a) Will there be generalization to the same clusters, i.e. /sp, st, sk/ in word initial speech production?
(b) Will Rachel's online motor-programming and planning have improved so that she is able to accurately produce non-words which contain the treated consonant clusters?
(c) Will generalization extend to other untreated [s] consonant clusters?
(d) Will singleton [s] production improve as a result of the [s] cluster intervention?
(e) Will production of other fricatives improve as a result of the fricative [s] treatment?
(f) Will auditory discrimination of closely related non-words improve generally?
(g) Will improved speech output result in improved written forms, and are Rachel's speech difficulties reflected in her spelling?

These questions led to the development of controls words not targeted in therapy, shown in Table 9.4.

We generated many questions and many associated control words. In some situations and with some children it would not be possible or appropriate to investigate each of these areas. Getting Rachel to name each of the treated (Table 9.3) items and untreated control items (Table 9.4) was time consuming. If we had not been able to investigate all of these many areas it would still have been helpful to pose selected questions together with selected appropriate stimuli, albeit on a smaller scale. Figure 9.3 summarizes the design of Rachel's intervention programme.

Baseline evaluation took place prior to intervention at T1 when Rachel was 7 years, 7 months. T2 assessment took place after completion of the

Table 9.4: Rachel's control stimuli for assessment pre- and post-intervention, to be used to answer a range of research questions

Question	Controls items used to answer questions		
(a) Will there be generalization to the same clusters in word-initial speech production?	[sp]	[st]	[sk]
	SPECK	STEAK	SKETCH
	SPIKE	STAFF	SKUNK
	SPACE	STAR	SKI
	SPANNER	STOOL	SKIRT
	SPADE	STAIN	SKATE
(b) Will Rachel's online motor programming and planning have improved so that she is able to accurately produce non-words which contain the treated consonant clusters?	[sp]	[st]	[sk]
	[mʊsp]	[dɛst]	[bɒsk]
	[fɪsp]	[gɛɪst]	[dæsk]
	[pisp]	[nɛʊst]	[kɒsk]
	[bæsp]	[vist]	[maɪsk]
	[tɛsp]	[bɪst]	[faʊsk]
(c) Will generalization extend to other untreated [s] consonant clusters?	[sn]	[sm]	[sl]
	SNORE	SMASH	SLIME
	SNAIL	SMOKE	SLIT
	[sw]	[skw]	[str]
	SWITCH	SQUIRREL	STRAWBERRY
	SWAN	SQUARE	STRONG
	[scr]	[spl]	[spr]
	SCRATCH	SPLIT	SPRAY
	SCRUB	SPLASH	SPRING
(d) Will singleton [s] production improve as a result of the [s] cluster intervention?	Word-initial	Within-word	Word-final
	SOCK	PERSON	CASE
	SADDLE	ASSEMBLY	MOUSE
	SALAD	BASKET	CROSS
	SEAL	BISCUIT	ADDRESS
	SALT	PLASTER	CLASS
(e) Will production of other fricatives improve as a result of the fricative [s] treatment?	[z]	[θ]	[f]
	Word-initial	Word-initial	Word-final
	ZOO	THIEF	LEAF
	ZEBRA	THIN	ROOF
	ZED	Within-word	GIRAFFE
	ZERO	TOOTHBRUSH	CALF
	ZIP	TOOTHPASTE	KNIFE
	Within-word	Word-final	
	MUSIC	MOTH	
	EASEL	TEETH	
	POISON		
	PIZZA		
	RAISIN		
	Word-final		
	MAZE		
	SIZE		
	BANANAS		
	ROSE		
	BUZZ		

Table 9.4: *Continued*

Question	Controls items used to answer questions		
(f) Will auditory discrimination of closely related non-words improve generally?	[sp]	[st]	[sk]
	[hʊsp] [hʊps]	[dɪst] [dɪts]	[gɒsk] [gɒks]
	[vʊsp] [vʊps]	[kɛst] [kɛts]	[fɪsk] [fɪks]
	[bɛsp] [bɛps]	[fɒst] [fɒts]	[mɛsk] [mɛks]
	[tisp] [tips]	[nust] [nuts]	[pusk] [puks]
	[kɜsp] [kɜps]	[θʊst] [θʊts]	[disk] [diks]
(g) Will improved speech output result in improved written forms, and are Rachel's speech difficulties reflected in her spelling?	Control items from (a), (c), (d) and (e) above		

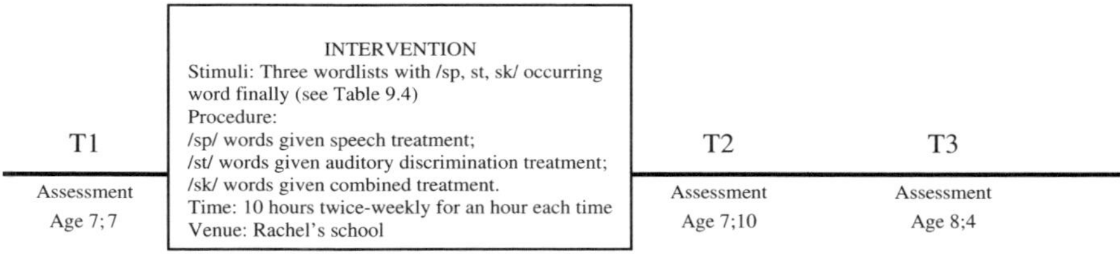

Figure 9.3: The design of Rachel's intervention programme.

intervention (aged 7 years; 10 months), and longer term follow-up after 6 months with no intervention at T3, aged 8 years, 4 months.

Outcomes: Some Answers

Treated Words

Rachel's spoken production, auditory discrimination and spelling of treated consonant clusters improved significantly over the course of the intervention. Her performance on speech, spelling and auditory discrimination tasks pre-intervention (T1) was compared with scores obtained on completion of the programme at T2, and at T3, six months later using paired samples t-tests (see Pring, 2005, for further details of this statistical test). The difference in change between the three wordlists was not significant, despite the fact that they had been treated using different interventions. By the final assessment Rachel was obtaining scores of 90–100% accuracy in her production of the treated words.

Untreated Controls

We returned to the questions posed initially about generalization. Let us consider each of these in turn.

(a) Will there be generalization to the same clusters, i.e. /sp, st, sk/ in word-initial speech production, e.g. SPOON, SKIRT, STOOL?

Yes. Rachel was able to generalize from the clusters targeted in word-final position in intervention, to untreated items where the clusters appeared in a different word position.

(b) Will Rachel's online motor programming and planning have improved so that she is able to accurately produce non-words which contain the treated consonant clusters, e.g. [mʊsp], [bɪst], [θɪsk]?

Yes, Rachel made significant gains in her production of the non-words. At the final assessment (T3) she was able to produce all the non-word items with 100% accuracy, suggesting that her online motor programming had improved.

(c) Will generalization extend to other untreated [s] consonant clusters, e.g. /spr/ in SPRAY, and /sn/ in SNORE?

No. Rachel's performance on the control words with /s/ clusters in word-initial position did not differ significantly between pre- and post-intervention. She was able to accurately produce the two-element /s/ clusters, i.e. /sn, sm, sl, sw/, at T1 and thus the intervention had little impact on these clusters, except perhaps to consolidate them at a conversational level. Three-part /s-/ clusters, e.g. /skw, str, skr, spl, spr/, were not accurately produced in the pre-intervention phase, or following intervention.

(d) Will singleton [s] production improve as a result of the [s] cluster intervention, e.g. SOCK, PERSON, CASE?

Yes. A significant difference was found between Rachel's T1 performance on the /s/ singleton words and her performance post-intervention. At T1 Rachel found word-initial /s/ production slightly, but not significantly, more challenging than /s/ in word-final position or within words. At T2 assessment she was scoring 100% for each of the three word positions. This was supported by observations from Rachel herself and from her teachers that she could now say /s/.

(e) Will production of other fricatives improve as a result of the fricative [s] treatment, e.g. THIN, ZOO?

Yes. Rachel improved in her ability to accurately realize non-treated fricatives and was approaching ceiling (i.e. 100% accuracy) by the end of the intervention.

(f) Will auditory discrimination of closely related non-words improve generally?

Yes and no. Rachel's auditory discrimination was assessed by asking her to make same/different judgments about non-word pairs such as [hʊsp]/[hʊps]. There was no significant change in Rachel's auditory discrimination of /sk/ from pre- to post-intervention. /sk/ words received the combined speech and auditory discrimination intervention. However, discrimination of /sp/ and /st/ did improve significantly from pre- to post-intervention.

(g) Will improved speech output result in improved written forms?
Yes. Rachel's spelling of the treated words improved significantly from pre- to post-intervention. However, no significant changes were noted for the control words from pre- to post-intervention. It should however be noted that Rachel's spelling of the control items at T1 was significantly better than her spelling of the treatment words which meant that there was less scope for making gains with the control words.

What Did We Learn from Rachel's Intervention?

Rachel's intervention informs us about generalization patterns that can occur in a school-age child with PSDs. Rachel's intervention was effective in bringing about significant gains in her production of the three targeted /s/ clusters. However, practitioners typically strive for greater gains extending beyond the specific words addressed in intervention. In Rachel's case we had carefully selected a range of control stimuli which would allow us to answer specific questions about the extent of generalization. The patterns of change observed in the control stimuli informed our knowledge of the two major types of generalization, introduced earlier in the chapter: across-item generalization and across-task generalization. We consider each of these areas in turn.

Across-item Generalization

We found that working on word-final /s/ clusters resulted in significant changes in Rachel's production of word-initial clusters. In general, research suggests that generalization from a segment treated in one word position to another word position can occur (e.g. Elbert and McReynolds, 1975). However, the question has not been specifically investigated for clusters, and has been minimally investigated with older children with PSDs. Similarly, generalization was noted from the treated words to untreated non-words. This supported our original hypothesis that addressing stored motor programs through intervention would shake up online motor programming of new words.

Generalization did not extend to other untreated /s/ clusters such as /sm/ and /spr/. Research into /s/ clusters – and particularly /s/ + stop clusters – has suggested that this group of sounds should be treated differently from other clusters since they are fundamentally different from other clusters. In Chapter 5 we reviewed evidence about the /s/ + stop clusters. For example, in words with initial /sp, st, sk/ consonant clusters the sonority sequencing principle is not adhered to as the more sonorous fricative precedes the less sonorous stop, e.g. consider words like SPOT and SPOON. The vowel forms the sonorous peak but the /p/ in the onset cluster is the lowest point, rising again for the /s/ that precedes it. It is for this reason that /s/ clusters have sometimes not been considered true clusters but rather adjunct clusters where /s/ is regarded as an adjunct (or attachment) to the rest of the syllable, which will then follow the rules of sonority. Rachel's intervention addressing /s/ + stop clusters did not lead to gains in other /s/ clusters, but did result in improvements in words with singleton /s/ as well as other fricatives. These findings support the work of Hodson (1997, and see Chapter 5). She suggests that /s/ clusters be incorporated as primary potential targets in her cycles approach for children with highly unintelligible speech. She suggests that /s/ clusters should be targeted before singleton stridents such as /s/ because working on the /s/ clusters will involve working on stridency - the forceful airflow striking the back of the teeth - and may have greater overall effects on a child's intelligibility overall.

Across-task Generalization

Rachel received three different treatments for three different stimuli lists. This makes across-task generalization fairly difficult to evaluate. Nevertheless, there was some evidence for across-task generalization.

- The /sp/ words received a speech treatment. For these words, Rachel's auditory discrimination had improved although this was not directly addressed with these words, e.g. she showed improved ability to distinguish between words such as RASP/RAPS.
- The /st/ words received an auditory treatment. For these words, Rachel's speech production had improved although speech work was not directly done on these items, e.g. she produced words like HASTE and WEST with increased accuracy.
- Rachel's spelling of the treated /sp, st, sk/ words improved as a result of intervention. Spelling was not the direct focus of the intervention for any of these wordlists, although Rachel was exposed to written stimuli during the intervention.

Rachel received a dual speech and auditory treatment for the /sk/ words. Her ability to make same/different auditory discrimination judgments did not improve for contrasts involving /sk/ (e.g. WHISK/WICKS), although her speech production of these words did. We suggest that the combined speech and auditory treatment may have been confusing for Rachel and did not allow her to consolidate her auditory discrimination ability with these specific stimuli.

The intervention described with Rachel provides some interesting insights into generalization patterns that occurred with one child with PSDs. The findings need to be contextualized within the body of literature that already exists on the topic of generalization. Rachel is clearly just one individual child and the results for other children may be very different. The extent of the generalization that occurred with Rachel was fairly large compared to other studies. One of the reasons for this may be methodological: a very wide range of control stimuli was selected to give the greatest chance of observing such effects. Glogowska (2001) has noted, 'what shows up in terms of change . . . largely depends on what you chose to measure and how you measured it in the first place' (p. 7).

Generalization: Suggestions for Intervention

- Achieving generalization involves careful planning, especially for children with PSDs.
- Be clear about the aspects of the speech processing system you are targeting in intervention, and use this and your knowledge of theoretical models (e.g. the speech processing model shown in Figure 2.3 in Chapter 2 and referred to in Rachel's case in this chapter) to determine the extent of generalization that might feasibly occur.
- Develop questions about generalization that you would like to be able to answer on completion of intervention. Use these questions to guide the development of appropriate stimuli, as we did in Rachel's case.
- Refer to the evidence base that already exists on generalization, bearing in mind that children with speech difficulties are part of a heterogeneous population.
- Consider both main types of generalization: across-item and across-task, bearing in mind that to evaluate across-item generalization you need to design and select stimuli carefully, and to evaluate across-task generalization you will need to keep your stimuli constant.
- Ensure that any changes noted can be attributed to your intervention rather than general effects such as maturation. This can be done by achieving a stable pre-intervention baseline; evaluating performance on tasks that are not related to tasks addressed in therapy and thus where generalization would not feasibly be expected to occur.
- Choose as many control items as possible and practical for your circumstances. In doing so you will be able to answer a range of questions about generalization and be able to contribute to the evidence base in a valuable way.

Summary

The key points are as follows.

- Generalization is the extent to which a targeted area addressed in intervention results in changes beyond the specific aspect addressed.
- Across-item generalization is where generalization occurs from treated stimuli to matched but untreated stimuli.
- Across-task generalization is where generalization occurs from a treated task (e.g. speech) to an untreated task (e.g. spelling).
- Evidence exists about the nature and extent of generalization that can arise from phonological intervention, but findings are not consistent and vary widely from child to child.
- Across-item generalization may be more readily achieved than across-task generalization, although this may be because the latter is not always measured.
- Rachel's case gave an example of how to evaluate generalization and its extent to untreated stimuli and tasks.
- Three different interventions were carried out with Rachel, each addressing a wordlist with specific /s/ clusters in word-final position.
- Intervention was shown to be effective as Rachel made significant gains in her speech production, auditory discrimination and spelling of the treated words.
- A range of control items were used to evaluate generalization.
- Rachel showed generalization to a range of control items including words with the /s/ clusters in word-initial position, matched non-words, words with singleton /s/ in all word positions and words with other fricatives.
- Generalization was not found to extend to other untreated /s/ clusters such as /sm/ and /sn/.
- Rachel showed across-task generalization from her speech production to her spelling and auditory discrimination of closely related words.

KEY TO ACTIVITY 9.1

(a) Does Rachel experience any difficulties with input? Outline the levels of input processing at which any difficulties occur.

Yes, Rachel has some difficulties with input. Specifically she experiences difficulty with the auditory discrimination of closely related non-words (Level B) in the Bridgeman and Snowling (1988) task, e.g. VOST/VOTS. She also experiences difficulties with the same test where real words are used, e.g. LOST/LOTS (Level D) although the difficulties are not as severe as for non-words, as indicated by the three XXXs at level B and one X at Level D indicative of standard deviations below the mean for her age. For more details of the Bridgeman and Snowling (1988) task see Chapter 5 (Table 5.4) and also Stackhouse *et al.*'s (forthcoming) compendium of psycholinguistic tests for children.

(b) Does Rachel have any difficulties with output? Compare her performance at various levels of speech production.

Rachel also experiences output difficulties. She has difficulties at Levels G, I and J of the output part of the profile with picture naming tasks, real word and non-word repetition. However, at each of these levels of the profile there are tasks where Rachel performs in an age-appropriate way, e.g. at Level I she performs below age on the Constable repetition test (Constable *et al.*, 1997) but in an age-appropriate way on other repetition tests such as the Aston Index blending subtest (Newton and Thompson, 1982). This suggests that she has basic skills at each of these levels but some of the more challenging tasks reveal weaknesses.

(c) Are there any links that you might be looking for between her input and output?

The Bridgeman and Snowling (1988) auditory discrimination tasks involve discrimination of /s/ and /t/ segments in words such as LOT and LOSS, as well as the discrimination of /st/ and /ts/ clusters in words such as LOTS and LOST (See Chapter 5, Table 5.4). Given Rachel's difficulties in hearing the difference between such closely related words, she might have difficulties in the production of words involving segments such as /s/, /t/ or /s/ clusters, although this will not necessarily be the case.

KEY TO ACTIVITY 9.2

(a) What aspect of Rachel's phonological system would you choose to target in intervention?

We chose to target Rachel's /s/ + stop clusters: /sp, st, sk/ because she has specific difficulties with these rather than general difficulties with clusters.

(b) Why would you select the target?

Evidence from intervention studies suggests that /s/ clusters appear to be different to other clusters in their response to intervention. In particular, treatment of /s/ + stop clusters (i.e. /st, sp, sk/) has been shown to result in little generalization to other clusters suggesting that they may not be a good starting point if hoping to affect all clusters through intervention. However, Rachel has difficulties specific to /s/ clusters rather than affecting all clusters, and there is evidence from the literature that working on /s/ clusters may result in improvement in these sounds as well as improvements in singleton /s/ (Hodson, 1997).

KEY TO ACTIVITY 9.3

(a) What questions would you want to ask about generalization arising from the intervention programme as planned above?

The questions we asked were as follows.

1. Will there be generalization to the same clusters, i.e. /sp, st, sk/ in word-initial speech production?
2. Will Rachel's online motor programming and planning have improved so that she is able to accurately produce non-words which contain the treated consonant clusters?
3. Will generalization extend to other untreated [s] consonant clusters?
4. Will singleton [s] production improve as a result of the [s] cluster intervention?
5. Will production of other fricatives improve as a result of the fricative [s] treatment?
6. Will auditory discrimination of closely related non-words improve generally?
7. Will improved speech output result in improved written forms and are Rachel's speech difficulties reflected in her spelling?

(b) For each question, give an example of the stimuli you would use to evaluate this.

1. Will there be generalization to the same clusters, i.e. /sp, st, sk/ in word-initial speech production? Control words: SPECK, STEAK, SKETCH.
2. Will Rachel's online motor programming and planning have improved so that she is able to accurately produce non-words which contain the treated consonant clusters? Control words: [mʊsp], [dɛst], [bɒsk].
3. Will generalization extend to other untreated [s] consonant clusters? Control words: SNORE, SWITCH, SLIME.
4. Will singleton [s] production improve as a result of the [s] cluster intervention? Control words: SOCK, PERSON, CASE.
5. Will production of other fricatives improve as a result of the fricative [s] treatment? Control words: ZOO, THIN.

6. Will auditory discrimination of closely related non-words improve generally? Control words: [hʊsp] v. [hʊps].
7. Will improved speech output result in improved written forms and are Rachel's speech difficulties reflected in her spelling? Control words: Words from 1, 3, 4 and 5 above.

(c) What additional control measures would you employ so that you can make claims for the effectiveness and specificity of your intervention, i.e. how will you prove that she was not just improving anyhow or through classroom work?

We carried out assessment of Rachel's mathematical and general language abilities. If we could demonstrate that Rachel did not make significant gains in these areas, then it would be reasonable to conclude that our specific intervention had resulted in the specific speech processing changes. We also obtained a stable pre-intervention baseline, and carried out longer-term follow-up after intervention had ceased. A stable pre-intervention baseline demonstrates that a child is not improving before intervention starts. Long-term follow-up provides information about the long-term effects of the intervention, i.e. whether any changes have been maintained or whether these were lost due to a recency effect.

Note

1. http://www.psy.uwa.edu.au/mrcdatabase/uwa_mrc.htm.

Chapter 10
Linking with Literacy

In the same way that spoken language comprises different skills (e.g. vocabulary development, comprehension, expression, appropriate use of language for a given context, speech), written language also has its own related skills (e.g. word recognition, decoding text, abstraction of meaning, expressive and functional writing, spelling). Problems with any one or more of the skills comprising spoken language can have an impact on the development of written language. In turn, delayed written language development inhibits later development of language skills derived from reading texts, e.g. more advanced vocabulary and understanding. Children with spoken language difficulties are at risk of developing problems with written language early on because they have a shaky foundation on which to build their literacy skills, and if not resolved can enter a downward spiral as they are not being exposed to the same language and experiences embedded in printed material as their peer group. However, it can be difficult to predict precisely how children's problems with spoken language skills will impact on the nature of their written language development: '. . . pure reading disorders are rare; different language skills interact to produce a spectrum of reading outcomes' (Snowling and Stackhouse, 2006, p. 320).

Whatever the cocktail of language problems a child with PSDs presents, one robust finding is that children with PSDs are particularly at risk for difficulties with phonological awareness and spelling. Further, these difficulties can be associated with problems not only at the output level but also with input (e.g. auditory discrimination of similar sounding words or words containing segments that they have trouble producing), and in the lexical representations (e.g. fuzzy storage of items). However, with appropriate ongoing support at school and home, children with PSDs can make progress with both their spoken and written language difficulties and not necessarily face insurmountable problems academically (Nathan and Simpson, 2001) and psychosocially (Nash, 2006). A positive attitude by all involved is an essential ingredient. Take Ben for example, a boy aged 9;2 with PSDs, who commented:

> Reading and spelling are very important at school . . . for learning . . . For example if you are learning about animals you read a book on animals. I don't like reading at school because the books are hard but I like reading at home. I have to practise spelling . . . I want to get a prize in assembly.

Later in this chapter we will tell you more about Ben's intervention and how we tried to involve both spoken and written stimuli. We will share suggestions based on working with other children with speech and literacy difficulties and examine the role of the speech and language therapist in the light of this. But first, let us examine further the links between speech, literacy and phonological awareness.

Speech, Spelling and Phonological Awareness

Speech

A basic premise of the psycholinguistic approach to children's speech difficulties is that their difficulties arise from problems at one or more points in their underlying speech processing system. Such problems, however, do not just impact on speech and intelligibility; clear and consistent speech production is particularly important for spelling or when learning new vocabulary. Typically, when asked how many syllables there are in a word (an important phonological awareness skill), children repeat the word, segment it out loud or in a whisper and then count the beats on their fingers. We do this task with children in order to help them reflect and rehearse the structure of words so that when exposed to new vocabulary or when asked to spell a word they have the strategies necessary to achieve new word learning or spelling. If they are not able to produce the right number of syllables in the word or if they cannot say the word in the same way on more than one occasion then they will not be able to rehearse and store the new word or spell it correctly. For example, when trying to spell a multi-syllabic word, Kevin, a 12-year-old boy with apraxia of speech and dyslexic difficulties said exasperatedly: 'If I can't say it I can't split it up!' (from Stackhouse, 1996, p. 19).

In a longitudinal study by Nathan, Stackhouse, Goulandris and Snowling (2004a) 47 children, who had been referred for speech and language therapy at 3 years of age because of concerns about their speech development, were followed up between the ages of 4 and 7 years and compared to matched controls without speech difficulties. Approximately 25% of the children with speech difficulties resolved their speech difficulties by the end of the study when the children were around 7 years of age. Those children whose speech difficulties persisted generally had more severe speech difficulties, speech input processing problems (auditory discrimination difficulties) and delayed language skills. The PSDs were associated with poorer literacy outcome in which spelling was a particular difficulty (see following section).

However, not all speech difficulties impact on written language performance in the same way and it is important to consider the nature of a child's speech difficulties when evaluating risk for literacy difficulties. Studies of children with motor execution difficulties (arising from cleft lip and palate or cerebral palsy) affecting only Level K on the speech processing profile (bottom right of Figure 2.1 in Chapter 2) suggest that such speech difficulties are not necessarily linked to spelling problems (e.g. Stackhouse, 1982; Bishop and Robson, 1989). Similarly, children with isolated articulation difficulties (e.g. lisps) are not necessarily at an increased risk of having literacy problems provided that they have no language difficulties and that their articulation difficulties are not severe (Bishop and Clarkson, 2003). Type of speech difficulty may however influence outcome. Dodd, Gillon, Oerlemans, Russell, Syrmis and Wilson (1995) found that children described as having 'disordered phonology' were more at risk of spelling difficulties than children with 'delayed phonology' or 'articulation difficulties'. This finding has some support from a follow-up study of 14 children with speech difficulties at age 12–13 years who had been tracked since they were around 5 years of age (Leitao and Fletcher, 2004). It was those children with an original diagnosis of 'non-developmental speech errors' – rather than those with a 'developmental delay' – who performed less well on phonological awareness and literacy measures (see Dodd, 2005, for further discussion of speech subgroups and literacy outcome).

Bishop and Clarkson (2003) investigated the speech, language and literacy skills of 161 normally-developing control children aged from 7.5 to 13 years and 75 twin children of the same age who either had specific speech–language impairments, or were co-twins of affected children. Written narratives were elicited from children using a sequence of five photographs depicting a simple story. This is a challenging task for children with speech and language difficulties and an appropriate way of tapping into higher level language and literacy skills. The children's narratives were analysed for grammatical complexity and accuracy, intelligibility, and semantic content. Only 42 of the twin children could spell well enough to attempt the narrative task. Some co-twins of affected children had deficits in written language, despite normal performance on oral language tests. Their literacy difficulties were less obvious than those of children with overt PSDs. Most children with language impairments found the writing task difficult with particularly marked deficits on measures of spelling and punctuation. The children with language impairments made a relatively higher proportion of phonologically inaccurate spelling errors when compared to younger children at a similar vocabulary level. Those with a poor performance on a non-word repetition test were especially likely to have poor written language. Non-word repetition tests are particularly challenging for children with PSDs (see Rachel's speech processing profile in Figure 9.1, Chapter 9) and can be used to identify children whose difficulties are persisting even when they appear to have resolved their difficulties in familiar everyday speech.

In summary, authors agree that speech difficulties impact on literacy outcomes when they are more severe, are characterized by atypical speech errors, persist beyond the age of five and a half years, and co-occur with language difficulties (Stackhouse, 2006).

Spelling

Bishop and Clarkson (2003) note that literacy research has focused more on reading than spelling, and that it has often been argued that spelling performance can be deduced from reading performance since the two are typically highly correlated. However, this is not necessarily the case, particularly for children with PSDs where there are more likely to be dissociations between the skills comprising literacy performance.

A study by Clarke-Klein and Hodson (1995) revealed that children with histories of speech difficulties made more phonologically deviant misspellings than their normally-developing peers. Speech sound errors do not necessarily map directly onto spelling errors (Snowling and Stackhouse, 1983; McCormack, 1995; Gillon and Dodd, 2005), but rather difficulty with speech may result in imprecise phonological representations of words in the lexicon (Treiman, 1985; Stackhouse, 2006), resulting in inconsistent erroneous spellings. Phonological knowledge is the bridge linking speech and spelling. Children with speech sound disorders at preschool may be at risk for later spelling difficulties due to poor phonological awareness and difficulties in phonological coding in verbal memory. Bishop and Adams (1990) contrasted literacy outcomes for two groups of 8-year-old children: a group whose speech difficulties had resolved and a group whose speech difficulties remained. They found that a significant number of the children with persisting speech problems had literacy difficulties, while their resolved counterparts did not. The proposed critical age hypothesis suggests that if children can resolve their speech and language difficulties by the age of five-and-a-half years then literacy problems are less likely to ensue. However, defining and recognizing a resolved speech difficulty is not straightforward. There are some indications that a history of speech and language difficulties may still put a child at risk for spelling difficulties in particular, even when the speech difficulties seem to be no longer present. Nathan, Stackhouse, Goulandris and Snowling (2004b) followed up the literacy outcome at around 7 years of age of children from their longitudinal study reported above (Nathan *et al.*, 2004a). They examined the performance of 39 children from their original group of children with speech disorders and 35 matched normal controls on national *Statutory Assessment Tests* (SATs) of reading, reading comprehension, spelling, writing and maths. On comparing the performance of two groups, there were more children scoring below average in the group with speech disorders compared to the controls. Their performance was particularly poor on spelling and reading comprehension (a finding replicated by Leitao and Fletcher, 2004). Further examination of the group with speech disorders revealed that 11 out of the 39 children appeared to have resolved their speech difficulties by 7 years of age, leaving 28 with PSDs. The PSD subgroup performed significantly less well than the normal controls on all of the tests, but were particularly poor at spelling. The 11 children in the resolved subgroup performed significantly better than the children in the PSD subgroup on all of the measures and did as well as the controls on all tasks except spelling where they still had significant difficulties.

This suggests that speech processing difficulties persist and that speech and spelling share underlying phonological skills (Lewis, Freebairn and Taylor, 2002; Gillon and Dodd, 2005). A corollary of this is that as a later acquired but related skill, spelling offers an important window into a child's developing speech processing and phonological systems and should be included routinely in investigations of the nature of speech difficulties in children.

Phonological Awareness

Phonological awareness is the ability to reflect on and manipulate the structure of spoken language (e.g. into words, or syllables, or sounds). Popular phonological awareness tasks include rhyme, syllable and sound segmentation, blending and spoonerisms. Phonological awareness tasks vary widely and may include input tasks, i.e. where a child does not need to give a spoken response and could point or nod to respond to the task, e.g. rhyme judgment: Do CAT and MAT rhyme? An example of an output task involving rhyme is in rhyme generation tasks, e.g. 'Say as many words as you can that rhyme with CAT.' Phonological awareness tasks can be categorized at various levels of phonological unit, e.g. rime, syllable and segment (see Stackhouse and Wells, 1997 Chapter 3).

Children need to develop phonological awareness in order to make sense of an alphabetic script such as English. For example, children have to learn that the segments (the consonants and vowels) in a word can be represented by a written form – letters. When spelling a new word, children have to be able to divide the word into its segments before they can attach the appropriate letters. When reading an unfamiliar word, they have to be able to decode the printed letters back to segments and blend them together to form the word. Thus, it is not surprising that phonological awareness skill is associated with reading and spelling performance and, along with letter knowledge, is a strong predictor of reading outcome.

Investigations of the predictors of literacy, however, confirm that it is the phonological awareness tasks that focus at the level of the phoneme rather than the rhyme that are the best predictors of later literacy performance in both typically developing children (Muter, Hulme, Snowling and Taylor, 1998; Muter, 2006) and children with speech and language difficulties (Nathan *et al.*, 2004a). This does not mean that rhyme is not a useful skill to investigate or teach, but that in itself it is not a clear indicator of literacy performance or outcome (Stackhouse, 2001). Articulatory skill is also emerging as a predictor of literacy outcome in normally-developing children (Carroll and Snowling, 2004) particularly when dealing with complex sequences such as clusters, e.g. /spr/ (Griffiths, 2005).

It is not always possible to predict what the relationship between phonological awareness skills and literacy might be in individual children. Single-case studies have shown that children can read normally in the presence of severe phonological difficulties (Temple, Jeeves and Vilarroya, 1990; Stothard, Snowling and Hulme, 1996). Stothard *et al.* (1996) describe a girl, aged 6;6, who experienced severe difficulties with phonological awareness tasks as compared to control children, but showed normal reading and spelling development. Closer investigation of her reading did, however, reveal deficits in her non-word reading, similar to those described in the child investigated by Hulme and Snowling (1992). The two children are contrasted in terms of their phonological processing difficulties, and it is suggested that in some cases, as for the girl in Stothard *et al.*'s paper, phonological difficulties may not be sufficiently severe to constrain reading of real words. The girl was found to have some auditory perceptual difficulties, which resulted in poor performance on many phonological awareness tasks, but her phonological representations – in contrast to many other children – were normal and thus gave her the basis to develop reading and spelling in the normal way.

Other children with language difficulties, particularly those with comprehension or 'semantic–pragmatic' difficulties may appear to have intact phonological skills and decode text perfectly well. However, if stored phonological representations are not linked with semantic representations, children may read well but not understand what they have read. Such children are often described as 'hyperlexic'. This term indicates that a child can read print mechanically better than they can understand it, i.e. decoding ability extends beyond what is expected given the children's comprehension and cognitive skills (Grigorenko, Klin, Pauls, Senft, Hooper and Volkmar, 2002). However, an investigation of children with hyperlexia found that the children's phonemic awareness skills were not commensurate with their word-reading skills, and that wide inter- and intra-individual variations existed on all the phonemic awareness measures (Sparks, 2001).

Individual cases remind us that the relationship between phonological processing and literacy is not as clear-cut as it may seem. They suggest that there is not only one path of development and that the ways that children may compensate for areas of weakness need to be investigated and incorporated into intervention plans (see Gillon, 2004, for a comprehensive review of phonological awareness, literacy and intervention).

Relationship between Speech, Phonological Awareness and Literacy

There has been a tendency in both research and practice to regard phonological awareness as a completely distinct area rather than another product of the speech processing system. Phonological awareness tasks require a range of speech processing skills if they are to be completed successfully, e.g. listening; discriminating; remembering; segmenting or deleting or swapping sounds; and speech production. It is not only necessary for literacy to develop but also helps children to reflect on new words and phrases they hear and store them for use as required. Thus, difficulties within the speech processing system can lead to both speech and phonological awareness difficulties that interact to impede the development of literacy. However, this relationship is not just a one-way street: young children developing their reading and spelling become more skilled in phonological awareness and this is turn helps to refine their speech processing skills. For normally-developing children speech, literacy and phonological awareness develop together in a mutually supportive way. This is often not the case for children with PSDs who may require specific support to develop their speech, phonological awareness and literacy skills in harmony with each other.

Figure 10.1 summarizes the relationship between speech, phonological awareness and literacy, and how an intact speech processing system is the basis for development of all three areas. The speech processing system (depicted in Figure 2.3) exists to allow a child to deal with and develop spoken language. It could stay as just that if we did not expect our children to be literate as well as good conversationalists. Because of the demands made on children to develop literacy, they need to adapt and apply their spoken language skills to deal with and develop reading and writing skills. To do this they need to be aware of how print represents spoken language and its segments. Thus, it is via phonological awareness that children move their spoken language skills across (from left to right in Figure 10.1) to the literacy domain.

ACTIVITY 10.1

Consider Figure 10.1 below, which shows how the speech processing system gives rise to speech, phonological awareness and literacy. You will note the double-ended arrows linking speech and phonological awareness; and phonological awareness and literacy, which indicate the way in which

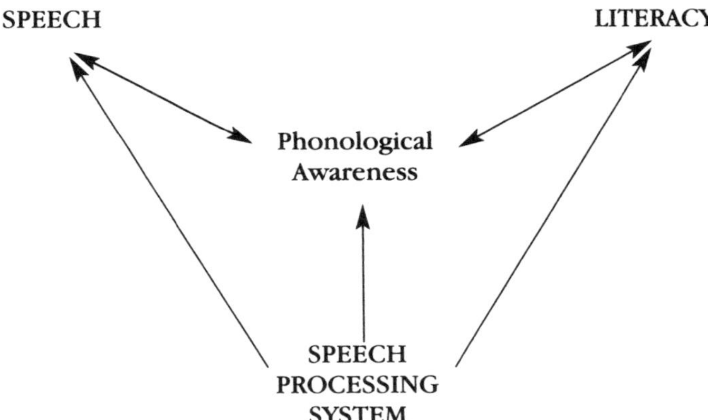

Figure 10.1: The relationship between speech, phonological awareness and literacy. (Reproduced by kind permission of Whurr Publishers from Stackhouse and Wells, 1997.)

these areas mutually support each other. Now answer a–d below, giving examples of tasks from your own experience as an adult (or if you prefer from your experience with children's development of these skills).

Give an example of a task in which:

(a) speech helps promote phonological awareness;
(b) phonological awareness supports speech;
(c) phonological awareness is used to aid literacy;
(d) literacy aids phonological awareness.

We have provided our own examples in the Key to Activity 10.1 at the end of this chapter. Read on for further development of these concepts and ideas.

Models of Literacy Development

In the UK the *National Literacy Strategy* is part of the *National Curriculum*, which all children follow at school. The *National Literacy Strategy* aims to unite the important skills of reading and writing with speaking and listening. Literacy is a main key to accessing all aspects of the curriculum; hence reading, writing, speaking and listening skills are of utmost importance. Literacy involves many different reading and spelling skills depending on the demands of the task (see Activity 1.4 in Stackhouse and Wells, 1997, pp. 20–22). For example, as adults we are able to decode nonsense or non-English words. We can also read single words, sentences, and narratives either silently or out loud. Most importantly we can understand what we read most of the time. We can make reasonable attempts at spelling nonsense words or unfamiliar words from dictation (e.g. when an unusual name is given over the telephone) and we can write sentences and narratives where our knowledge of spelling interacts with our knowledge of sentence construction, vocabulary and the broader structure and conventions of the narrative form. These sentences are often original (rather than copied or remembered) and convey meaning. Of course, none of this would have happened if we had not got a grasp of spoken language, been exposed to print and been taught the explicit links between the sounds of our language and the written forms of print (see Hatcher, 2006, for further discussion about teaching letter–sound links).

Young literacy learners have to learn how to decipher the symbols of the written language pertinent to them. For English-speaking children or adults these symbols are in the form of an alphabetic code. Their task is to learn which written symbols represent the particular sounds of a language in the process of grapheme–phoneme (i.e. letter–sound) conversion. With increased exposure to written material, orthographic representations of written words are established in the lexicon, enabling readers to recognize familiar words and bypass the mechanics of grapheme–phoneme conversion. Thus, many researchers have suggested 'dual route' models of reading: (a) grapheme–phoneme conversion taking place using the sub-lexical route to decode unfamiliar words, and (b) recognition of familiar words stored in and retrieved from the lexicon (Harley, 2001). Similarly, for writing, we need to retrieve the written representation from the orthographic lexicon, if we know the word, or alternatively to carry out phoneme–grapheme conversion in order to attempt spelling. In many cases there are no obvious rules to predict how particular words should be written (e.g. consider the rime of words such as YACHT versus POT), yet adults and children learn how to recognize and write these words through building up their orthographic knowledge – but how do they do this?

Stage models of literacy development have helped to understand not only how children progress with their reading and spelling development but also how to pinpoint when they are failing to progress. For example, Frith (1985) suggested that children with literacy difficulties are best understood by considering their development to be arrested at a particular developmental point. Frith's (1985) model is a developmental model used to conceptualize three stages of typical literacy acquisition: a logographic or whole-word recognition phase; an alphabetic phase in which grapheme–phoneme conversion is relied upon; and an orthographic phase in which stored representations can be drawn on and irregular orthography has been learnt.

- Stage 1: The iogographic phase. This is a visual phase in which children rely on whole-word recognition of words they know. They are not able to decode unfamiliar words. They recognize familiar words such as their name or the word <STOP> appearing in a road sign. Children at this stage may be able to write their own name, but in general their spelling will be non-phonetic, i.e. there will be little or no logical sound–letter correspondence, e.g. MUMMY might be spelt as <mmmnntp> or <rhdpbs>. The incidence of this type of spelling soon diminishes in young normally-developing children, but it can persist in many children with a history of speech difficulties (Dodd *et al.*, 1995).

- Stage 2: The alphabetic phase. When children are able to apply letter–sound rules to decode new words they are able to break through into the alphabetic stage. When reading they will now be able to sound out individual segments and then blend them together to make a word. Spelling may initially be semi-phonetic in this stage with children showing some logical letter–sound matches but also omitting vowels, and using some consonants to represent syllables, e.g. TELEPHONE → <tlf> and sounded out as [tɛ lə fəʊ]. Gradually children learn how to fill in these gaps and spelling becomes more logical and phonetically based, e.g. TELEPHONE → <telafon>. Target words are recognizable even if the spelling is not conventional. Children segment the word successfully and apply their letter knowledge but have yet to learn the conventions of English spelling (see Activity 1.2 in Stackhouse and Wells (2001, p. 8) for an analysis of emergent spelling skills in a 6-year-old girl's writing of a popular nursery rhyme).
- Stage 3: The orthographic phase. In this phase, the child acquires the conventions of English orthography. They are able to recognize larger chunks of words such as prefixes like <un> and <non> in words like UNHAPPY and NON-SMOKER, as well as suffixes such as <ion> in words like ADDITION and VISION. Having this knowledge means that children can read similar words by analogy, which means more efficient reading.

Frith's stage-based model of literacy fits well with Stackhouse and Wells's (1997) developmental phase model of speech development summarized in Chapter 2 (see Figure 2.4). In this phase model, children's speech development progresses through five successive phases:

(1) pre-lexical
(2) whole word
(3) systematic simplification
(4) assembly
(5) metaphonological.

It is proposed that children who move through these phases smoothly have the phonological skills to support their literacy development. In particular, children need to enter the systematic simplification phase, characterized by consistent use of simplification processes, in order for them to begin to reflect on their speech and develop phonological awareness skills typical of the later metaphonological phase. In contrast, children who are arrested at the whole word stage where speech may be inconsistent, or show atypical features particularly as the child gets older, will have trouble developing phonological awareness and associated literacy skills. The premise of this model is that difficulties within any one of these phases, or with moving from one phase to another, will result in both speech and literacy difficulties. However, it is the phase(s) at which a child's speech development is problematic or arrested that will determine the nature of the associated speech difficulties and the likelihood of associated literacy problems (see Chapter 2, Figure 2.5).

We can now map these speech phases onto Frith's literacy phases (see Figure 10.2). Both models assume a necessary pre-lexical stage where children are developing early language skills. At the whole-word level of speech production, children experience a parallel phase in literacy - the logographic phase - where they can recognize familiar words as wholes (e.g. name of their favourite cereal) but cannot read or recognize unfamiliar words. Children may be able to write a known word at this stage, e.g. their own name, but generally spelling may appear to be a random string of letters and it is not always easy to guess what the target is. They then become increasingly sensitive to the components of words. This is marked in speech by the increased and consistent use of simplifying processes as they attempt to master the sound structure of their language and learn to assemble the components into connected speech (the assembly phase). In the metaphonological stage children are able to reflect on the sound structure of their language in an abstract way. At this point they are able to break through to the alphabetic stage of literacy development and read unfamiliar words by sounding them out and spelling in a more logical way by using letter-sound knowledge even if the result is not conventionally correct. Mastering these skills means that children will have acquired the foundations of speech and literacy. Further stages of development involve refinement of the skills and experience of irregular and unusual forms. They will go on to apply their morphophonological knowledge to recognize chunks of words, e.g. <tion> in ADDITION and to spell these. However, even in normally developing children with no obvious speech or literacy difficulties, this progression through a series of stages of literacy development does not occur in all cases. Individual children have been described who omit the alphabetic phase but still go on to establish a well-developed orthographic system (e.g. see Campbell and Butterworth, 1985; Stothard *et al.*, 1996). Further, this proposed sequence of development may well be language specific and different patterns have been described in different languages (Wimmer, 1996). Adopting this devel-

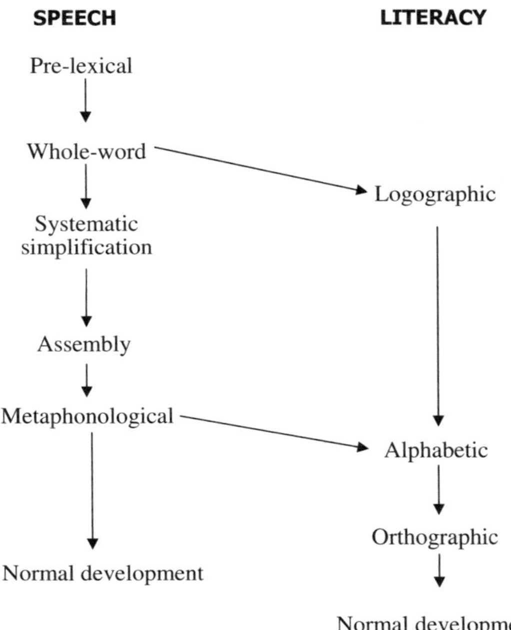

Figure 10.2: The relationship between the phases of speech and literacy development. (Reproduced with kind permission of Whurr Publishers from Stackhouse and Wells, 1997.)

opmental perspective allows us to understand more about the relationship between speech and literacy and in particular between speech and spelling (see Activity 10.2).

ACTIVITY 10.2

Aim: To examine spelling errors from a developmental perspective.

Consider the following spelling attempts from Ben, aged 8;9.

Target	Spelling
STAMP	sramp
STRING	sring
CHEESE	tees
JAM	jam
FRIDGE	frith
SHARP	sarp
MASH	mas

Now answer the following questions.

(a) At which stage of Frith's model of literacy development (shown in Figure 10.2) is Ben at?
(b) What questions do you have about Ben's speech and spelling?

We suggest answers to these questions in the Key to Activity 10.2 at the end of this chapter. Further details of Ben and his speech and spelling are presented in the case section of this chapter.

Integrated Approaches to Speech, Phonological Awareness and Literacy

Some phonological interventions can be considered on a continuum with phonological awareness interventions (see Stackhouse, Wells, Pascoe and Rees, 2002, for a review). For example, Gillon (2000) used a phonological awareness intervention approach with children (ages 5;6–7;6) with spoken language impairments and matched control children. Children with spoken language impairment were allocated to three different treatment groups: (a) an integrated phonological awareness program, (b) a traditional program that focused on improving articulation and language skills, and (c) a minimal intervention control group. The phonological awareness tasks in this study aimed to improve children's awareness of sound structure in spoken language and to develop explicit knowledge of the links between spoken and written word forms. The traditional therapy involved a phoneme-oriented, articulatory approach and, in some severe cases, activities from the *Nuffield Centre Dyspraxia Programme* (Connery, 1992; revised by Williams and Stephens, 2004) were used. This is a program of graded sessions to teach articulatory placement and coordination of motor speech sequences. The study found that children who received phonological awareness training obtained age-appropriate levels of literacy performance, and in addition their speech articulation improved. Gillon concluded that the presence of a severe phonological impairment does not restrict a child's access to the benefits of phonological awareness training.

Following on from this, Gillon (2005) set up a three-year longitudinal study of 12 children with moderate to severe speech difficulties. These children received therapy targeting speech and phonological awareness and their performance was compared with 19 normally developing controls and with a group of matched children who also had speech difficulties but who did not receive specific phonological awareness training. The results suggest that children as young as 3–4 years of age can benefit from phonological awareness training and that phonological awareness can be incorporated into a speech and language therapy programme which also targets intelligibility.

Intervention studies (e.g. Harbers, Paden and Halle, 1999; Hesketh, Adams and Hall, 2000; Denne, Langdown, Pring and Roy, 2005) have been more cautious in their interpretation of the benefits of phonological awareness training on speech output performance. Harbers *et al.* found that the rate and degree of change in phonological awareness did not always parallel production performance. Similarly, Denne *et al.* (2005) caution against using phonological awareness therapy in isolation from therapy that targets speech production more directly. They randomly assigned 20 children (age range 5-7 years) with 'expressive phonological disorder' to either a treatment or a non-treatment group. The children in the treatment group received 12 hours of phonological awareness therapy. The results revealed that the treated group did indeed improve their phonological awareness skills but that there was no difference between the treated and non-treated groups on speech or literacy outcome. A comparison of phonological awareness therapy and articulatory training approaches for children with phonological disorders (aged 3;6–5;0) was carried out by Hesketh *et al.* They found both types of therapy effective in enhancing phonological awareness skills and speech output, when contrasted with speech and phonological awareness gains made in a control group of normally-developing children over the same period. However, no effect of therapy type was found in this study. Such comparisons of articulation vs. metaphonological therapies are problematic in that conventional articulation therapy can often be seen to require and encourage metaphonological awareness, although to a lesser extent than the pure phonological awareness training condition.

Stackhouse *et al.* (2002 p. 15) note:

> the threads of a therapy program need to be knitted together for an individual child in order to take into account individual differences. Phonological awareness runs throughout the program and should not be something tagged on to therapy or pulled out when the child is having literacy difficulties.

This means that clear-cut comparisons between different therapies targeting speech output are difficult to make. However, the indications are that successful literacy outcome is dependent on both phonological awareness and speech training being combined and integrated into a therapy programme from an early age. Further, what is necessary to include is an analysis of the intervention tasks to establish the levels of speech processing involved and the degree of implicit/explicit phonological awareness involved. Rees (2001b) presents a procedure for doing this by addressing the issue of 'What Do Tasks Really Tap?' She poses seven questions that need to be asked about a therapy activity in order to understand its psycholinguistic properties (see Chapter 3, Book 2,

Stackhouse and Wells, 2001). Question 4 of these relates to the metaphonological demands of an intervention task and has four components.

(a) Does the child have to reflect on his or her speech production?
(b) Does the child have to show awareness of the internal structure of phonological representations or of spoken stimuli?
(c) If so, what kind of segmentation is required?
(d) Does the child have to manipulate phonological units?

We will return again to these important questions in Activity 10.4 but first let us look at Ben, a boy with PSDs and associated literacy difficulties.

Case Study: Ben Aged 8;8

Ben had a normal developmental history with the exception of delayed speech. Socially and emotionally, he was experiencing some difficulties when we first met him, which may have been related to his parents' recent divorce as well as his speech difficulties. Academically Ben required additional support to maintain his position in the class. Increasingly, his speech errors had been observed in his spelling, and there were concerns about his literacy progress in general. Ben's speech difficulties at CA 8;8 were subtle but persisting. He was referred late to speech and language therapy (at CA 6;3) but in the past two years had received intervention that had had a positive effect on his phonology. However, difficulties remained and there was concern that Ben was at risk for experiencing further reading and spelling difficulties linked to his persistent speech problems.

Assessment: Speech Processing

The speech processing profile was used to organize the data from this part of the assessment. At each level of the profile at least one assessment was carried out. A range of assessment materials was used; this included data already obtained from standardized tests, as well as unpublished, non-standardized tests or subtests from standardized materials. Ben's speech processing profile at 8 years, 8 months is shown in Figure 10.3. The ticks and crosses shown on the profile indicate Ben's performance in relation to other children of his chronological age, with one tick indicating age-appropriate skills, and the number of crosses showing the number of standard deviations below the mean.

√ = age-appropriate performance
X = 1 standard deviation below the expected mean for his age
XX = 2 standard deviations below the expected mean for his age
XXX = 3 standard deviations below the expected mean for his age

INPUT

F Is the child aware of the internal structure of phonological representations?
√ – Picture rhyme detection (Vance *et al.*, 1994)
√ – Picture onset detection (PhAB picture alliteration subtest, Frederikson *et al.*, 1997)

E Are the child's phonological representations accurate?
√ – Auditory detection of speech errors (Constable *et al.*, 1997)

D Can the child discriminate between real words?
XXX – Minimal pair auditory discrimination of clusters (Bridgeman and Snowling, 1988)
√ – Aston Index discrimination subtest (Newton and Thompson, 1982)

C Does the child have language specific representations of word structures?

Not tested

B Can the child discriminate speech sounds without reference to lexical representations?
XXX – Minimal pair auditory discrimination of clusters in non-words (Bridgeman and Snowling, 1988)
√ – Aston Index discrimination subtest – non-words (Newton and Thompson, 1982)

A Does the child have adequate auditory perception?
√ – audiometry. But has history of middle ear infections as a baby.

OUTPUT

G Can the child access accurate motor programmes?
X – Single word naming test (Constable *et al.*, 1997)
X – Word-finding vocabulary test (Renfrew, 1995)
X – Edinburgh Articulation Test (Anthony *et al.*, 1971)

H Can the child manipulate phonological units?
√ – PhAB spoonerism subtest (Frederikson *et al.*, 1997)
√ – PAT rhyme fluency subtest (Muter *et al.*, 1997)

I Can the child articulate real words accurately?
X – Real word repetition subtest (Constable *et al.*, 1997)
√ – Aston Index blending subtest – real Words (Newton and Thompson, 1982)

J Can the child articulate speech without reference to lexical representations?
√ – Aston Index blending subtest – non-words (Newton and Thompson, 1982)
X – Non-word repetition subtest (Constable et al., 1997)

K Does the child have adequate sound production skills?
√ – Nuffield Motor assessment; Oral examination and DDK
Finds it hard to produce [ʃ]

L Does the child reject his own erroneous forms?
Inconsistently – informal observation

Figure 10.3: Ben's speech processing profile at age 8;8.

ACTIVITY 10.3

Consider Ben's speech processing profile shown in Figure 10.3 and answer the following questions.

(a) Outline Ben's strengths and main areas of difficulty.
(b) What questions do you have about his speech processing skills and what further assessments would you carry out in order to answer these questions?

Read the descriptions of the tasks we carried out in the Key to Activity 10.3 at the end of this chapter and compare your answers to (a) and (b).

Overview of Ben's Speech Processing Profile

In casual conversation with Ben, his surface speech deficits were relatively minor. However, examination of his speech processing profile revealed that he had many specific difficulties. His difficulties are spread throughout the profile with both speech input and output affected.

Strengths

Ben's speech processing profile showed a range of strengths: He had age-appropriate phonological representations as tested by specific sorting games focusing on his error sounds, as well as the auditory detection of speech errors (Constable *et al.*, 1997) which required him to make judgments about whether words were correctly produced or not. He had age-appropriate awareness of the internal structure of phonological representations and equally good skills in the manipulation of phonological units.

Ben's ability to devise online motor programmes was relatively good. When presented with the written word BISCUITS he did not recognize the word. He was able to sound it out by grapheme–phoneme conversion, and then blend the sounds and accurately devise an online motor programme. At first he rehearsed this new motor programme in a whispered voice: he was heard to say the word accurately: [ˈbɪskɪts]. However, having carried out this rehearsal, he then recognized the word as a familiar one after all, and produced it at normal volume using his stored motor programme: [bɪsɪts]. Examples such as this were key in planning the intervention programme.

Ben had age-appropriate semantic knowledge and was aided by the use of pictures. His online motor programming skills were variable: when faced with more challenging non-words he performed at a lower level than one might expect for a child of his age, e.g. on the non-words from Constable *et al.* (1997, Level J) such as HELIKOPKA (derived from real word

HELICOPTER). However, online motor programming was a relative strength when compared to his access of stored motor programmes.

Weaknesses

Ben had two core areas of difficulty: one on the input side and one on the output side of his speech processing profile. Input difficulties were mainly with his auditory discrimination of closely related real words (Level D) and non-words (Level B). Ben performed variably on the discrimination tasks for both real word and non-word items. On standardized tests such as the auditory discrimination subtest from the *Aston Index* (Newton and Thompson, 1982) he scored age-appropriately for both real and non-words. However, the more challenging items in a cluster sequence discrimination task (Bridgeman and Snowling, 1988) were problematic, and Ben scored significantly below the mean for his age. This test requires children to distinguish between [st] and [ts] using a same/different paradigm with word pairs such as [fɪts] and [fɪst]. The rationale behind this procedure is to investigate whether children who make sequencing errors in their speech output also have difficulties discriminating sequences in their speech input. Ben's difficulty with the Bridgeman and Snowling tasks suggested that sound sequencing - both for input and output - was problematic for him.

Output difficulties were centred on his stored motor programmes where it seemed that frozen motor programmes have not been updated, despite improved online motor processing, as illustrated by the BISCUIT example above. Ben found repetition of real and non-words hard: especially when these were longer, low frequency and more phonetically complex words. It was hypothesized that his discrimination difficulties and frozen motor programmes were working together to affect his speech processing: if children are not processing all the linguistic information encoded in a word, then they will not be able to create accurate motor programmes and produce these appropriately. Ben had a history of input difficulties (Level A - auditory perception) when he was younger. Although these problems with his hearing appeared to have resolved, the effect may be more lasting on his speech processing system. Both auditory discrimination and motor programming needed to be addressed in order for change to be brought about in Ben's speech processing.

Assessment: Speech and Spelling

The PACS procedure (*Phonological Assessment of Child Speech*, Grunwell, 1985) was carried out to provide information on Ben's speech production system. Severity indices have been introduced in previous chapters and are useful measures for encapsulating the degree of difficulty children experience with their speech. PCC (percentage of consonants correct), PVC (percentage of vowels correct) and PPC (percentage of phonemes correct) were used. The severity of Ben's speech difficulties was estimated at two points before the intervention, separated by about 6 weeks. The difference between these scores at the two pre-intervention points was not a significant one indicating a stable pre-intervention baseline. The severity indices suggest that Ben's speech difficulties are mild. Nevertheless, he did have some specific difficulties:

- [ʧ] was reduced to its stop component, e.g. CHEESE → [tiz];
- [ʤ] was fronted to [s] or [d], e.g. JAM → [sæm] or [dæm];
- [f] was typically substituted for [θ], e.g. THUMB → [fʌm];
- [ʃ] was fronted to [s], e.g. FISH → [fɪs];
- [r] was glided to [w] for approximately 20% of the time, e.g. RAKE → [weɪk].

Ben was stimulable for each of these segments in isolation, although [ʃ] was extremely hard for him to produce and required many attempts. While Ben had generally mastered all consonant clusters, he found it difficult to produce [st] and [str] in all word positions typically deleting [t]. Word-initially [str] was produced variably as [sw], [s] and [sr]. A summary of Ben's speech data is presented in Table 10.1.

Table 10.1: Summary of Ben's speech data at CA 8;8

Assessment	Comments	
Severity indices	Percentage of consonants correct (PCC): 86% Percentage of vowels correct (PVC): 99% Percentage of phonemes correct (PPC): 90.3%	
Phonetic inventory	Word initial position: all segments except [ʧ], [ʤ], [θ], [ʃ] Word medial position: all segments except [θ], [ʃ] [ʒ] Word final position: all segments except [ʧ], [θ], [ʃ], [ʒ]	
Stimulability	All segments stimulable except [ʃ]	
Phonological processes analysis (% use)	Developmental processes: cluster reduction (30%); fronting of [ʧ], [ʤ] and [ʃ] (87.5%); gliding [r] to [w] (20%)	
Single word speech sample	CHEESE → [tiz] JAM → [sæm] THUMB → [fʌm] FISH → [fɪs] RAKE → [weɪk]	BIRTHDAY → ['bɜfdeɪ] BRIDGE → [bwɪs] ESKIMO → ['ɛksɪməʊ] SHELL → [sæl] STROKE → [səʊk]
Connected speech sample	HOW MUCH → [aʊ mʊts] I HAD A LITTLE → [aɪ hæd ə lɪtəl] IT GOT BROKEN → [i gɒʔ ' bwəʊkɪn] HE WERE LATE FOR WORK → [ɪ wɜ leɪ fɔ wɜk]	

Ben's letter knowledge was assessed by asking him to write all graphemes to dictation. He was able to do this with 100% accuracy. However, his phoneme–grapheme links were inaccurate in a single-word dictation task leading us to conclude that his spelling development was arrested early on in the alphabetic stage. Qualitative analysis of his spelling showed that his difficulties in representing consonants accurately were limited to a small set of sounds. *The Schonell Graded Word Spelling Test* (in Newton and Thompson, 1982) was administered, and results from this test qualitatively analysed. In this test children are required to write increasingly hard single words, e.g. TIME; YOLK; INSTITUTION. In addition, we devised further items incorporating Ben's speech production errors and presented these to him in a dictation task. In general the speech errors were replicated in his spelling, although with varying degrees of consistency, e.g. [θ] was always correctly represented by the grapheme <th> in real words, [ʃ] was variably represented as <sh>, occasionally being omitted or represented by <s>. Table 10.2 compares spoken and written productions of Ben's errors.

Table 10.2: Comparison of Ben's spoken and written productions

Target underlined	Spoken production	Written production
[st], e.g. STOP, STAMP	[s] e.g. STOP → [sɒp]	st, sr, s e.g. STOP <stop> STAMP <samp>
[str], e.g. STRAIGHT, STRIPE	[s], [sw], [sr], e.g. STRIPE → [swaɪp] STRAIGHT → [seɪt]	str, sr e.g. STRIPE <strip> STRAIGHT <srate>
[tʃ], e.g. CHEESE, CHIPS	[t], [ts] e.g. CHEESE → [tis]	ch, t e.g. CHEESE <teese> CHIPS <chips>
[dʒ], e.g. JOIN, BADGE	[dʒ], [s], e.g. JOIN → [dʒɔɪn] BADGE → [bæs]	j, t, th e.g. JOIN <thon> BADGE <baj>
[θ], e.g. THINK, THIN	[f], e.g. THINK → [fɪnk]	th e.g. THINK <think> THIN <thin>
[ð], e.g. THIS, MOTHER	[θ], e.g. MOTHER → [mʊθə]	th e.g. THIS <this> MOTHER <mother>
[ʃ], e.g. SHELL, FISH	[s], e.g. SHELL → [sæl] FISH → [fɪs]	sh, s e.g. SHELL <shell> FISH <fis>
[r], e.g. RED, RABBIT	[r], [w] e.g. RED → [wɛd]	r, w e.g. RED <red> RABBIT < wabit>

Intervention Planning

Intervention planning focused on the two key areas of psycholinguistics and phonology. From a psycholinguistic perspective we aimed to answer the question, 'What aspects of Ben's speech processing system should be worked on?' From a phonological perspective we wanted to answer the question, 'Which aspects of the sound system should be addressed?' Because speech, literacy and phonological awareness are all overlapping skills we also asked, 'How can we integrate work on speech, literacy and phonological awareness into our intervention programme?'

We designed a hierarchy of tasks to be carried out in intervention. Early tasks in the hierarchy were designed to tap one of Ben's areas of weakness (i.e. either output or input) while later tasks tapped both of these aspects. Each step in the hierarchy was designed to be increasingly challenging for Ben, although the increments between tasks were very small, e.g. Task 1 was a non-word reading task while Task 2 was the same task but slightly more challenging for Ben in its use of real words. This hierarchy was designed to focus first on each of Ben's weak points individually and to support them with relative strengths (e.g. pictures, online motor programming) and then to bring them together working on both input and output. Tasks involved a combination of literacy, phonological awareness and speech activities using the same set of stimuli. Ben's intervention task hierarchy is presented in Table 10.3.

ACTIVITY 10.4

Consider Task 1 (non-word reading) of Ben's intervention task hierarchy in Table 10.3. Now answer the following questions from Rees (2001b) to determine the metaphonological demands of the task.

(a) Does Ben have to reflect on his speech production?
(b) Does Ben have to show awareness of the internal structure of phonological representations or of spoken stimuli?
(c) If so, what kind of segmentation is required?
(d) Does Ben have to manipulate phonological units?

Now turn to the Key to Activity 10.4 at the end of this chapter to check your answers, then read the following.

With the intervention tasks outlined, we now needed to decide on the targets to be used in intervention. Ben's difficulties were limited to a small group of segments [ʃ, ʤ, ʧ, θ] and clusters [str, st]. Four targets were selected from these [st, ʃ, ʧ, θ] in order to carry out minimal work to

Table 10.3: Ben's intervention task hierarchy

Task 1 = easiest; 9 = most challenging	Description	Part of the speech processing system tapped	Phonological awareness and literacy skills tapped
Task 1	Non-word reading task	Taps output: the relative strength of online motor programming and bypasses auditory discrimination	Requires alphabetic knowledge of grapheme–phoneme links, i.e. decoding; blending skills
Task 2	Real word reading task	Taps output: online motor programming and/or stored motor programmes – bypasses auditory discrimination	Requires access of stored orthographic representation (top-down approach) OR alphabetic knowledge of grapheme–phoneme links, i.e. decoding (bottom-up approach)
Task 3	Listening and picture matching task, e.g. therapist produces word and Ben required to indicate matching picture stimulus from a selection of pictures	Taps input: pictures are provided to give top-down support but bypasses output weaknesses	Requires a tacit level of phonological awareness only

Table 10.3: *Continued*

Task 1 = easiest; 9 = most challenging	Description	Part of the speech processing system tapped	Phonological awareness and literacy skills tapped
Task 4	Listening and real word matching task, e.g. therapist produces word and Ben required to indicate matching written word from selection	Taps input: relies on phoneme–grapheme conversion and orthographic knowledge – bypasses output, no picture support available	Requires access of stored orthographic representation (top-down approach) OR alphabetic knowledge of phoneme–grapheme links (bottom-up approach)
Task 5	Non-word listening and word matching task, e.g. therapist produces non-word and Ben required to indicate matching written word from selection	As above but non-word discrimination is more challenging	Alphabetic knowledge of phoneme–grapheme links, (bottom-up approach)

Task 6	Real word listening and written output, i.e. writing to dictation	Taps input and written output	Requires access of stored orthographic representation (top-down approach) OR alphabetic knowledge of phoneme–grapheme links, (bottom-up approach)
Task 7	Non-word listening and written output, i.e. writing to dictation	As above, but more challenging with non-words	Alphabetic knowledge of phoneme-grapheme links, (bottom-up approach)
Task 8	Real word listening and repetition	Taps input and spoken output	Requires a tacit level of phonological awareness only
Task 9	Non-word listening and repetition	As above, but more challenging with non-words	Requires a tacit level of phonological awareness only

achieve maximal generalization. It was hypothesized that improvement of this set of items would generalize to other problematic sounds (see Chapter 9 for suggestions for maximizing generalization). Each target was randomly allocated to four phases of intervention: [st] was addressed in intervention Phase I, [ʃ] in Phase II, [θ] in Phase III and [ʧ] in Phase IV and a set of stimuli designed for each target (see next section). Each phase of intervention comprised nine one-hour sessions, i.e. working through the nine tasks of the task hierarchy in Table 10.3. focusing on one particular target, giving Ben a total of 36 hours of intervention. Baseline evaluation took place prior to the intervention at T1, and then following each of the four phases of intervention. On completion of the programme (T5), re-assessment took place, and at T6, longer-term follow-up evaluation took place. See Figure 10.4 for the design of Ben's intervention programme.

Stimuli Design for Each of the Four Targets

Four lists of stimuli were devised with each list representing one of the four target segments. The requirements for each of the four treatment lists are set out below:

(a) each list to consist of 10 monosyllabic words;
(b) each list to represent a different target:
  - list A = [st]
  - list B = [ʃ]
  - list C = [θ]
  - list D = [ʧ]

(c) each of the lists to have half the items with the target in word-initial position, and the other five with the target in word-final position;
(d) items to be matched across the groups by Thorndike-Lorge written frequency (from the MRC Psycholinguistic database)[1] and for spelling irregularities.

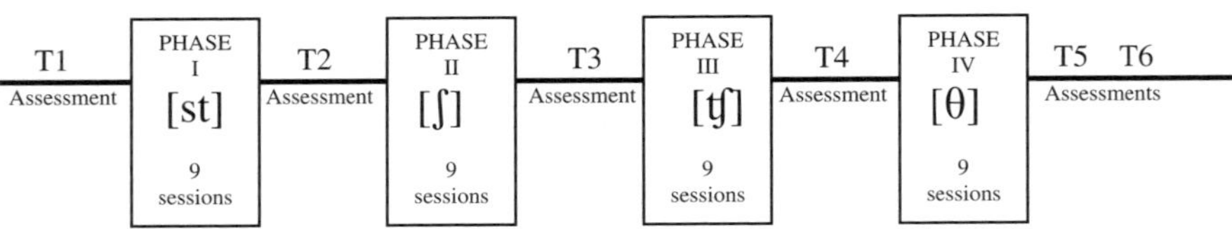

Figure 10.4: The design of Ben's intervention programme.

ACTIVITY 10.5

(a) Using the requirements in (a) to (c) above, devise a list of stimuli for one of Ben's targets: [st, ʃ, tʃ, θ]. The list will need to consist of 10 monosyllabic words. Five of the words will need to have the target in word-initial position and five of the words will need to have the target segment or cluster in word-final position. If you were devising all four lists of words you would need to ensure that the words on each list are balanced in terms of frequency and spelling irregularity as in (d) above, however you do not need to do this for this activity.
(b) You will also note from Ben's task hierarchy shown in Table 10.3, that non-words were an important part of intervention. Based on your list of 10 real words, create a set of 10 matched non-words which could be used in intervention. This could be done by keeping the target (e.g. /st/) in the same word position as for the real word, and altering the medial vowel and remaining consonant to produce a phonotactically acceptable non-word, e.g. real word: STACK ~ STIP.

Read on to see the words that we selected for each of Ben's four lists.

Ben's four treatment real word stimuli lists are presented in Table 10.4.

The task hierarchy in Table 10.3 shows that for each target, real word and non-word tasks were carried out. For each of the real words listed in Table 10.4, a matched non-word was created by keeping the target segment and altering the medial vowel and remaining consonant to produce a phonotactically acceptable non-word (SHIP ~ SHAN). These non-words are presented in Table 10.5 together with the real word targets from which they were derived.

In order to evaluate generalization effects, lists of untreated stimuli were created. These stimuli lists allowed Ben's progress to be measured. Each of the assessments involved the following tasks:

(a) picture naming of treatment stimuli words (see Table 10.4);
(b) repetition of untreated, matched non-words (see Table 10.5);
(c) picture naming or repetition of all untreated, control words;
(d) spelling of both real and non-words from dictation.

Outcomes

The following questions were asked.

Table 10.4: Ben's four treatment stimuli lists

		List A	List B	List C	List D
		[st]	**[ʃ]**	**[θ]**	**[ʧ]**
(1)	Word-initial target	STACK	SHEET	THAW	CHAIR
(2)		STAY	SHELL	THIN	CHOKE
(3)		STEAL	SHIP	THORN	CHAP
(4)		STOLE	SHOCK	THANK	CHILL
(5)		STUCK	SHORE	THICK	CHEEK
(6)	Word-final target	PAST	DISH	MOTH	CATCH
(7)		MIST	CASH	MOUTH	COACH
(8)		TEST	PUSH	PATH	MATCH
(9)		NEST	BASH	DEATH	PEACH
(10)		GUST	LASH	BATH	BENCH

Table 10.5: Ben's four treatment stimuli lists showing real words and matched non-word stimuli

		List A		List B		List C		List D	
		[st]		**[ʃ]**		**[θ]**		**[ʧ]**	
(1)	Word-initial target	STACK	[stip]	SHEET	[ʃɔp]	THAW	[θiz]	CHAIR	[ʧɒk]
(2)		STAY	[stɔ]	SHELL	[ʃɪg]	THIN	[θɒs]	CHOKE	[ʧup]
(3)		STEAL	[stɔg]	SHIP	[ʃæn]	THORN	[θɑb]	CHAP	[ʧɪd]
(4)		STOLE	[stɑb]	SHOCK	[ʃʌb]	THANK	[θɪp]	CHILL	[ʧəʊb]
(5)		STUCK	[stɒn]	SHORE	[ʃim]	THICK	[θud]	CHEEK	[ʧɒs]
(6)	Word-final target	PAST	[dɛst]	DISH	[pɪʃ]	MOTH	[sæθ]	CATCH	[bɑʧ]
(7)		MIST	[kist]	CASH	[bɛʃ]	MOUTH	[gaʊθ]	COACH	[fiʧ]
(8)		TEST	[maɪst]	PUSH	[fɒʃ]	PATH	[wəʊθ]	MATCH	[weɪʧ]
(9)		NEST	[tʌst]	BASH	[nʌʃ]	DEATH	[tɛθ]	PEACH	[bɛʧ]
(10)		GUST	[bæst]	LASH	[vaʃ]	BATH	[dəʊθ]	BENCH	[suʧ]

(a) Is the intervention effective in bringing about improvements in Ben's speech production of treated items beyond chance level? If the intervention is effective, does the success of the intervention vary across the four targets, and why?

(b) Is the intervention effective in bringing about improvements in Ben's spelling of treated items beyond chance level? If the intervention is effective for spelling, does the success of the intervention vary across the four targets, and why?

In this section we focus on these questions in turn.

(a) Is the intervention effective in bringing about improvements in Ben's speech production of treated items beyond chance level? If the intervention is effective, does the success of the intervention vary across the four targets, and why?

Ben's intervention was effective in bringing about statistically significant improvements in his speech production of targeted words. We carried out a statistical procedure called two-way mixed between-within subjects ANOVA (see Pring, 2005, for further details of this procedure). We found a statistically significant main effect for time for speech [$F(5, 145) = 11.746$, $p < 0.001$]. This meant that Ben was able to realize more of the targets accurately at the single-word level after the intervention. The scoring procedure we used focused specifically on the target segments and not on the remainder of the word. One point was awarded for each correct target (i.e. [ʃ, θ, ʧ, st]). Raw scores were converted into percentages. Improvements had occurred not only for the treated words (from 40% accuracy to 70% accuracy) but also for the non-words (from 32% accuracy to 70% accuracy). The matched untreated items followed a similar pattern of improvement (from 40% to 70%) showing that some generalization had taken place. Ben's speech performance over the course of intervention from T1 (pre-intervention) to T6 (long-term follow-up) is shown in Figure 10.5 in which we have collapsed the results of the four targets.

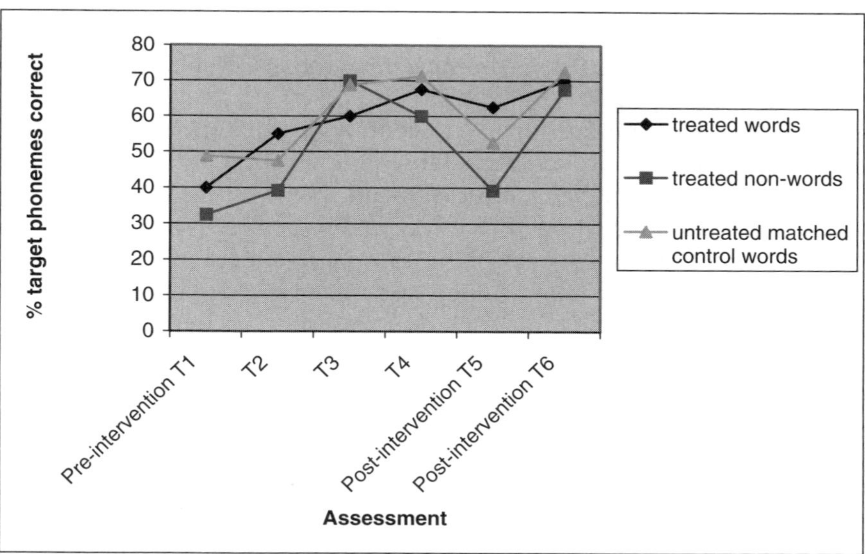

Figure 10.5: Comparison of Ben's stimuli groups over the course of intervention for speech.

From this collapsed data in Figure 10.5, it is not clear whether Ben made greater gains with some of the targets than others. When we considered the four individual targets addressed in intervention, we found that it was mainly [θ] and [ʧ] which contributed to the positive changes in Ben's speech shown in Figure 10.5. These were different from the target [st] in that [st] was approaching ceiling at the start of intervention and had little scope for significant gains, whereas [θ] and [ʧ] were much harder for Ben to produce and the scope for improvement was much greater. The target that was most challenging for Ben to produce was [ʃ], and thus this had the greatest scope for improvement. However, the gains made for this target were small. One explanation is that Ben had very limited productive phonological knowledge (PPK) of this segment (see Chapter 3, and Table 3.2 for an explanation of this term). It was easier for him to make gains with targets that he had at least some knowledge about, such as [θ] and [ʧ]. Another explanation might be that the therapy programme met the needs of the targets [θ] and [ʧ], but [ʃ] may have required more direct articulatory work. Ben had difficulty raising his tongue – see Level K on Ben's speech processing profile (Figure 10.1). This affected his production of [ʃ], which he could produce in isolation only with considerable difficulty. Although, to some extent the intervention did involve assisting Ben with his articulation of this sound, it could have been more specifically targeted at this level for [ʃ] in particular. Very often, children with PSDs need different approaches for different targets within the same intervention programme

(b) Is the intervention effective in bringing about improvements in Ben's spelling of treated items beyond chance level? If the intervention is effective for spelling, does the success of the intervention vary across the four targets, and why?

Ben's spelling was significantly more accurate than his speech at the start of the intervention. However, Ben's intervention was effective in bringing about statistically significant improvements in his spelling of targeted words. Again, we carried out a two-way mixed between–within subjects ANOVA and found a statistically significant main effect for time for spelling [$F(5, 145) = 9.862$, $p < 0.001$]. Ben was able to spell more of the targets accurately at the single word level after the intervention, although the change was not as great as for speech. Our scoring procedure for spelling focused specifically on the target segments and clusters and not on the remainder of the word, with one point awarded for each appropriately written target. Raw scores were converted into percentages. Improvements had occurred not only for the treated words (from 70% accuracy to 90% accuracy) but also for the non-words (from 70% accuracy to 90% accuracy) and the matched untreated items (from 62% to 85%) showing that some generalization had taken place. Ben's spelling performance over the course of intervention from T1 (pre-intervention) to T6 (long-term follow-up) is shown in Figure 10.6.

Examining the individual segments and clusters addressed in intervention, it was found that:

1. Ben seemed to be mastering [st] by the start of the intervention. He was accurate in his written and spoken realizations of this segment, and this did not change in any significant way for speech or spelling.
2. [tʃ] was effectively modified in both speech and spelling, responding in similar ways over the course of the programme. Initially [tʃ] was challenging for Ben in both speech and spelling. However, consistent improvements were noted throughout the programme. Ben's productions – both written and spoken – changed hand-in-hand for both modalities.
3. [θ] was challenging for Ben in both speech and spelling. His initial low scores improved significantly over the course of intervention.
4. A notable mismatch between speech and spelling occurred for [ʃ]. Ben's ability to represent [ʃ] in written forms was 90% accurate, but his ability to produce the sound was limited by his articulatory difficulties. This pattern was maintained over the course of the intervention: [ʃ] remained near ceiling for spelling, and although some significant gains were noted in his speech production, he required further intervention to improve production of [ʃ] beyond an accuracy level of approximately 15%. This pattern of performance suggests that Ben's phonological representations were accurate for [ʃ].

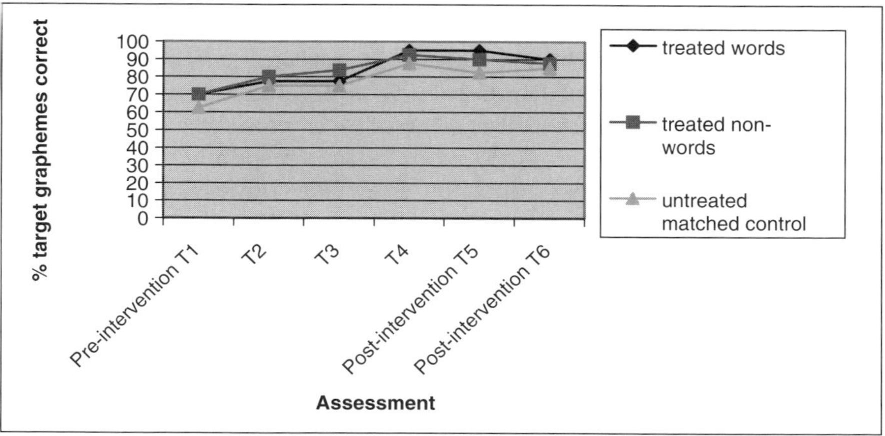

Figure 10.6: Comparison of Ben's stimuli groups over the course of intervention for spelling.

> In contrast, his phonological representations were not accurate for [ʧ] and [θ]. Intervention targeted this and resulted in parallel gains for speech and spelling. Comparing speech and spelling performance in this way can inform our understanding of a child's speech processing difficulties.

From a broader perspective, limited change was observed in Ben's speech processing skills. The speech processing profile revealed no significant change, either on the input or output side of the profile. PACS (Grunwell, 1985) revealed some changes in the use of particular targets. Standardized literacy tests revealed that although Ben had made gains in his spelling following the intervention, the gap between Ben and his age-matched peers was widening on both reading and spelling. Some positive comments were made by Ben himself, his teachers and his father about the effects of the intervention. To some extent these may have reflected the fact that Ben was now emotionally more settled and more confident.

Ben's Intervention: Next Steps

Ben's intervention was successful in addressing his use of specific segments such as [ʧ] and [θ]. However, it was not as effective in addressing his articulation difficulties with [ʃ]. Ruscello (1995) and Dagenais (1995) suggest that children like Ben with PSDs might respond to visually oriented treatment such as biofeedback techniques when more traditional speech production and auditory techniques have failed to work. Much speech intervention - like Ben's - relies heavily on the auditory modality. For children with auditory processing difficulties, this may be inappropriate, and alternative approaches required. Ben did experience some auditory discrimination difficulties and these were taken into account in the intervention planning although they were not the main focus of intervention. Examples of visual biofeedback interventions are provided by Dagenais (1995) and Dent (2001). Dent describes intervention for two older children (CA 8;6 and 10;5) who had not responded to traditional therapy, but for whom electropalatography (EPG) intervention was successful. A next step for Ben might be the use of EPG specifically for his [ʃ] production. This might not just improve his speech directly but also scaffold his auditory discrimination difficulties.

Literacy Difficulties: The Role of the Speech and Language Therapist

Implicit throughout this chapter, and all the books in this series, is the message that speech and language therapists do need to be knowledgeable about normal and atypical literacy development, and in particular the relationship between spoken and written language. However, this does not mean that they are expected to teach reading and spelling; indeed, they are not trained to do this. They are, however, well placed to identify children at risk for literacy problems early on, explain these difficulties to all involved, and incorporate skills like phonological awareness and letter knowledge into their routine therapy programmes with school-age children (e.g. see Nathan and Simpson, 2001). Thus therapists have a supportive, training and collaborative role in a child's literacy development (Scott and Brown, 2001) as well as a direct role in promoting literacy skills routinely through their intervention programmes with children with speech and language difficulties. Snowling and Stackhouse (2006 p. 326) note:

> . . . The role of the speech and language therapist however, does not include *teaching* reading and spelling which is traditionally and rightly the teacher's domain. Rather, the therapist's role is one of ensuring that the underlying oral language skills that contribute to literacy development are in place, and if not, in promoting these.

In summary, written and spoken language should not be regarded as two separate areas, each tackled by different professional groups. An understanding of the links between the two areas and their subskills arising from a common speech processing system will enable therapists, teachers and others to design and deliver comprehensive intervention packages.

Speech and Literacy: Practical Suggestions for Intervention

- In terms of assessment, both standardized and non-standardized, qualitative assessments should be used to evaluate skills in spoken language, reading, writing and spelling. The literacy assessment and intervention carried out with Ben was at a single-word level. Narrative writing and reading tasks would have provided additional insights into his ability to process and produce larger pieces of text. Bishop and Clarkson (2003) note that single-word spelling and continuous writing can yield very different pictures.
- Speech, phonological awareness and literacy are all overlapping skills that are underpinned by the speech processing system. When working with children with PSDs this overlap will often be apparent. Interventions with this client group need to address the speech processing system as a whole and offer integrated management of

each of these areas – as attempted in our intervention with Ben and as described by Watson and Gillon (1999).

- An integrated intervention is one in which speech processing and production, phonological awareness and reading/spelling are included. The same set of stimuli can be used in speech, phonological awareness and literacy tasks. As for Ben's intervention, therapy tasks should use a child's areas of strength to support areas of weakness.
- Clearly, when SLTs are including written stimuli in intervention there is an opportunity for collaborative working with teachers. Popple and Wellington (2001) describe this process of collaboration in a school setting, while Nathan and Simpson (2001) describe the integrated speech and literacy intervention that took place in a school setting with Luke, a 7-year-old boy with subtle PSDs. Therapists may work on the spoken and written production of words that are part of the school curriculum, or can focus on aspects of the curriculum that pose particular problems for children with PSDs, e.g. new word learning.
- Risk factors for literacy difficulties include having persisting speech difficulties beyond the age of 5;5, having severe speech difficulties and having difficulties that affect many aspects of the speech processing system (e.g. Nathan *et al.*, 2004a). Part of the SLT's role is identifying at-risk children and communicating these risk factors to teachers and parents, and working with them to develop programs to help children acquire age-appropriate skills and strategies for reading and writing development.

Summary

Some key points are as follows.

- Children with PSDs are at risk for literacy problems, particularly with spelling.
- Longitudinal studies show the links between unresolved speech problems and literacy development.
- These links are dynamic and influenced by factors such as teaching, intervention and general oral language abilities.
- The speech processing system is the shared foundation for normal speech, phonological awareness and literacy development.
- Given the close links between these domains, literacy is an integral part of any intervention programme addressing persisting speech problems in the school-age population.
- Although therapists are not literacy teachers, they have an important role in integrating and including written stimuli in interventions with children with PSDs.

- The developmental phase model from Stackhouse and Wells can be linked to Frith's (1985) model of the phases of literacy development.
- Phase models are helpful in capturing the dynamic nature of children's development and allow us to consider how a child's development has become arrested at a particular phase.
- Children with PSDs may need different treatment plans for different segments.
- Ben's intervention aimed to address residual errors in his speech, as well as improving his spelling of these words. Single-word stimuli were selected based on his difficulties, and used in a task hierarchy which involved integration of speech, spelling and reading.
- Overall Ben's intervention was effective for both speech and spelling, but he made minimal improvement with words containing the target segment /ʃ/ for which he had articulatory difficulties compared to the targets /tʃ/ and /θ/.
- A child's lack of progress in therapy, e.g. with a particular segment compared to others, can inform our understanding of the nature of the speech difficulties and enable a more tailor-made therapy phase to follow.
- Comparing speech and spelling performance, e.g. of the same target in words (or connected speech), can inform our understanding of the nature of a child's speech processing difficulties.
- Speech and language therapists have a key role in identifying literacy difficulties and in promoting literacy skills as an integral and routine part of their therapy programmes.
- Intervention based on collaboration between professionals and carers, and shared training is essential.

KEY TO ACTIVITY 10.1

(a) Give an example of a task in which speech helps promote phonological awareness.

If you are asked how many syllables there are in a low frequency spoken word like ENDOCRINOLOGIST you may well reproduce the word out loud (or silently articulate the word) while counting the syllables on your fingers.

(b) Give an example of a task in which phonological awareness supports speech production.

When experiencing a word-finding problem, i.e. you are unable to think of someone's name or a particular word you require, many people are able to provide information about the initial sound of the word, the number of syllables or another word that is phonologically similar. Once you have got some sound cues, e.g. I think it starts with a /b/ and it has two syllables, this phonological knowledge can trigger the access and production of the correct word.

(c) Give an example of a task in which phonological awareness is used to aid literacy.

When attempting to read an unfamiliar word, you will draw on your knowledge of grapheme–phoneme links in order to first sound out the word, then blend the sounds into a word or you will recognize by analogy with known words familiar sound/grapheme chunks.

(d) Give an example of a task in which literacy aids phonological awareness.

You are asked to make a spoonerism from a phrase like ROAD LAMP, i.e. you are being asked to swop around the initial sounds in both words. Many adults will carry out this task either by writing down the words and physically crossing out and swopping the initial letters, or visualizing this swop in their head to give the answer LOAD RAMP.

KEY TO ACTIVITY 10.2

(a) At which stage of Frith's model of literacy development (shown in Figure 10.2) is Ben at?

Based on the limited spelling data presented, Ben appears to have moved out of the logographic stage of literacy development into the alphabetic phase. His spellings would be described as 'semi-phonetic' indicating that he can use letter–sound knowledge but has not yet learned all spelling conventions.

(b) What questions do you have about Ben's speech and spelling?

- (i) **Affricates** (in CHEESE, JAM, FRIDGE). Does he have difficulties producing the affricates 'ch' and 'j' in his speech? As he wrote <th> for 'j' at the end of FRIDGE does he have any interdental articulation that might be confusing him when spelling? Can he discriminate between and produce affricates perfectly well but does not know how to write them down? Is <jam> a whole word learned response of a familiar item?
- (ii) Digraphs (<sh> in SHARP, MASH). On both occasions Ben transcribed these as <s>. Can he discriminate the difference between 's' and 'sh'? Does he have fuzzy representations stored of words including 's' and 'sh'? Does he produce 's' for 'sh' in his speech? Does he know about digraphs in spelling, and particularly about <s> vs. <sh>?
- (iii) **Clusters** (in STAMP, STRING, FRIDGE). As he wrote the cluster at the beginning of FRIDGE accurately does he only have difficulties with 's' clusters? Does he represent all 's' clusters as <sr>? Is

there a difference between his spelling of two- vs. three-element clusters in other examples of 's' clusters and in the full range of English clusters? Can he detect the difference between words with singleton 's' and words with 's' clusters, e.g. SAY vs. STAY vs. STRAY? Does he have fuzzy representations of these words? Can he produce 's' and 's' clusters clearly in his speech? Is it true that he can spell nasal clusters at the end of words as he did here in STAMP and STRING?

KEY TO ACTIVITY 10.3

(a) *Ben's strengths.* No obvious hearing loss (A); can discriminate between simple CVC non-words (B) and real words (D); adequate stored phonological representations for the items tested (E); some awareness of the internal structure of these representations (F); could manipulate some phonological units (H); can blend real (I) and non-words (J); has adequate sound production skills (K).

Ben's main areas of difficulty. The profile shows two core areas of difficulty, one on the input side and one on the output side. He had difficulties discriminating between non-words and words which differed only in the sequence of the cluster, e.g. VOST ~ VOTS; LOST ~ LOTS (Levels B and D). Output difficulties were centred on his stored motor programmes where it seems that many frozen motor programmes have not been updated (Level G), despite improved online motor processing (Level J). Ben found repetition of both real and non-words hard: especially when these were longer, low frequency and more phonetically complex words suggesting difficulties with both stored motor programmes for familiar words (I) and assembling new motor programmes for unfamiliar words (J). His errors may be compounded by inconsistent self-monitoring of his speech output (L).

(b) What questions do you have about his speech processing skills and what further assessments would you carry out in order to answer these questions?
   - We asked: Are Ben's speech production errors because he is unable to distinguish between his own error sounds and target productions? In order to answer this question, an auditory lexical decision task was devised comprising 50 items based on Ben's output errors (see Stackhouse *et al.*, forthcoming, for guidelines on this). Ben performed poorly on this task, unable to distinguish between sound pairs such as [tʃ] and [t]; [ʃ] and [s] in both real and non-word items, and in all word positions. We concluded that Ben's auditory

lexical/discrimination skills affect his speech production and should be addressed in intervention.

- We asked: Is there a link between Ben's spelling and speech difficulties? Using speech data already gathered, we asked Ben to spell the words so that comparisons could be made. Then, using spelling data already obtained from Ben, we asked him to produce the same words in a naming task, once again allowing for comparisons to be made between the two. Some links were found between his speech and spelling with difficulties affecting particular segments. These are discussed in greater detail in the text.

KEY TO ACTIVITY 10.4

(a) Does Ben have to reflect on his speech production?
No, not to produce the non-word initially. However, yes, if he wants to check that his production of the non-word is what he meant to produce (Level L on the speech processing profile).

(b) Does Ben have to show awareness of the internal structure of phonological representations or of spoken stimuli?
Yes, if he reads non-words by analogy with known words, e.g. STIP is like CHIP but with 'st' at the beginning instead of 'ch'. However, no, if he builds up the word by grapheme–phoneme conversion though he will need to draw on a tacit knowledge of what are legal combinations of sounds and letters in English.

(c) If so, what kind of segmentation is required?
Phonemic segmentation if reading letter by letter. However if using analogy strategy, segmentation may be at the level of onset and rime or other familiar chunks.

(d) Does Ben have to manipulate phonological units?
Yes, he has to remember the segments in the right sequence and then blend them together to produce a word.

Note

1. www.psy.uwa.edu.au/mrcdatabase/uwa_mrc.htm.

Chapter 11
Intelligibility

Intelligibility is a term commonly used when describing children's speech, but one that is rarely defined and challenging to measure. It has been described as 'the understandability of speech' (Yorkston, Dowden and Beukelman, 1992), 'the match between the intention of the speaker and the response of the listener' (Schiavetti, 1992) and, the ability to use speech to communicate effectively in everyday situations (Osberger, 1992). It is the immediate criterion by which communicative attempts are judged, and is closely linked to communicative competence. It is clear that improving intelligibility is an important aim for many speech interventions. Dodd and Bradford (2000) note, 'Intelligible speech is the long term goal for most intervention approaches for children with speech disorders' (p. 191).

This chapter aims to review the literature on intelligibility, and to focus practically on how intelligibility might be measured and used as an outcome measure when working with children with PSDs. The chapter is divided into three main sections.

- Measuring intelligibility. How do we measure intelligibility? What are the advantages and shortcomings associated with each technique?
- Explaining intelligibility. What do we know about the factors that influence intelligibility? This section introduces a review of research papers that have had intelligibility as their focus.
- Intelligibility as a clinical outcomes measure. How has intelligibility been used as an outcomes measure to evaluate the effects of intervention?

We conclude the chapter with some suggestions for best practice in the assessment of intelligibility, and for including intelligibility in intervention.

ACTIVITY 11.1

Make a list of factors that contribute to intelligibility, and that make speech unintelligible. It may be helpful to group these under speaker factors, listener factors, and environmental factors. In carrying out the task, think of speakers (children or adults) who you find it challenging to understand - why? Think of your own weak points as a listener, which means that you find some speakers easier than others to understand. Think of situations in which your understanding of speech is compromised. Now turn to the Key to Activity 11.1 at the end of the chapter before reading what follows.

Measuring Intelligibility

Intelligibility levels are frequently used in making clinical decisions. For this reason measurements need to be reliable and valid. A reliable measurement is one that yields consistent results over repeated observations or measurements under the same conditions each time. A valid measurement is one that measures what it purports to measure. A starting point is to be clear about what one is attempting to measure. Intelligibility and severity are related concepts that overlap considerably, and are both likely to be affected by many of the same factors (Yorkston and Beukelman, 1981; Gordon-Brannan and Hodson, 2000). Methods devised to quantify severity levels include percentage of consonants correct (PCC) (Shriberg and Kwiatkowski, 1982), percentage of vowels/diphthongs correct (PVC) (Shriberg and Kwiatkowski, 1982) and percentage of phonemes correct (PPC) (Dodd, 1995). These are typically calculated from a connected speech sample, but can also be obtained from single-word tasks. They focus on the intended consonants, vowels or phonemes, expressing the total number correct as a percentage of the total number intended. Severity indices have been used when introducing children in our case studies throughout this book. In a study by Shriberg and Kwiatkowski (1982), experienced practitioners rated recorded samples of children's speech in terms of intelligibility, and these percentage ratings were then linked to PCC measures. It was found that their judgments of mild difficulties with intelligibility correlated with PCC scores of 85%; judgments of mild-moderate difficulties with intelligibility correlated with PCC scores between 65% and 85%; judgments of moderate-severe difficulties correlated with 50-65%, and scores less than 50% were considered severe.

Although intelligibility may be closely related to severity the two are different indices of speech (Kent, Miolo and Bloedel, 1994). Intelligibility is word or utterance recognition in natural communication situations. True measures of intelligibility should thus involve listeners attempting to discern meaning from an individual's speech in a way that approximates a real-life environment. Severity indices typically involve carrying out counts based on transcribed or recorded data.

ACTIVITY 11.2

What tools do you have at your disposal for evaluating intelligibility? Consider:

- assessments that may not specifically be designed for this purpose, but could be adapted to provide information on intelligibility;
- assessments designed specifically for assessing intelligibility;
- any experimental approaches that you might use to evaluate a child's intelligibility.

Now read the following for further discussion of ways of evaluating intelligibility.

Three approaches typically used for measuring intelligibility are:

- word identification tasks;
- listener rating scales;
- formal assessments which make use of one or both of these methods and are normally designed to be used with a specific speech-disordered population.

Each of these approaches to the evaluation of intelligibility is discussed in further detail in the following sections, followed by an evaluation of the approaches.

Word Identification Tasks

Word identification tasks require the listener, or a panel of listeners, to write down what the speaker says. An open response format is most commonly used with the listener instructed simply to write down the word or words they hear. In some cases closed-set tasks are used, where listeners are given a range of multiple-choice alternatives from which to select their responses. In this case, Kent, Weismer, Kent and Rosenbek (1989) suggest that the possible multiple-choice responses should reflect the potential speech production errors in the target population. The speech sample may consist of single words or sentences, typically pre-recorded onto an audiotape and randomized. While single-word tests are easier to administer and score, connected speech intelligibility tests have more contextual validity as measures of what happens in the real world. Scoring procedures vary but typically involve sentences being scored on the number of key words correct or by the total number of words correctly identified.

Listener Rating Interval Scales

Listener rating interval scales require listeners to make judgments about the speaker's intelligibility using a technique such as interval scaling or direct magnitude estimation. Interval scaling requires the listener to assign a number to each recorded stimulus, e.g. on a four point scale where 1 = completely unintelligible and 4 = completely intelligible, as shown in Figure 11.1 below.

Direct magnitude estimation requires an estimate - typically a percentage - of parts of a sentence which are understood, e.g. 100% would indicate that a listener understood the entire sentence, whereas 50% would suggest understanding of only about half of the words. The technique is typically used with a standard, or reference stimulus, chosen as a good exemplar of midrange intelligibility (Weismer and Laures, 2002). The listener is required to come up with an estimate of the percentage of the utterance understood, e.g. writing 20% or 25% if he or she had only discerned the first word in a short sentence.

Formal Tests

Some formal tests of speech intelligibility have been developed. An early example of such a test is Tikofsky's (1970) revised list for the estimation of single-word intelligibility in adults with dysarthric speech. More recent tests, also devised for quantifying dysarthric speech, include the *Frenchay Dysarthria Assessment* (Enderby, 1983) and Yorkston and Beukelman's (1981) *Assessment of the Intelligibility of Dysarthric Speech*. Two computerized tests, the *Sentence Intelligibility Test* (SIT) (Yorkston and Beukelman, 1981) and the *Computerized Assessment of Intelligibility of Dysarthric Speech* (CAIDS), (Yorkston, Beukelman, and Traynor, 1984) are available for Macintosh and Windows platforms.

For children, the *Children's Speech Intelligibility Measure* (CSIM) (Wilcox and Morris, 1999) has been devised for the assessment of single-word intelligibility. Fifty words are randomly selected from given sets of words and the child repeats these onto an audiotape. Two to three listeners are then required to listen to the tape, either transcribing the

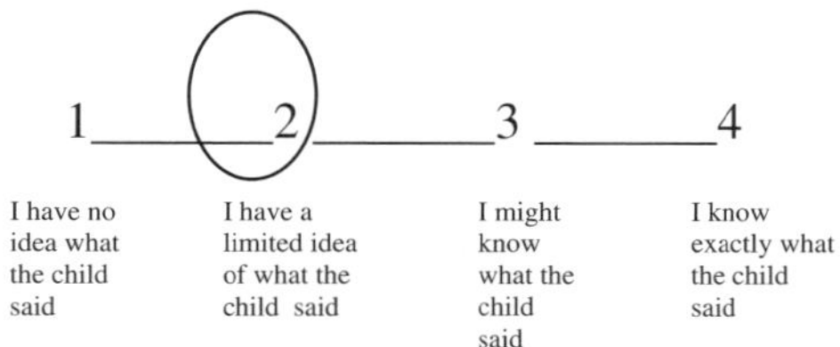

Figure 11.1: Example of a listener rating interval scale.

words or using a multiple-choice format. Alternatively the *Weiss Comprehensive Articulation Test* (Weiss, 1980) includes a section for transcribing a 200-word speech sample, followed by a calculation of the percentage of words understood. The *Beginners Intelligibility Test* (BIT) (Osberger, Robbins, Todd and Riley, 1994) was developed specifically for use with young children with hearing impairment and speech and language delays. Scoring is based on the percentage of words correctly determined.

Word identification tasks have the advantage of having high validity (Samar and Metz, 1988; Schiavetti, 1992; Konst, Weersink-Braks, Rietveld and Peters, 2000). Calculating the percentage of words understood from a continuous-speech sample is thought to yield the most valid measure of intelligibility (Kent *et al.*, 1994; Gordon-Brannan and Hodson, 2000). In addition, the metric of speech intelligibility produced - typically a percentage of words correctly heard - is readily usable by practitioners and researchers. The disadvantage is that data collection and analyses are time consuming and not always practical in clinical situations. Furthermore, the method of scoring whole words as either correct or incorrect is a fairly gross one, imparting no information about parts of words that are intelligible and providing limited opportunities to reflect on qualitative changes that may have occurred within words as part of a pre–post intervention design. For children with severe speech difficulties, this may be a particular problem.

An intelligibility study by Pascoe and Tuomi (2001) used a write down paradigm to evaluate the understandability of adult, second language speakers of English with non-standard dialects in South Africa. At the first level of analysis, whole words were scored as correct or incorrect. At a further level of analysis, the percentage of consonants and percentage of vowels/diphthongs correctly identified, were considered for each participant. Error matrices (also called confusion matrices) were used to determine the consonants and vowels that were accurately perceived, and those that resulted in listener confusion. An error matrix is a grid in which target consonants (on one axis) are compared to listeners' perceptions on the other, as shown in Figure 11.2.

		Perceived as				
		p	b	t	k	s
Target	p		X			
	b		X			
	t			X		
	k				X	
	s					X

Figure 11.2: Example of an error matrix where /b, t, k, s/ are perceived correctly as the target but /p/ is perceived as /b/.

When all targets are accurately perceived, a diagonal line should run from one corner of the matrix to the other. In Figure 11.2, it can be seen that all of the consonants are accurately perceived with the exception of /p/ being perceived as /b/. It was argued that in the case of non-standard dialects, speech and language therapists need to be able to distinguish between characteristics of the accent that do not compromise intelligibility, and those features which lead to miscommunication. The study was able to conclude by offering some intelligibility-driven suggestions for intervention targets for South African therapists working with this specific client group.

The use of rating scales is frequently cited as a fast and easy method that does not require particular tools or training, and is practical for severely unintelligible speech when target words are not known. However, the reliability and validity of this approach are questionable (Schiavetti, 1992; Konst *et al.*, 2000) and if it is used it should be with awareness that its validity is unproven. Formal tests are clinically useful, and have been used with a range of client groups including people with motor speech disorders, laryngeal cancer, foreign dialect, and cleft palate. Their development and use has been important in increasing awareness of intelligibility issues. However, they have been criticized due to design difficulties, e.g. Kent *et al.* (1989) comment on the stimuli used in the *Frenchay Dysarthria Assessment* (Enderby, 1983) noting that it contains word items that are highly variable with respect to syllable number and shape thus making it difficult to understand the sources of variability in an intelligibility score.

The indices used for severity (e.g. PPC, PCC) are practical for practitioners to use: they do not require a panel of listeners and speech samples are relatively easy to obtain. However, with connected speech samples, difficulties may occur with children with very unintelligible speech when one does not know the desired target. Flipsen (2002) suggests that these indices should be obtained from spontaneous connected speech if they are to be valid. A further criticism of all the measurement techniques is the fact that although they may be able to index the intelligibility or severity of disordered speech, they are typically limited in their explanatory power, and thus in their ability to inform and monitor intervention. This important point is developed in the following section. It seems most likely that since intelligibility is not a unitary phenomenon, there is not likely to be a single adequate measure for research and clinical purposes. Kent (1992) suggests that data be triangulated or verified using a variety of different measures, e.g. by using word intelligibility tests, sentence intelligibility tests and rating scales.

Explaining Intelligibility

Research has suggested that intelligibility measures should transcend mere indexing of severity of speech disorder and attempt to seek explanations for intelligibility deficits (Kent *et al.*, 1989; Weismer and Martin, 1992). For example, individuals with dysarthria may obtain identical scores on a single-word intelligibility test, but qualitative perception of their speech may differ, and analysis of error matrices may reveal different strengths and weaknesses. A comprehensive model of intelligibility needs to account for these differences, which can then be used in treating speech disorders and monitoring progress. An explanatory model must relate overall intelligibility to underlying variables associated with

- the speech produced by the speaker;
- its transmission in the environment;
- its perception by the listener.

Any work on intelligibility needs to quantify parameters in each of these areas as well as considering interaction between them (Schiavetti, 1992). Chin, Finnegan and Chung (2001) caution that in the case of children with hearing impairment this distinction cannot be so clearly made. For such children deafness is an important audiological concern but questions of language acquisition, speech production and environment itself are equally important, typically involving professionals from a range of different, but overlapping backgrounds, e.g. speech and language therapy, audiology and education.

Much of the research into intelligibility has focused on adults with acquired neurogenic speech deficits, e.g. Parkinson's disease (Weismer, Jeng, Laures, Kent and Kent, 2001; Kempler and Van Lancker, 2002), amyotrophic lateral sclerosis (Riddell, McCauley, Mulligan and Tandan, 1995; Weismer *et al.*, 2001), dysarthria (Garcia and Dagenais, 1998; Whitehill and Ciocca, 2000; Hustad and Beukelman, 2001; De Bodt, Hernandez-Diaz and Van De Heyning, 2002; Hustad, Jones and Dailey, 2003; McHenry, 2003) as well as a fairly substantial amount of research into the speech and voice of laryngectomy patients (e.g. McColl, Fucci, Petrosino, Martin and McCaffrey, 1998; Searl, Carpenter and Banta, 2001; Prosek and Vreeland, 2001; Eksteen, Rieger, Nesbitt and Seikaly, 2003) and hearing impaired individuals (e.g. Cienkowski and Speaks, 2000; Kvam and Bredal, 2000). Studies such as these have informed our understanding of the variables that underlie intelligibility, as well as ways of measuring them, including the use of formal assessments. In terms of speaker factors we know that both segmental and supra-segmental factors influence intelligibility. Speech sound production seems to be the single most important factor in influencing intelligibility, but it is not likely to account for more than 50% of what makes an individual understandable (De Bodt *et al.*, 2002). It is likely that the interaction of segmental and supra-segmental factors is an essential aspect of understanding speech intelligibility. Segmental characteristics strongly associated with reduced intelligibility include omission of word-initial consonants, voicing errors (Miralles and

Cervera, 1995), errors of consonant clusters, consonant substitutions and unidentifiable distortions. Clearly the types of errors will depend on the speech disorders of the population under study, although within this population there will also be individual variation. Research with individuals with dysarthria (e.g. Weismer and Martin, 1992) has found that although intelligibility involves a number of potential phonetic dimensions, only a small number of these may be needed to predict a speaker's level of intelligibility. Kent, Kent, Rosenbek, Weismer, Martin, Sufit, *et al.* (1990) investigated single word productions of individuals with amyotrophic lateral sclerosis and listeners' responses to these productions. Error profiles revealed that the intelligibility deficit does not uniformly affect all phonetic contrasts. Rather, certain contrasts seem to contribute more heavily than others to the word identification errors that define an intelligibility deficit. It seems that speakers with few segmental errors may still be unintelligible and speakers with many errors may be quite intelligible (Konst *et al.*, 2000).

Supra-segmental features are thought to constitute about 20% of intelligibility in the speech of people with dysarthria (De Bodt *et al.*, 2002), and include rhythm, duration of speech sounds, stress, fundamental frequency and intonation. An excessively fast or slow rate may reduce intelligibility. Studies of adults with acquired motor speech disorders show that intelligibility increases when rate is slowed to more normal levels (e.g. Yorkston and Beukelman, 1981; Pilon, McIntosh and Thaut, 1998). Atypical stress patterns may also reduce intelligibility since listeners use stress as an automatic language processing strategy and have certain expectations. For example, consider the normal stress pattern used in a word like TOMATO where the second syllable receives primary stress (xXx): [tə ˈmɑ teʊ]. Now produce TOMATO with atypical stress, e.g. (xxX) [tə mɑ ˈteʊ]. It sounds like an entirely different word! It is not hard to imagine the difficulties experienced by second language speakers when attempting to master stress patterns in another language, and the difficulties first language speakers may have in understanding them. Speech perception does not simply involve recording a sequence of sounds as the speech signal enters the auditory system, but attending preferentially to certain aspects of the signal. These strategies are well practised and natural, having been shaped by the predictable structure of the incoming signal. Listening to the unusual speech signal produced by someone with speech difficulties challenges normal perception abilities, making it an effortful process. Yorkston and Beukelman (1981) suggest that the positive effect of slowed rate on intelligibility may occur as speakers have more time to achieve accurate articulatory placement.

In terms of voice quality, a harsh or hoarse voice adds noise to the signal making it harder to understand. High-pitched voices have fewer harmonics and are more susceptible to reduction in intelligibility. Voice quality may be a factor secondary to articulation and is thought to contribute no more than 30% of the intelligibility of dysarthric speech (De Bodt *et al.*, 2002). Hyponasal speech, e.g. as when one has a blocked nose, can be harder to understand because of the loss of oral–nasal contrasts, and hypernasal speech, typical of cleft palate, is thought to have a slightly more serious impact on intelligibility. However, overall nasality is thought to be one of the least dominant contributors to intelligibility, estimated at about 5% in dysarthric speech (De Bodt *et al.*, 2002). De Bodt *et al.*'s (2002) study on perceptual ratings of dysarthric patients showed that the impact of articulation on intelligibility is dominant, but inclusion of other dimensions, such as prosody and voice, results in a more balanced estimation of intelligibility. These authors caution that voice quality and nasality may be more important contributors for other client groups such as the hearing impaired or cleft palate populations.

In terms of the speech material used, we know that sentence intelligibility scores are higher than when single words are used (Osberger, 1992). Thus, a single-word intelligibility estimate should not be considered a good predictor of sentence or connected discourse intelligibility (Weismer and Martin, 1992) since speech perception is a highly complex process. In general, it seems that use of short, syntactically simple and semantically predictable sentences will increase intelligibility (Garcia and Dagenais, 1998).

Findings related to the listeners used to evaluate intelligibility are less clear. It is frequently noted that listeners who have had experience in listening to disordered speech give higher intelligibility ratings than naïve listeners without this experience (e.g. Osberger, 1992; Liss, Spitzer, Caviness, and Adler, 2002). Experienced listeners do not require personal knowledge of a speaker but rather the ability is generalized across all individuals with the same type of disorder (Osberger, 1992), and thus experienced speech and language therapists are generally better at understanding disordered speech than non-SLTs (see Bridges, 1991). However, Fujimoto, Madison and Larrigan (1991) and Ellis and Fucci (1992) found no significant differences between the ratings given by the SLTs and naïve listeners in their studies. Higher intelligibility scores are typically obtained when listeners are able to both see and hear speakers. The average improvement in the intelligibility of a hearing impaired talker's speech between the listener only and look-plus-listen condition has been reported to be roughly 15% (Monsen, 1983). When other visual cues (e.g. gestures, pictures, or initial letters) are used in addition to auditory signals of severely disordered dysarthric speech, intelligibility has been found to significantly increase (Hunter, Pring and Martin, 1991; Garcia and Dagenais, 1998; Hustad and Beukelman, 2001).

Compared to the adult studies above, there have been relatively few intelligibility studies that focus on children with speech difficulties. Much of the work in this area relates to children born with cleft palates (e.g. Van Lierde, De Bodt, Van Borsel, Wuyts, and Van Cauwenberge, 2002) or those with hearing impairment and cochlear implants (e.g. Chin *et al.*, 2001, 2003; Allen *et al.*, 2001), with fewer papers on autism (e.g. Koegel, Camarata, Koegel, Ben-Tall and Smith, 1998), cerebral palsy (e.g. Pennington and McConachie, 2001) and Down syndrome (Kumin, 1994). Whitehill (2002) provides an interesting review of the literature on intelligibility measures of cleft palate speech. Although intelligibility measures are being increasingly used for this population, concerns about the reliability and validity of the type of measures used were expressed as well as a reiteration of the need to use intelligibility as an explanatory factor rather than a simple index of acceptability, i.e. we need to understand the factors contributing to and resulting in intelligibility levels rather than merely stating what the intelligibility level is.

There have been even fewer studies of the intelligibility of children with phonologically disordered or delayed speech. Kwiatkowski and Shriberg (1992) studied the intelligibility of children with speech delays by asking caregivers to observe a simultaneously videotaped and audiotaped sample of a child engaged in conversation with a practitioner, and write down (gloss) what they thought their child was saying. Caregivers were correct with 78% of the utterances and 81% of the words, suggesting fairly high levels of intelligibility due to familiarity with the speakers. Weston and Shriberg (1992) used listeners' glosses of children's intended words to provide data for their studies of the potential influence of selected contextual and linguistic variables on word intelligibility. They found that intelligibility outcomes were associated with utterance length and fluency, word position, intelligibility of adjacent words, phonological complexity and grammatical form. Flipsen (1995) studied parents' intelligibility ratings of their children with phonological difficulties, and contrasted these with the ratings given by unfamiliar adults. Mothers understood significantly more words than fathers or unfamiliar adults. This is not surprising since it was noted that mothers in the study spent more time with their children than the fathers. Gordon-Brannan and Hodson (2000) carried out an investigation of pre-school children's intelligibility by comparing the scores obtained for a range of severity and intelligibility measures. The children ranged in phonological proficiency from adult-like to severely disordered. They suggested that any child above the age of four years with a speech intelligibility score of less than 66% (i.e. less than two thirds of utterances understood by unfamiliar listeners) should be considered a candidate for intervention. Their study also underlined the complexity – and importance – of measuring intelligibility.

Regarding the normal development of intelligibility, it is known that greater intelligibility is associated with increased chronological age. By three years of age, a child's spontaneous speech should be at least 50% intelligible to unfamiliar adults. By four years of age, a child's spontaneous speech should be intelligible to unfamiliar adults, even though some articulation and phonological differences are likely to be present. There remains a great deal of research to be done in determining individual factors that affect the intelligibility of children with persisting phonological difficulties.

ACTIVITY 11.3

1. Close your eyes and listen to the speech of a young child, approximately two-and-a-half years of age. How easy is it to understand his or her speech? What makes it easy or hard to understand? Consider both segmental and suprasegmental factors.
2. If possible, make a recording of the child's connected speech. Gather together a small group of listeners (either therapists, people familiar with the child or other naïve listeners). Give them the opportunity to listen to the child's speech. How easy is it to understand? What makes it easy or hard to understand? How does visual information - or lack thereof - influence a child's 'understandability'?
3. Consider similarities and differences between listening to the young child talking in your own language, and listening to a competent adult speaker of a foreign language unfamiliar to you.

Now turn to the Key to Activity 11.1 at the end of this chapter to review the list of factors which may affect intelligibility. Then read the following for further discussion of how intelligibility has been used as an outcomes measure.

Intelligibility as an Outcomes Measure

Intelligibility may be regarded as the *sine qua non* of spoken language, however it has been used as an outcome measure in a very limited number of clinical efficacy and effectiveness studies in the field of speech and language therapy to date. Outcomes measures are discussed in greater detail in Chapter 12. An outcome is the result of an intervention. Outcomes measures provide information for answering questions about clinical practice, and give an indication of treatment success. Robey and Schultz (1998) have described a systematic method for developing a treatment via a five-phase outcome research model that is employed in many scientific disciplines. We first introduced this model in Chapter 2, and it is discussed further in Chapter 12. Phase I of the model focuses on discovery, developing hypotheses about intervention to be tested in later phases; Phase II tests effectiveness; Phase III evaluates efficacy; Phase IV examines efficiency; and the final phase determines cost effectiveness, cost-benefit, and cost-utility. Specific research designs are appropriate for each phase in the model, and the evidence about a treatment's outcome, as tested in each phase, can be rated by a level, or quality, of evidence scale.

We carried out a literature search for published research focusing on intelligibility. Just 15 papers were found where intelligibility had been used as an outcomes measure following intervention. There may have been some weaknesses in our search strategy as some outcomes studies will have used intelligibility as one of many secondary measures. However, different search strategies and a common consensus in the field suggest that this is in fact the case (e.g. ASHA Special Emphasis Panel in Treatment Efficacy, 2002). Because intelligibility is a difficult concept to report reliably and accurately, many researchers may prefer to use well established standardized tests instead. Intelligibility has been used with varying degrees of validity and reliability as an outcomes measure in several surgical and medical papers (e.g. Rieger, Wolfaardt, Jha, Seikaly, 2003; Sinha, Young, Hurvitz and Crockett, 2004) suggesting that for professionals not directly involved in speech and language therapy, intelligibility seems an important and, misleadingly, 'easy-to-get-at' concept. The fact that it has been used to a limited extent to evaluate SLT interventions is unfortunate since it is a key outcomes measure for much SLT work, and a factor which unites many SLTs working with disparate client groups. However, this limited usage may suggest that SLTs are aware of the difficulties in measuring intelligibility.

Of the 15 studies using intelligibility as an outcomes measure, 11 were considered to be in Robey and Schultz's (1988) Phases III–IV, which are concerned with the efficacy, effectiveness and/or cost effectiveness of specific interventions. Of these 11 papers, six focused on dysarthric clients (Yorkston, Hammen, Beukelman and Traynor, 1990; Hunter *et al.*, 1991; Keatley and Wirz, 1994; Pilon *et al.*, 1998; Hustad *et al.*, 2003; Sapir, Spielman, Ramig, Hinds, Countryman, Fox and Story, 2003), two were with clients post-laryngectomy (Christensen and Dwyer, 1990; Max, De Bruyn and Steurs, 1997) and one focused on children with autism (Koegel *et al.*, 1998). An interesting paper by Furia, Kowalski, Latorre, Angelis, Martins, Barros, *et al.* (2001) used intelligibility as an outcome measure for a package of treatment for oral cancer patients. Patients were divided into three groups based on extent of tongue resection (total, subtotal or partial glossectomy). All patients then received speech therapy to activate articulatory adaptations, compensations, and maximization of the remaining structures for 3 to 6 months. Speech therapy was found to be effective in improving speech intelligibility, even after major resection. Improvement of speech intelligibility was noted in two of the groups. The improvement of speech intelligibility in the third group was not statistically significant, and this was attributed to the small and heterogeneous sample.

Flipsen (1995) notes that in working with children who have significant speech delays, the ultimate goal is to improve a child's ability to communicate effectively and from this point of view it is surprising that not more studies of this client group have included intelligibility data. While intervention studies concerned with addressing children's phonology have not used intelligibility measures (i.e. word identification tasks; listener-rating scales or formal intelligibility assessments), use has been made of speech severity indices. Dodd and Iacano (1989) included percentage of phonological processes (PPP) from a spontaneous language sample as a means of evaluating gains in speech production following intervention. Holm and Dodd (1999) used PCC (percentage of consonants correct) as one of several outcomes measures for the child in their study. Almost and Rosenbaum (1998) included a conversational measure (PCC - based on a conversational speech sample rather than single words) with the participants of their randomized control trial, showing that not only did their treatment group of children improve in terms of single-word production but that they went on to show gains in their conversational speech. Although measures such as PCC are not strictly intelligibility measures, they are an important bridge between impairment-based measures and intelligibility evaluations, and can provide a concise way of encapsulating the outcomes of interventions.

Intervention Case Studies and Intelligibility

In this section we consider intelligibility as an outcome measure in five school-age children with PSDs presented in this book. Before describing how we evaluated changes in the children's intelligibility, let us turn our attention to Activity 11.4.

ACTIVITY 11.4

Have you ever evaluated changes in a child's intelligibility occurring as a result of intervention? Consider how you did this, or ways that would be practical and quick to do. Bear in mind some of the points made in this chapter about outcomes measures and carrying out reliable and valid measures. Once you have reflected on these points, read on to find out how we evaluated intelligibility changes occurring in a small number of children with PSDs.

How Did We Evaluate the Children's Intelligibility?

Oliver, Joshua, Katy, Rachel and Ben are five children with PSDs described in chapters throughout this book. Because these children were very different, each child was viewed as a single case. We wanted to measure each child's intelligibility before and after intervention, so that we would know whether our intervention had brought about any changes at this very functional level. For each child we obtained measures of intelligibility from a group of unfamiliar listeners in identical conditions. Pre- and post-intervention intelligibility scores were compared, and any changes were related to other outcomes measures. Speech severity indices (PCC, PVC and PPC) were also calculated for each child before and after intervention, so that severity and intelligibility could be contrasted.

The Participants

Because intelligibility is about both speaker and listener, the participants in our intelligibility evaluation included the children (as speakers) and then a larger group of listeners. Further details follow below.

Children

The five school-aged children between the ages of 5;6 and 9;5 have been introduced in previous chapters. The children attended the same mainstream school where they received individual speech and language therapy on a twice-weekly basis with the same therapist. The children received therapy for a period of four to nine months. Therapy was based on psycholinguistic principles following a careful analysis of each child's underlying strengths and weaknesses. The therapy activities consisted of some traditional table-top therapy as well as computer-based sessions. The children were monolingual English speakers who have ongoing speech and language difficulties that have not resolved despite previous intervention. The children differed in terms of age, nature and severity of speech difficulties, concurrent problems and educational attainment. Each of the children received intervention tailor-made to their specific needs, as part of a single case study design.

Listeners

Naïve (i.e. untrained listeners with no special knowledge of language) and unfamiliar (i.e. they did not know the children) listeners were used to judge the children's speech. First year speech and language therapy, and speech sciences students were invited to participate as listeners in the study. These students had:

(a) limited experience of children with speech disorders;
(b) lived in Britain for the past three years and had English as their first language;
(c) normal speech and hearing.

This information was obtained by means of a written questionnaire. Responses from students who did not meet all three criteria were excluded from the analysis, e.g. students who had worked for more than 6 months' duration with a child or children with speech difficulties were excluded. In total, 33 students participated in the study.

Materials

All the assessment and intervention sessions with the children had been audio-taped. The children and their guardians had given informed consent for the recordings to be made and for these to be used anonymously for research and teaching purposes. From this body of data, a sample of speech was compiled for each of the five children pre- and post-intervention, consisting of 10 sentences and 20 single words spoken on two occasions, pre- and post-intervention. Intelligibility is typically found to be higher when sentences are used, although the relationship between single words and sentences might vary from child to child. Including both single words and sentences was thought to allow for a representative sample of each child's speech while also giving the opportunity to compare the relationship between the single-word and sentence conditions. Sentences between 5 and 15 syllables were used. These had been obtained using repetition tasks. Oliver, the youngest child (see Chapter 4), was not able to carry out the repetition tasks due to concentration and/or memory difficulties, and for this reason there was no repeated sentence data for him. Because of the single case design, and the fact that the children varied in terms of age and mean length of utterance, different items were selected for each child. This also reduced any learning effects within the listener group. We aimed to choose single words and connected speech that were representative of normal everyday speech, and did not focus specifically on the words or segments addressed in therapy. For example, Joshua's intervention focused specifically on consonant clusters but his single-word speech sample was based on a random selection of words, only a small number of which contained clusters.

The inclusion of spontaneous speech posed a problem. Spontaneous, connected speech is important for valid measures of intelligibility (Kent *et al.*, 1994). However, by definition it is unlikely that one will obtain the same spontaneous utterances on two separate occasions, i.e. pre- and post-intervention. However, in an attempt to include spontaneous speech, four further speech samples were included for each child. These consisted of two spontaneous sentences spoken before intervention and two (other, different) spontaneous sentences for each child post-intervention. An attempt was made to match these spontaneous items in terms of length and content.

The audio recordings of all the speech samples were put in a randomized order onto CD-ROMs. For each child 10% of the utterances were repeated so that the reliability of listeners' responses could be calculated. This is termed intra-judge or intra-rater reliability and can be measured using a statistical procedure: Pearson's product moment correlation (for more information see Pallant, 2001). We found a strong positive correlation between the scores, which means that most of the 33 raters were being reasonably consistent in how they responded to identical items. Inter-rater reliability was also calculated using another statistical procedure called Cronbach's alpha (α). Inter-rater reliability is the extent to which two or more individuals agree, i.e. it evaluates the consistency of the responses across all raters. Using this procedure we found a lower inter-rater reliability, however Pallant (2001) suggests that where a limited number of test items is used, a lower score is considered acceptable. These measures are important for demonstrating that a study is evaluating what it claims to measure and is doing so in ways that are replicable. Practitioners carrying out less formal intelligibility assessments with smaller groups of listeners may not necessarily have the time to quantify reliability in this way.

Procedure

The word-identification or write-down paradigm in which words intended by the speaker are compared with words understood by the listener is consistent with definitions of intelligibility. It has also been shown to be a valid, reliable measure of intelligibility and was thus chosen as the criterion measure in this study. The procedure was piloted with a group of 60 speech and language therapists to refine the procedure before being used in the study.

Each of the students was given an evaluation booklet. The cover of the booklet contained written instructions for reference, as well as a brief questionnaire designed to elicit information about the student's eligibility to participate. Sheets inside the booklet consisted of consecutively numbered blank answer blocks. Instructions were given verbally, as well as in written form on the evaluation sheets for reference. Instructions given were as follows.

> I am going to play you some samples of children's speech. Listen carefully and then write down what you think each child is saying. Don't use phonetic transcription. All the children are saying proper English words and I want you to guess what they are. They are all children from the north of England.
>
> If you don't know what the child is saying try to make a guess. Remember there is no right or wrong answer. The important thing is to guess at what you hear.

> Let me show you what I mean. (Plays the tape and a child says: 'Critmit'.) Now, I have clearly heard 'critmit' but that is not a real, English word so I can't write that. What does it sound like? It does sound a bit like 'Christmas' so I'll guess that it's Christmas. I'll write CHRISTMAS in next to the relevant number.
>
> I can only play each sample for you once. If you have a problem or I'm going too fast, please put your hand up or just shout STOP as I can stop the tape at any time for you and help you with your questions. If you do get left behind - just put a dash and move on to the next numbered item you hear.

The recordings were played to the group using a laptop computer and speakers. Four practice items were given initially to familiarize students with the task.

Analysis

Two levels of analysis took place. Initially, whole words (the single words in isolation and in sentences) were the focus of the evaluation. A more fine-grained analysis then took place, looking within words at segmental features. Each of these analyses is outlined in turn.

Whole-word Analysis

Single words were marked as correct where a listener's written response matched the child's target production. They were marked as incorrect where the listener's written response differed from the child's target production or where they indicated that they did not know what the child had meant. In cases where students suggested two possible 'answers,' i.e. writing <tusk> or <task> for TUSK, a point was awarded as long as the target item appeared. In cases where plural forms were omitted or extraneously included, i.e. writing <dogs> for DOG, or <cat> for CATS, points were awarded irrespectively. The repeated sentences and spontaneous speech were marked on a word-by-word basis with points given for any correctly matching words, again slight differences in morphology were discounted. The percentage of total words transcribed correctly in each of the 10 samples (pre- and post-intervention for each of the five children) was calculated. Next, the percentage of single words in isolation, and single words in sentences, transcribed correctly was calculated to yield separate single words and sentence scores for each child pre- and post-intervention. Finally, spontaneous speech scores were considered for each child.

The main objective was to evaluate any changes in intelligibility that occurred within each child, from the pre-intervention assessment to the post-intervention assessment. Repeated measures t-tests were used for this purpose, with each child regarded as a single case. Results were calculated for all utterances to yield overall intelligibility scores, as well as for single words, repeated sentences and spontaneous speech.

Within-word Analysis

The within-word analysis was based closely on the methods outlined by Bryan and Howard (1992, pp. 362–3) for comparing a stimulus with a response. For each target item (single words and sentences), the number of consonants[1] was counted, i.e. there are three consonant targets in the single word item GASP and nine in a standard British English production of the following sentence:

THE MAN LIKED THE GIRL.

The listeners' responses were re-evaluated by converting each grapheme into the corresponding phoneme, and then comparing it to the target consonant. Each consonant was awarded between 0 and 3 points (1 point for correct voicing, 1 point for correct manner of articulation, and 1 point for correct place of articulation). Matched consonants were awarded 3 points, and where consonants were omitted 0 points were given. For example, a listener who wrote <cusp> when Rachel produced GASP, received 8 (out of a possible 9) points. He was given 2 points for the correct place and manner features of the word initial [k], and 3 points each for the correct [s] and [p] segments. Another listener who wrote <boo> for GASP, received 1 point (from the possible 9) for the shared manner feature of the initial stop.

Bryan and Howard (1992) outlined two versions of this scoring procedure: strict and lenient scoring. The lenient method was used for the purposes of this study. This meant that consonants in a word response did not have to occur in the same syllabic position as in the stimulus word to score for feature similarity, i.e. when comparing a CVC response such as <cap> with the CVCV stimulus CAPER, full points were awarded for the matching [k] and [p]. For sentences, this lenient procedure was again adopted, with an attempt made to match response words with stimulus words, e.g. for the stimulus THE MAN LIKED THE GIRL, the written response <like a girl> was matched, not sequentially with the first three words but logically with the last three words of the utterances. If, as in many cases, it was not possible to discern which part of a sentence had been attempted, then response and stimulus words were matched in a one-to-one, sequential way. Repeated measures t-tests were used to compare mean scores for each child's pre- and post-intervention results. Results were again calculated for all utterances to yield overall intelligibility scores, as well as for single words, repeated sentences and spontaneous speech. The design is summarized in Table 11.1.

Severity indices (PCC, PVC and PPC) were also calculated for each child, before and after intervention and are included for comparative

Table 11.1: Design of intelligibility evaluation showing comparisons made between pre- and post-intervention for each child

	Level of Analysis			
	Whole-word analysis		Within-word analysis	
Single words	pre	post	pre	post
Repeated sentences	pre	post	pre	post
Spontaneous speech	pre	post	pre	post

purposes. These indices were based on a random sampling of 50–100 utterances before and after intervention, following procedures outlined by Shriberg and Kwiatkowski (1982) and Dodd (1995).

ACTIVITY 11.5

Consider the single-word sample of Joshua's pre- and post-intervention data presented below, together with the written response from one of the listeners.

Single words:

Target	Listener writes (pre)	Listener writes (post)
YELLOW	hello	yellow
BROTHER	brother	brother
SCARF	car	calf

Now complete the table of Joshua's pre- and post-intervention intelligibility scores for single words based on the results for this one listener. You may need to refer to the description of the two levels of analysis given previously.

	Level of Analysis			
	Whole-word analysis		Within-word analysis	
	Pre	Post	Pre	Post
Single words				

Turn to the Key to Activity 11.5 on completion of the table. Then read the following for more information about how the five children's intelligibility changed over the course of intervention.

What Were the Results?

Oliver

Oliver's intelligibility did not change significantly over the course of the intervention. His single-word intelligibility was extremely low both before and after intervention, e.g. at the whole-word level 0% of single words were correctly identified pre-intervention, increasing to 2% post-intervention. From a qualitative perspective it was noted that while none of the listeners correctly identified Oliver's targets for pre-intervention utterances, 25% of them were able to identify his production of some single word targets post-intervention, e.g. CAT – /k/ and /t/ were both segments that were addressed in therapy. Oliver was not able to carry out the repeated sentences task due to memory and concentration difficulties, and thus there were no data from him in that section. Oliver's spontaneous speech intelligibility was low and again showed no significant difference from pre- to post-intervention. Nevertheless a significant difference was found when comparing his intelligibility at the single word level, with the scores obtained for spontaneous speech ($t(16) = -2.25$, $p < 0.05$). This may reflect the fact that Oliver is a skilled communicator in other ways, using supra-segmental cues such as pitch variation to help convey his messages. Oliver's speech severity indices revealed severe difficulties with his consonant production, and moderate difficulties with vowel production. Significant changes in these severity indices did not occur when comparing pre- and post-intervention results. Oliver's intelligibility scores are summarized in Table 11.2.

Joshua

Joshua's intelligibility did not change significantly over the course of the intervention. At the single-word level his intelligibility was greater than children such as Oliver and Katy. However, the difference between his scores pre- and post-intervention was not significant. Joshua's intelligibil-

Table 11.2: Oliver's intelligibility scores showing percentage of items correct from pre- to post-intervention

	Level of Analysis			
	Whole-word analysis		Within-word analysis	
	Pre	Post	Pre	Post
Single words	0	2	16	22
Repeated sentences	Not tested			
Spontaneous speech	13	19	27	36

ity for sentences also showed no significant change from pre- to post-intervention evaluation. For spontaneous speech, Joshua's results suggested the highest level of intelligibility for all the children. A substantial (but not significant) decrease was noted in his spontaneous intelligibility from T1 to T2 (85% pre-intervention to 68% post-intervention). This may have been due to the selection of the spontaneous utterances: the fact that they were not appropriately matched in some way, and that only two spontaneous utterances were selected for each time period. Despite the many processes still occurring in his speech and the immature quality of his speech outlined in Chapter 6, his intelligibility in spontaneous speech was relatively high. A significant difference was noted between his single word intelligibility and his spontaneous speech intelligibility ($t(10) = -2.26$, $p < 0.05$). Severity indices revealed a mild–moderate level of difficulty for Joshua, with this again remaining constant over the course of the intervention. Joshua's intelligibility scores are summarized in Table 11.3.

Katy

Katy's intelligibility did not change significantly from pre- to post-intervention. Her single-word intelligibility was very low, both before and after intervention, e.g. at the whole-word level 5% of single words were correctly identified pre-intervention, increasing to 6% post-intervention. Katy's speech intelligibility at the sentence level similarly did not show a significant change from pre- to post-intervention despite the fact that her intervention had specifically addressed connected speech. Katy also made no significant changes in her intelligibility at the spontaneous speech level when comparing pre- and post-intervention scores. Unlike Oliver, her scores for the single word and sentence tasks were consistent, with no significant differences noted between the tasks using different stimuli. Katy was the only child to show significant gains in her speech severity indices. She made significant gains with her overall PPC ($t(99) = -4.662$,

Table 11.3: Joshua's intelligibility scores showing percentage of items correct from pre- to post-intervention

	Level of Analysis			
	Whole-word analysis		Within-word analysis	
	Pre	Post	Pre	Post
Single words	22	28	54	59
Repeated sentences	45	40	48	49
Spontaneous speech	85	68	91	65

$p < 0.001$) which changed from 41.9% to 58.2%. Significant gains were also noted for her PCC scores from 22% (pre-intervention) to 49% (post-intervention), $t(99) = -6.051$, $p < 0.01$. Her PVC did not change significantly from pre- to post-intervention. Final consonant production formed the focus of her intervention, and this was a 'drop in the ocean' given the pervasiveness and severity of her speech difficulties. Interestingly, her teachers and parents commented on her improved intelligibility, which was not demonstrated in our intelligibility procedure, but may have been noticed in the 'real world' due to increased confidence and willingness to try and rephrase her speech when misunderstood. Table 11.4 summarizes Katy's intelligibility scores.

Rachel

Rachel's intelligibility improved significantly over the course of the intervention. For single words, the whole-word analysis revealed no significant change, however the within-word analysis revealed significant improvements in intelligibility from 56% (pre-intervention) to 74% (post-intervention), $t(19) = -2.31$, $p < 0.05$. No significant gains were noted for the repeated sentences and spontaneous speech at either level of analysis. The difference between her single-word and connected speech intelligibility was not a significant one. Rachel's intelligibility was relatively good, and her severity indices mild, in comparison to the other children. This is not surprising given the descriptions of her speech in Chapter 9: her surface speech difficulties were more specific and less severe than the other children. Her speech severity scores were approaching ceiling at pre-intervention, e.g. PCC of 96%. Table 11.5 summarises Rachel's intelligibility scores.

Ben

Ben's intelligibility improved significantly over the course of the intervention, following a similar pattern to Rachel. Like Rachel, his surface speech

Table 11.4: Katy's intelligibility scores showing percentage of items correct from pre- to post-intervention

	Level of Analysis			
	Whole-word analysis		Within-word analysis	
	Pre	Post	Pre	Post
Single words	5	6	38	40
Repeated sentences	10	6	19	16
Spontaneous speech	8	11	17	18

Table 11.5: Rachel's intelligibility scores showing percentage of items correct from pre- to post-intervention

	Level of Analysis			
	Whole-word analysis		Within-word analysis	
	Pre	Post	Pre	Post
Single words	28	40	56	74
Repeated sentences	60	64	63	78
Spontaneous speech	38	50	48	62

Table 11.6: Ben's intelligibility scores showing percentage of items correct from pre- to post-intervention

	Level of Analysis			
	Whole-word analysis		Within-word analysis	
	Pre	Post	Pre	Post
Single words	34	40	65	74
Repeated sentences	64	73	69	76
Spontaneous speech	24	50	24	62

difficulties were more specific and less severe than the other children. For single words, the whole-word analysis revealed no significant change, however the within-word analysis revealed significant improvements in intelligibility from 65% (pre-intervention) to 74% (post-intervention, $t(31) = -2.61$, $p < 0.05$). No significant gains were noted for the repeated sentences and spontaneous speech at either level of analysis. The difference between his single-word and connected speech intelligibility was not a significant one. Ben's severity indices showed a mild level of difficulty, approaching ceiling pre-intervention and not demonstrating a significant change post-intervention. Table 11.6 summarizes Ben's intelligibility scores.

Discussion

Katy and Oliver were children with extremely high severity indices pre-intervention. Low levels of intelligibility were noted both before and after intervention for these children. These levels of less than 10% indicate profoundly unintelligible speech. As such it is unlikely that significant intelligibility gains would be made after one episode of intervention. Intelligibility should not be used as the main or only outcome for children with PSDs as they may never reach high levels of intelligibility, and other less obvious changes in their speech may be lost. Intervention was specific in targeting certain aspects of their speech difficulties. In Katy's case it is not surprising that overall intelligibility did not improve given the range of simplifying processes still occurring in her speech, and the fact that her speech intervention was very specifically addressed to one particular process. Similarly, Oliver received intervention for four specific consonants, but almost all consonants were potential candidates as targets and will need to be addressed in the future.

Two levels of analysis were carried out: one focusing on whole words, and the other looking within words at the accuracy of consonantal features. At the first level, the intelligibility evaluation did not reveal any significant changes in intelligibility for any of the children. At the more fine-grained level of analysis, significant improvements in intelligibility were found for two of the children: Rachel and Ben. Previous studies have evaluated intelligibility using only the whole-word method. Our evaluation suggested that this method may be too gross to reveal differences, and that a more detailed analysis of results can show gains that would otherwise go undetected. For example, Katy made significant gains in her ability to produce final consonants (see Chapter 8, and Pascoe, Stackhouse and Wells, 2005). The intervention aimed to get her to produce any final consonant, rather than the specifically correct segment. One of Katy's stimuli in the intelligibility task was NOTE. In the pre-intervention sample she produces [neʊ]. Most of the listeners wrote <no> in accordance with what they heard. The post-intervention sample had Katy producing [neʊd], and most of the listeners duly wrote <node> or <nod>. The whole-word scoring system was not able to credit this improvement, but the within-word level was able to take this into account. It is clear that improvements had been made as she was now using final consonants, yet there is still likely to be a great deal of confusion for her listeners until she is able to voice final plosives appropriately and mark phonological contrasts in this position: possible next steps for intervention. It would be valuable to monitor intelligibility with children receiving ongoing intervention to determine at which point in the intervention programme intelligibility significantly improves. This perspective ties in well with a cycles approach to intervention (Hodson and Paden, 1991) where a child is exposed to more than one isolated sound over the course of intervention and has the opportunity for making rapid progress with some sounds and slower progress with more challenging segments as they are cycled and recycled in intervention sessions.

The within-word feature analysis is not without problems. Listeners participating in the evaluation were asked to write down what they thought the children were saying. They were also instructed to guess at words or to indicate parts of words or sentence in cases where they were unsure what the entire utterance was. When listeners provided partial information (e.g. writing <c ?> or <something ending with 'b'> this was useful for the feature analysis. However, in many cases listeners entirely omitted a response providing no information about parts of the word they might have heard. Instructions to listeners should emphasize the importance of giving a response.

The fact that limited changes were noted for some of the children may be due to the method used to evaluate intelligibility. In this study listeners unfamiliar with the children were required to discern what the children were saying from audio samples of the children's speech, many at a single-word level. Many of the listeners described the task as extremely challenging, and mentioned reasons such as accents, lack of visual information and context, as reasons that made it so. It has been found in previous research that listeners who have had experience in listening to disordered speech give higher intelligibility ratings than naïve listeners without this experience (e.g. Osberger, 1992; Liss *et al.*, 2002). Results from our evaluation carried out with speech and language therapists could not be directly compared to the results obtained from the student listener group, but the comments from both groups suggested that the task was challenging for the SLTs too. Removing some of the constraints (e.g. presenting both audio and video recordings) may have meant that the children's intelligibility increased, and would be more representative of a real life situation. The listeners could then have picked up on a wider range of cues that may have made the evaluation a more sensitive one. As it was, children such as Oliver and Katy who had made gains in their speech production (see Chapters 4 and 8 respectively) were not able to demonstrate these in the intelligibility task at either level of analysis.

Higher intelligibility scores are typically found when listeners are able to both see and hear speakers. The average improvement in the intelligibility of hearing impaired talker's speech between the listener only and look-plus-listen condition has been estimated as approximately 15% (Monsen, 1983). When other visual cues (e.g. gestures, pictures, or initial letters) are used in addition to auditory signals of severely disordered dysarthric speech, intelligibility has been found to significantly increase (Hunter *et al.*, 1991; Garcia and Dagenais, 1998; Hustad and Beukelman, 2001). Konst *et al.* (2000) cautioned that visual cues were absent in the experimental situation in their study. Clearly such cues provide important contextual support in real life interaction. If you were working specifically to improve intelligibility, you would be bringing this in to your therapy and training the speaker in the full use of cues as appropriate, e.g. including AAC (alternative and augmentative communication). Our intelligibility evaluation gave information about the children's speech pre- and post-intervention but it does not reflect any changes in their broader competence as interactive communication partners. Further, the lack of normative data has also been cited as a methodological difficulty: we do not know how normally-developing children and adults would perform on tasks such as these.

Spontaneous speech is central to the concept of intelligibility. In this evaluation single words and repeated sentences comprised the bulk of each child's speech sample. A very limited number of spontaneous items were included since they were difficult to match in terms of pre- and post-intervention production, and it is not always possible to know exactly what children with the severe speech problems were saying. Many of the children received higher intelligibility ratings for their spontaneous speech, and given that this is the most functionally relevant aspect of children's communication it is important that future studies of this kind include greater numbers of carefully matched spontaneous speech samples. For spontaneous speech, Joshua's results suggested the highest level of intelligibility for all the children. Despite the many processes still occurring in his speech and the immature quality of his speech outlined in Chapter 6, his intelligibility in spontaneous speech was high. Joshua often used an inappropriately loud voice. Although this is not always socially acceptable, it may have aided the listeners in the intelligibility task. Increased volume often comes about through deeper breathing and change of posture which in turn might help to produce clearer speech. This would explain Joshua's highest intelligibility score for the spontaneous items as compared to the single words or repeated sentences, as it was frequently noted when he was telling a story to the therapist that he would speak very loudly and emphatically.

Intelligibility and severity are closely related concepts affected by many common factors. The relationship between severity (as measured by PPC for single words) and intelligibility (for single words at a whole-word level) was investigated in our evaluation and a strong positive correlation between the two variables was found. This is consistent with the findings of Shriberg and Kwiatkowski (1982) who found similarly high correlations between the two measures. Most intervention studies that have attempted to include functional measures of changes in speech have incorporated the latter, using measures such as PCC, PVC and PPC (e.g. Almost and Rosenbaum, 1998; Holm and Dodd, 1999). These measures are relatively easy to obtain, do not require special equipment and unfamiliar listener groups, and can provide valuable information about a child's overall level of difficulty and progress. All the children's results are higher than their intelligibility ratings. This is not surprising given the different evaluation procedures used. Our results suggest that speech indices may not, however, always provide a full picture of a child's intelligibility. Rachel and Ben had PPC scores that suggested mild levels of severity, yet their intelligibility was only moderate, emphasizing that there are additional factors at play when evaluating intelligibility. Katy showed significant gains in her PCC score from pre- to post-intervention, yet this change did not yet have an effect on her intelligibility - at least within the stringent constraints of the evaluation that took place here. This discrepancy suggests that while PPC and related measures are concerned with individual segments, intelligibility measures move beyond this, incorporating supra-segmental and other features that can have a great effect on how poorly or well children with speech difficulties are able to make themselves understood. Rachel's intelligibility improved significantly from pre- to post-intervention, although her intelligibility was initially high. Intervention addressed one very specific aspect of her speech, yet her intelligibility improved for all words even those that did not contain the specific structures addressed in intervention. It was clear that Rachel gained a great deal of confidence as a result of the intervention and the change brought about in her speech. The initial recordings are quiet with Rachel's speech sounding generally unclear and mumbly. The final set of recordings show her speaking with a strong, louder voice and it was not surprising that her speech in general was considered more intelligible. This example highlights some of the difficulties in objectively measuring and explaining intelligibility. These factors are discussed in the following section which returns to intelligibility from a more general perspective.

A great many unanswered questions remain about children's speech intelligibility. First, the relationship between children's phonology and intelligibility remains unclear. Although factors such as loss of phonological contrasts, homonymy and consistency affect intelligibility, it is not clear how each of these factors contributes to intelligibility, and how the factors interact with each other. While we know that segmental phonology alone does not contribute to intelligibility, the other factors remain hard to access and measure. Work with adult clients with dysarthria by De Bodt *et al.* (2002) attempted to discern variables affecting intelligibility and to weight these in terms of relative percentage contributions. The clinical importance of such information is not hard to imagine: Yorkston *et al.* (1992) suggested that it is precisely the sort of information that is needed in order to move towards 'an intelligibility-based model of intervention'. For children with PSDs requiring long-term intervention, it would be helpful for practitioners to know which factors - segmental and otherwise - have the greatest effect on intelligibility, so that these could be prioritized in intervention. It may be that such factors vary from child to child, or that certain factors are linked to children of different ages, phases, sub-groups or speech processing profiles. Such information would be helpful in accounting for the persisting speech difficulties that some children experience despite having normal phonetic repertoires and performing age-appropriately on standardized measures.

From a psycholinguistic perspective there is much to be gained from linking the concept of intelligibility into one's understanding of a child's strengths and weaknesses. Intelligibility is clearly affected by speech processing at each of the output levels, but further work is needed to consider the contributions of levels such as motor programming, motor planning and self-monitoring of one's own speech. Intelligibility can seem a large and ungainly concept; tying it to a psycholinguistic framework may allow one to account for it more readily, and measure it more accurately. One way in which this might be done is by linking intelligibility measures to the developmental phase model from Stackhouse and Wells (1997) (see Figure 2.3 in Chapter 2). We know that normally-developing children's intelligibility increases with age, and that the same trend is likely to be followed by children with difficulties, although at a slower pace. It may be that at the whole-word level of development, intelligibility is low as children are concerned with meaning units in a fairly gross way. As children move through the systematic simplification phase and into the assembly phase of speech development, they may become more concerned with sound structures resulting in increased intelligibility. The dawning of the metaphonological phase may mean that they are now able to reflect on their speech in a more objective way, taking the listener's perspective into account and maximizing intelligibility through careful self-monitoring. However, while some children with severe speech difficulties may be able to make the leap into the metaphonological phase, they may still be unable to modify their speech production (and intelligibility) because of their motor problems in output.

It has been suggested here that intelligibility should be routinely included in evaluations of interventions for children with phonological difficulties. The inclusion of such measures will not only enhance our theoretical understanding of intelligibility, but also add to the armoury of outcomes measures that allow us to ensure interventions are socially and functionally relevant. Such evaluations are not without their difficulties, e.g. to measure changes in spontaneous speech intelligibility in ways that are reliable and valid may mean to lose what lies at the heart of intelligibility: spontaneity and 'real life' communication. When children with very severe difficulties are included in intelligibility evaluations with unfamiliar listeners, the task may become extremely challenging. In such cases, using visual information may allow for a task at a more appropriate level of difficulty in which subtle changes in children's communication can be more readily discerned.

The evaluation presented in this chapter attempted to devise a method for the reliable and valid measurement of intelligibility. The procedure was used successfully to this end, although suggestions have been made for future modifications. Intelligibility needs to be routinely evaluated both in intervention studies and in practice. Evaluations such as the one carried out here contribute to a body of knowledge about intelligibility and the factors that constitute it. Refinement of procedures for measurement of intelligibility will also inform our knowledge of these factors and ensure that our intervention outcomes are ultimately more valid, reliable and meaningful.

Intelligibility: Suggestions for Assessment and Therapy

This section draws together some suggestions for 'best practice' when using intelligibility in intervention and assessment.

- Intelligibility should routinely be used as a clinical outcome measure when working with children with PSDs.
- Intelligibility should not be used as the main or only outcome measure as doing so may mean that other important changes are disregarded.
- A range of outcomes should be used so that intelligibility can be contextualized together with other more specific changes that may have occurred.
- Word identification tasks are thought to have high validity and can be carried out using a small number of listeners (either familiar or unfamiliar with the child) and carefully selected recorded samples of the child's speech.
- In order for pre- and post-intervention comparisons to be meaningful, the conditions of the listening tasks and listeners used should be as similar as possible.
- Single words, repeated sentences and spontaneous speech should all be included in intelligibility evaluations.
- Spontaneous speech needs to be carefully matched for length of utterance, content and complexity.
- When carrying out intelligibility evaluations scoring needs to be sufficiently fine-grained to take into account the specific changes that may have occurred - especially for children with severe difficulties.
- Intelligibility evaluations including the group listening task in Activity 11.3 (No. 2), are useful for gathering information on all aspects contributing to intelligibility or lack thereof.
- This information can then be used to drive intervention where appropriate, e.g. if a fast rate is perceived as compromising intelligibility, intervention might focus on reducing rate.

Summary

The key points from this chapter are as follows.

- Intelligibility is widely held to be an important outcome when working with children with speech problems.
- It is however not well defined or understood and has been used as a clinical outcome measure in a fairly small number of studies.

- Intelligibility can be measured by means of word identification tasks, listener rating interval scales and formal tests.
- Intelligibility levels are frequently used in making clinical decisions, and therefore measurements need to be reliable, and valid.
- Word identification tasks have been shown to have the highest validity and reliability, but using a variety of methods for assessing intelligibility can also be helpful.
- Intelligibility needs to be explained and accounted for by considering the interaction of speaker, transmission system or environment, and listener.
- Speech sound production seems to be the single most important factor in influencing intelligibility, but it is not likely to account for more than 50% of what makes an individual understandable.
- The interaction of segmental and supra-segmental factors is an essential aspect of understanding speech intelligibility.
- There have been relatively few intelligibility studies that focus on children with speech difficulties.
- We used intelligibility as a clinical outcome measure by playing recordings of the children's pre- and post-intervention speech to unfamiliar listeners who carried out a word-identification task.
- Two of the five children showed significantly improved intelligibility as a result of the intervention.
- We suggest that this change needs to be viewed in the context of other, more fine-grained outcomes measures, but that the importance of intelligibility to drive intervention and as an ultimate outcome measure should not be underestimated.

KEY TO ACTIVITY 11.1

A speaker's intelligibility may be affected by:

- age: children may be harder to understand than adults;
- unfamiliar language/accents;
- very quiet/very loud speech;
- mumbly/slurred speech;
- being tired/ill;
- very fast/slow rate;
- articulation/phonology problems, e.g. sound substitutions, omissions, distortions;
- prosody;
- hyponasal speech/voice problems;
- hesitant/non-fluent speech.

Listeners may be affected by:

- hearing impairment/blocked ears;
- effect, e.g. if distracted, emotional;
- unfamiliarity with a language/dialect;
- unfamiliarity with listener.

Environmental factors:

- lack of visual information;
- no knowledge of context/topic;
- background noise.

KEY TO ACTIVITY 11.5*

	Level of Analysis			
	Whole-word analysis		Within-word analysis	
	Pre	Post	Pre	Post
Single words	1/3 (33.3%)	2/3 (66.6%)	15/24 (62.5%)*	21/24 (87.5%)

* We used standard British English to determine the number of targets. This may differ from readers' own pronunciation of some of the items, e.g. where /r/ is pronounced rhotically (as a consonant) in BROTHER

Worked Examples

Using Whole-word Analysis

Target	Listener writes (pre)	Listener writes (post)
YELLOW	hello	yellow
Whole-word scoring:	*0 (wrong)*	*1 (correct)*
BROTHER	brother	brother
Whole-word scoring:	*1 (correct)*	*1 (correct)*
SCARF	car	calf
Whole-word scoring:	*0 (wrong)*	*0 (wrong)*
TOTAL	1	2
For single words Using whole-word scoring, i.e. out of 3		

Using Within-word Analysis (× = wrong; √ = right/feature match with target)

Target	Listener writes (pre)	Listener writes (post)
<u>Y</u>E<u>LL</u>OW	<u>h</u>e<u>ll</u>o	<u>y</u>e<u>ll</u>ow
2 consonants: j, l		
each consonant has		
3 features:		
j: place: palatal	h: place: glottal ×	j: place: palatal √
manner: approximant	manner: fricative ×	manner: approximant √
voicing: voiced	voicing: voiceless ×	voicing: voiced √
l: place: alveolar	l: place: alveolar √	l: place: alveolar √
manner: approximant	manner: approximant √	manner: approximant √
voicing: voiced	voicing: voiced √	voicing: voiced √
<u>BR</u>O<u>TH</u>ER	<u>br</u>o<u>th</u>er	<u>br</u>o<u>th</u>er
3 consonants: b, r, ð		
each consonant has		
3 features:		
b: place: labial	b: place: labial √	b: place: labial √
manner: plosive	manner: plosive √	manner: plosive √
voicing: voiced	voicing: voiced √	voicing: voiced √
r: place: palatal	r: place: palatal √	r: place: palatal √
manner: liquid	manner: liquid √	manner: liquid √
voicing: voiced	voicing: voiced √	voicing: voiced √
ð: place: interdental	ð: place: interdental √	ð: place: interdental √
manner: fricative	manner: fricative √	manner: fricative √
voicing: voiced	voicing: voiced √	voicing: voiced √
<u>SC</u>AR<u>F</u>	<u>c</u>ar	<u>c</u>al<u>f</u>
3 consonants: /s, k, f/		
each consonant has		
3 features:		
s: place: alveolar	s: (omitted) ×	s: (omitted) ×
manner: fricative	×	×
voicing: voiceless	×	×
k: place: velar	k: place: velar √	k: place: velar √
manner: plosive	manner: plosive √	manner: plosive √
voicing: voiceless	voicing: voiceless √	voicing: voiceless √
f: place: dental	f: (omitted) ×	f: place: dental √
manner: fricative	×	manner: fricative √
voicing: voiceless	×	voicing: voiceless √
TOTAL:		
Potential features: 24	15 (√s)	21 (√s)

Note

1. Vowels were not included in this analysis because (a) they were not directly addressed in any of the children's intervention programmes, and (b) the results from PVC indices revealed that all children had relatively accurate vowel production. Vowels do not lend themselves so well to this type of feature analysis.

Chapter 12 Evaluating Intervention Outcomes

Evaluating intervention outcomes is arguably the most important part of the intervention process. Without this we cannot be sure we are doing the best for our clients and have no case in the argument for improved service delivery. There are constant calls in the literature and in our daily work for evidence to demonstrate that what we do works, and is a good investment of time and money. We also need to build and share evidence in order to develop the field: there is no point in each of us reinventing the wheel! Undoubtedly, an important goal in the study of children with specific speech, language and literacy difficulties is to enhance current knowledge of effective intervention. Without detailed studies of intervention, there can be no increase in knowledge about effective practice (Stackhouse and Wells, 2001). Evaluating intervention can also provide a sense of job satisfaction and motivation for individual practitioners. When we have evidence that what we do works, we are more confident and more secure in our attempts to develop further and build on that success. When intervention is carried out in a controlled way, the outcomes of the programme allow us to return to the theoretical starting point, and reconsider the nature of the speech and language processing system, and difficulties that may affect it.

Although we often believe that what we do works, we need to be able to demonstrate this in ways that move beyond the anecdotal and intuitive. Furthermore, whereas we are being increasingly asked to supply objective quantifiable evidence of the effectiveness of our procedures, it is not always clear how such evidence should be gathered and what it should consist of (Letts, 1995). In this chapter we attempt to pull together what is known about intervention outcomes and how to measure these. First, we focus on some commonly used terms such as outcomes, effectiveness, efficacy and efficiency, exploring what is meant by each term. Second, we provide a theoretical basis for conceptualizing outcomes measurements. Third, we turn our attention to what is known about outcomes of speech therapy intervention for school-age children with persisting speech difficulties and in what areas information is still needed. Fourth, focusing on case studies, we discuss the outcomes of intervention, as well as giving some practical pointers for ways in which intervention outcomes can be measured. Finally, we demonstrate how we can all contribute to these without making great changes to the ways in which we are already practising.

What are Outcomes?

An outcome is most simply defined as the result of intervention. The plural term 'outcomes' is often preferred since outcome is a multidimensional concept: it might be clinically, socially or functionally based. Frattali (1998) uses the term 'outcomes research' to cover all areas of outcomes measurement, management, efficacy and effectiveness (see Frattali, 1998, for a detailed discussion of temporal order, types, frameworks and operational definitions of outcomes). The terms effectiveness, efficacy and efficiency of intervention are often used interchangeably although in outcomes literature they do have distinct meanings which are reviewed here.

- Efficacy: the outcome of an intervention in an ideal situation. Does the intervention work in optimal circumstances?
- Effectiveness: the outcome of an intervention in a non-ideal, real-life situation. Does the intervention work in the real world?
- Efficiency: the outcome of an intervention as evaluated in terms of cost effectiveness and time effectiveness. Does X intervention bring about changes more rapidly or cost effectively than Y intervention?

These constructs are developed in further detail in the sections that follow. Cost effectiveness is covered briefly in this chapter, but is dealt with more comprehensively in Chapter 13 on service delivery.

ACTIVITY 12.1

Daisy, aged 8;9 with PSDs attends a mainstream school in the North of England. Imagine you will be seeing her for 1 : 1 speech intervention on a weekly basis for six sessions. Daisy's speech is generally intelligible to unfamiliar listeners but she persists in the inconsistent use of some immature and unusual speech processes. A sample of Daisy's speech is provided below:

Target	Daisy's production
STOP SIGN	[ˈtɒp saɪn]

MY STUPID COUSIN	[maɪ 'tju:pɪd kʊzɪn]
TANK TOP	[kæŋk 'kɒp]
BAT	[bæt]
LION AND TIGER	['laɪn ə 'kaɪgə]
FAST	[fæt]
SPOT THE DOG	['pɒʔ də dɒg]
SPOON	[pun]
MY SCHOOL	['maɪ gul]
STOP TALKING	[tɒp 'kɔkɪŋg]

You decide to devise a programme of intervention to improve Daisy's production of /s/ clusters and her backing of /t/ in word-initial position. Based on this information, answer the questions below about therapy outcomes.

(a) Define the outcomes by which you will evaluate the success of your intervention.
(b) How would you measure these outcomes?
(c) What other information would you gather post-intervention to evaluate outcomes?

Now turn to the Key to Activity 12.1 at the end of this chapter, then read the following.

Outcomes may be positive, negative or neutral. The outcomes one chooses to measure may be wide-ranging and should be carefully chosen for their relevance to the client and their intervention. Some intervention studies focus on one primary outcome measure (e.g. reading age) while others evaluate a broader range of measures, e.g. changes in speech, language and literacy using standardized assessments. Selecting and measuring therapy outcomes is no simple task. Van der Gaag (1993) describes the difficulties involved in trying to define a successful outcome for all groups of people involved in intervention: children, caregivers, teachers and therapists. Attempts have been made to define the outcome of intervention in ways that are meaningful, practical and coherent for these groups. Outcomes can potentially be diverse, including enhancing existing skills, teaching new skills, assisting with psychological adjustments and empowering carers. From a researcher's point of view, a wide variety of measures need to be included as this is likely to be most informative (Gallagher, 1998); however, the measures should not be so broad as to be meaningless. Generalization needs to be determined beyond the immediate context of the study, and measures should be carefully selected to evaluate this aspect (see Chapter 9). At the most simple level, studies aim to show that a new behaviour has been acquired, and more importantly that it has been

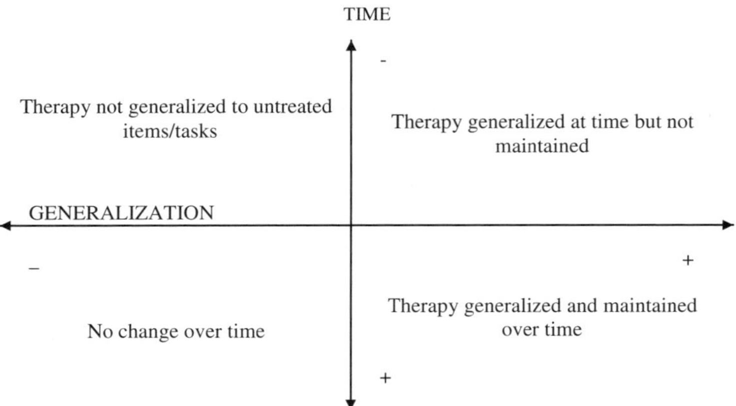

Figure 12.1: Two-dimensional model for measuring therapy outcome.

retained (long-term retention or maintenance) after the treatment has been completed. Figure 12.1 shows a two-dimensional model for measuring therapy outcome by considering the extent and maintenance of generalization over time. In Chapter 9 we introduced two types of generalization: across-item and across-task generalization. The two-dimensional model is a linguistic model when used in the light of across-item generalization, and a psycholinguistic model when used to evaluate across-task generalization. It is not a social model of functional communicative outcomes, although evaluation of such outcomes is also a vital part of the intervention evaluation process.

The model shows how generalization (on the horizontal axis) can vary from minimal to more substantial. At the same time, one can consider generalization in relation to time (on the vertical axis): over a short period (i.e. towards the top of the time arrow) therapy may or may not generalize initially, but maintenance over time (the right hand, lower quadrant) is the optimal outcome in terms of generalization.

ACTIVITY 12.2

Read the following brief descriptions of specific therapy outcomes for five children and place each one in the appropriate quadrant on the model in Figure 12.1.

- Joshua, CA 6;10, showed significant improvement in the accuracy of his consonant cluster production when control words were compared at pre- and post-intervention assessments. Longer-term follow-up showed that these gains had been maintained.

- Ben, CA 8;9, showed no significant improvement in his accuracy of /ʃ/ in treated words and untreated controls, when comparing pre- and post-intervention results.
- Katy, CA 6;5, made significant improvements in her ability to produce final consonants in single-word and connected speech. Two post-intervention assessments were carried out: one immediately post-intervention, which demonstrated significant gains for the pre-intervention baselines, and the second longer-term follow-up seven months later following a period of no intervention. This second assessment revealed that the gains in connected speech had been maintained.
- Rachel, CA 7;1, showed no generalization from the specific /s/ clusters addressed in her intervention (/sp, st, sk/) to other untreated /s/ clusters, e.g. /sm, spr/.
- Simon, CA 10;11, showed significant gains in his production of velars immediately post-intervention, with generalization noted to matched, untreated words. However, re-assessment following a two month break from therapy revealed that he was no longer using these sounds and his accuracy with velars was not significantly different from what it had been prior to intervention.

Now turn to the Key to Activity 12.2 at the end of this chapter before reading the following.

There is a wide range of standardized, norm-referenced speech and language assessment tools. These are frequently used as outcome measures for evaluating change following intervention. The advantages of using such tools to measure outcomes are numerous: they are readily available, easy to administer and allow one to compare an individual child to his or her normally-developing peers. There may, however, be difficulties when a child comes from a population not represented by the standardization sample. Single-case interventions where children can act as their own control get over this to some extent since each child's own individual performance is being compared across time. However, such tests are frequently designed, standardized and used with large groups of children to evaluate broad domains of their language and indicate whether or not intervention is warranted. Such tests as outcomes measures may not be sensitive to the subtle degree of change brought about, particularly for children with very severe difficulties. Ebbels (2000, p. 4) notes that:

> Standard tests of phonology . . . often measure changes in output phonology only. Improved output may be the end result of many changes within the speech processing system, for example improved discrimi-

nation, updated lexical representations and motor programs. These changes all represent progress and are only measured by standard tests if the changes have filtered right through to speech output. If the process is only partially complete, the progress could go unnoticed.

In Katy's case (Pascoe, Stackhouse and Wells, 2005, and see Chapter 8) significant changes were noted in her speech using specific stimuli linked to her intervention, however, gains could not be demonstrated on standardized tests of speech such as the *Edinburgh Articulation Test* (Anthony *et al.*, 1971) where Katy was still found to be severely delayed in relation to her age-matched peers. If one considers the fine-grained analyses and specific focus of intervention carried out in many single-case studies, the use of standardized tests as the sole form of outcomes measurement is not likely to convey the full picture of change. Stackhouse and Wells (1997) describe ways in which practitioners can devise their own specific probes for evaluating change in individual children. The cases presented in this book, e.g. Rachel's case in Chapter 9, illustrate this procedure.

The World Health Organization's (WHO, 2001) International Classification of Functioning, Disability and Health is a useful framework for setting intervention goals and addressing outcomes (see McLeod and Bleile, 2004, for detailed application of the framework to children with speech difficulties). Enderby and John (1999) developed an approach to evaluating outcomes of speech and language therapy, called the Therapy Outcome Measures (TOM), which is based on rating the dimensions of impairment, disability, handicap and well-being. In terms of the WHO's framework, it has been noted that research into phonological disorders has traditionally been focused largely at the impairment level (Goldstein and Gierut, 1998). Authors such as Enderby and Emerson (1995) and Seron (1997) urge that the way forward in terms of effectiveness research should involve more sensitive outcome measures, which can reflect the total impact of therapy including psychosocial change, e.g. self-esteem. An intervention study by Dodd and Iacano (1989) used a range of outcomes measures to evaluate change ranging from standardized assessments of phonology to more socially valid measures such as percentages of phonological processes used in a language sample. The randomized control trial of Almost and Rosenbaum (1998) included a conversational measure (percentage of consonants correct (PCC) in conversation) with these authors showing not only that their first treatment group of children improved in terms of single-word production, but that they went on to show gains in their conversational speech. Intelligibility is a key functional outcomes measure, yet there have been relatively few intervention studies with children with speech difficulties that have used intelligibility as an outcomes measure (see Chapter 11 for further discussion).

Benchmarking is a process used in management in which organizations evaluate various aspects of their own business processes in relation to best practice within their own industry. This allows companies to develop plans on how to adopt such best practice. Benchmarking has also been used in the evaluation of intervention outcomes, although to date to a fairly limited extent in the field of speech and language therapy. Authors such as John, Enderby and Hughes (2005a, b) have carried out benchmarking studies to evaluate intervention outcomes in the areas of dysphasia and voice work with adults. The type of information on service delivery that benchmarking studies can provide is well illustrated by John *et al.* (2005a). These authors investigated eight speech and language therapy services providing services to people with dysphasia. The TOM (Enderby and John, 1999) was the indicator or instrument used for evaluating change. It was found that access to services was equitable across the services. However, the effects of treatment varied from service provider to service provider as measured by the different dimensions of TOM, and there were significant differences between service providers on the TOM dimension of well-being at discharge. Each of the participating services was able to compare their own results with the others' and exchange information in order to achieve best practice in the field.

In summary, outcome measures need to be:

(a) numerous and sufficiently broad ranging to fully capture the effects of intervention and any generalization which occurs;
(b) selected on the basis of the individual child (or population of children) receiving intervention, and sufficiently sensitive to small and specific changes that may occur as a result of intervention;
(c) socially meaningful so that one is able to judge the functional effects of intervention on individuals' daily lives.

Outcome measures are designed to inform us about the effectiveness, efficacy and efficiency of intervention.

ACTIVITY 12.3

Consider the intervention that was carried out with Oliver in Chapter 4, and is briefly summarized below.

Child details: Oliver CA 5;6 attends a mainstream school. He has persisting speech difficulties. His speech is unintelligible to unfamiliar listeners, and he has severe difficulties with almost all aspects of input speech processing, stored representations and output.

Intervention: Oliver received a total of 28 hours of intervention. Intervention focused on four specific targets [k, dʒ, s, t], which were used in CVC and CV words such as COW, JAR, SUE and TWO. There were four phases of intervention with each focusing on use of the above targets in associated words. Intervention activities for each target followed a hierarchy that involved mainly input tasks, e.g. an auditory lexical decision task in which Oliver had to make judgments about whether the therapist's picture naming was accurate or not, e.g. Oliver was presented with a picture of a COW and asked to respond 'yes' or 'no' to questions such as: Is it a [zaʊ]? Is it a COW?

Outcomes: the intervention outcomes are described in Chapter 4 (p. 108) to which you should now refer. Once you have revised Oliver's outcomes answer the following questions.

(a) What were the intervention outcomes? How do you know?
(b) Can you comment on the intervention's effectiveness? What steps might have been taken to enable further comments to be made about this?
(c) Can you comment on the intervention's efficiency? How do you think it might compare to a different intervention (e.g. different procedures, aims, duration, intensity)?

Now turn to the Key to Activity 12.3 at the end of this chapter, then read the following.

Models and Frameworks for Outcome Measurements

Frattali (1998) outlines a hierarchical model outlining different levels of knowledge which might be addressed by intervention research shown in Figure 12.2. At Level 1, and forming the basis of the hierarchy is the following general question: Does speech and language therapy work? Intervention research at this most basic level is concerned with evaluating the outcome (successful or otherwise) of different types of speech and language therapy carried out with different client groups. Intervention studies focusing at Level 1 are important in giving other levels of outcomes research a solid foundation: there is no point in contrasting approaches or maximizing efficiency, if we do not yet know an approach works. Results of research have generally shown that speech and language therapy does work – especially for children with speech difficulties as reviewed in the following section.

Frattali (1998) suggested that what is needed at the next level of enquiry (Level 2) are insights into the *specificity* of treatment, i.e. what type of intervention works for what client group, under what conditions? These are studies that assume that intervention does work and aim to develop ways of improving the levels of success achieved. At this level,

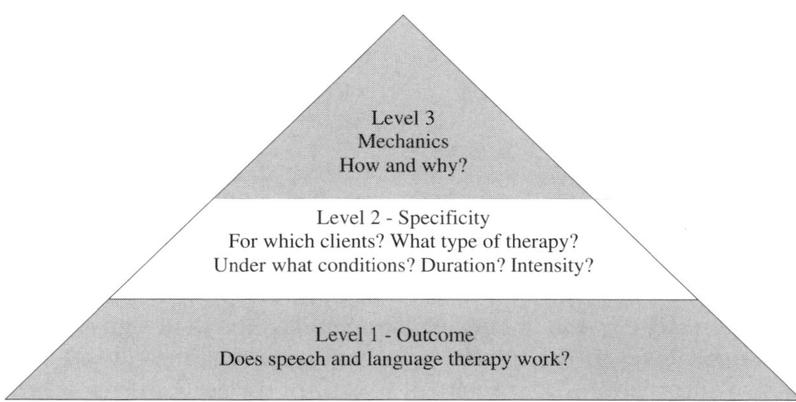

Figure 12.2: Levels of hierarchy in intervention research (based on Frattali, 1998).

we distinguish between interventions (e.g. as evaluated by Almost and Rosenbaum, 1998) and service delivery models (e.g. as evaluated by Glogowska *et al.*, 2000). Gallagher's (1998) review of treatment outcomes research reveals that most research has been carried out at the first and second levels of the hierarchy. However, her review of efficiency studies shows that while many efficiency studies have been carried out, we are still not able to answer many of the fundamental questions associated with this level.

The most in-depth but unresearched level of enquiry (Level 3) is concerned with understanding the mechanics of intervention: how does therapy bring about change? Authors such as Howell and Dean (1994), Frattali (1998) and Basso and Caporali (2001) consider that at this level of the theoretical framework we need to account not only for what is learnt but also how it is learnt. The process that constitutes therapy remains poorly understood and seldom considered. It is argued, that before we can begin to answer these Level 3 questions, we need to expand our knowledge of effectiveness (at Level 1) and of the specifics of therapy (at Level 2). The psycholinguistic approach and case studies are particularly well suited to providing detailed answers to these questions.

Another useful model for understanding intervention research is that of Robey and Schultz (1998). Their outcome research model has been mentioned throughout this book (see Chapter 2), and provides an outline of five systematic phases needed for intervention research. These are:

- Phase I: Develop a treatment;
- Phase II: Test its efficacy;

- Phase III: Test its effectiveness;
- Phase IV: Examine its efficiency;
- Phase V: Determine its cost effectiveness, cost-benefit, and cost-utility.

The authors suggest that specific research designs are appropriate for each phase in the model. Progression through the phases must occur in a sequential way with each phase building on the findings from the previous one. The first phase is about discovery, developing hypotheses about intervention to be tested in later phases. Single-subject designs are appropriate at this level. If this phase reveals that no harm is caused and the effects of intervention are positive, it is appropriate to proceed to the next phase. In Phase II single-subject designs remain appropriate, but are used more systematically to investigate efficacy: what is the ideal that an intervention might strive for? Once this question has been answered, Phase III investigations can occur. In Phase III, effectiveness is evaluated in real life conditions, and typically employing more powerful designs such as randomized control trials. RCTs are studies involving relatively large numbers of participants who are randomly assigned into two groups: one group receives a particular treatment or therapy, and another group receives no treatment. Assigning participants at random reduces the risk of bias (i.e. where individuals are aware that they are being treated and change in anticipation of the treatment) and increases the probability that differences between the groups can be attributed to the treatment (see Chapter 2). If the efficacy of the intervention is established in Phase III, it is appropriate to move on to Phase IV and examine efficiency. Here the intervention will be contrasted with other interventions in terms of outcomes. In the final phase, investigations take place into cost effectiveness, cost-benefit and cost-utility. Thus, it is suggested that while cost effectiveness may be at the forefront of managers' and purchasers' minds, it is the researcher's role to move through the five outcomes phases, concerned with building a solid foundation of evidence for a particular intervention and considering cost effectiveness at the appropriate point once a fairly substantial amount of outcomes data has been amassed.

What Do We Know about Therapy Outcomes for Children?

Speech and language therapy for children is generally held to have positive outcomes (Nye, Foster and Seaman, 1987; Gierut, 1998b; Law *et al.*, 1998; Goldstein and Gierut, 1998; Law and Garret, 2003). Results from studies of children with speech difficulties suggest that intervention typically brings about positive change (e.g. Nye *et al.*, 1987; Shriberg and Kwiatkowski, 1994; Gierut, 1998a; Law *et al.*, 1998; Goldstein and Gierut, 1998; Law and Garret, 2003; Joffe and Serry, 2004). Shriberg and Kwiatkowski (1994, p. 1100) summarize the positive benefits of intervention as follows:

> Children who receive phonological treatment exhibit improved intelligibility and general communicative functioning. There are no known risks involved in the treatment, and the long-term benefits for continued communicative, educational and social success are beginning to be documented.

Indeed, it is only in recent years that speech and language therapists have attempted to address the challenging task of documenting the outcomes of intervention for children with speech difficulties. However, this issue is not as clear-cut as it may seem since outcomes measures and criteria used to determine success can vary widely. Roulstone (2001) reported that 55% of articles in the *International Journal of Language and Communication Disorders* in the preceding two years focused on children. Of this number, only nine were intervention studies.[1] Law and Garret (2003) carried out a review of the effectiveness of speech and language interventions for children with primary speech and language delay/disorder. Twenty-five papers were found and used in the meta-analysis. The results suggest that speech and language therapy is effective for children with phonological or expressive language difficulties, but that there is less evidence that interventions are effective for children with receptive difficulties.

Many of the efficacy and effectiveness studies in the domain of developmental phonological difficulties have focused on pre-school children up to age five, rather than on the school-age child with persisting speech problems. Sommers *et al.* (1992) and Almost and Rosenbaum (1998) focused their surveys specifically on pre-school children. This is not surprising given the great emphasis that is rightly placed on early intervention. If children's speech and language difficulties can be identified and addressed at the earliest possible time, then the likelihood of preventing or at least minimizing negative academic and social sequelae is increased (Stackhouse, 2001). However, some children are appropriately identified from a young age and receive intervention to address their speech and language difficulties for many years but their difficulties do not resolve. Speech and language problems are often complex and require long-term management. The amount of intervention required to remediate children's complex difficulties is not yet known but the indications are that it should be regular and focused.

Approaches to Intervention Research

Efficacy Studies

Efficacy is defined as the outcome of an intervention in an ideal situation. Efficacy studies examine the outcome for children or groups of children who have received speech and language therapy, comparing them with children who have not and who therefore act as controls. Ethical dilemmas associated with withholding treatment are typically overcome by using delayed treatment, e.g. see Almost and Rosenbaum (1998) where all participants ultimately received intervention although the control children only received this at the end of the study. Delayed treatments are readily justified if children would in the normal course of events be subject to a period of time on a waiting list prior to receiving therapy.

The focus in group studies is on identifying children with broadly similar aetiologies or symptoms, by implication suggesting that the same treatment might be applicable to all members of the group. Randomized control trials (RCTs) are frequently cited as the gold standard of efficacy research (e.g. see Glogowska *et al.*, 2000). One of the first such group or RCT studies into the efficacy of articulation therapy was carried out with groups of school-age children (kindergarten, first and second grade, i.e. 5–7 years) using randomization techniques (Sommers, Cockerille, Paul *et al.*, 1961). Results from this pioneering work showed that direct and individual speech therapy was successful in reducing articulation errors, when compared to children who received only indirect classroom-based instruction. The randomized control trial carried out by Almost and Rosenbaum (1998) is one of the few to specifically address children with phonological difficulties, although focusing on pre-schoolers rather than school-aged children. Thirty children with severe speech difficulties were shown to have made significant gains in phonology when compared to the untreated group of children. Interestingly in this study, the expressive language measure (MLU) did not detect a difference between groups at any time suggesting that the benefits of phonological therapy were specific to speech and had no significant impact on language. This study was described in greater detail in Chapter 2.

While Almost and Rosenbaum (1998) were interested in the effects of phonological therapy on language production, Fey, Cleave, Ravida *et al.* (1994) investigated the reverse issue: would grammar facilitation affect the phonology of children with speech and language problems? They found that such a broad-based language approach was effective in improving children's grammar but did not significantly improve their speech production. They concluded that children between four and six years of age with phonological difficulties should have intervention directly addressed to their phonology. A recurring theme for many of these group studies is the great variability reported in the way individual participants respond to intervention.

Rvachew (1994) investigated the efficacy of auditory perception training as a means of improving speech production. Participants in the treatment group received systematic exposure to pairs of words minimally contrasted in terms of the children's error sounds (e.g. SHOE and MOO) while those in the control group received exposure to random words (e.g. CAT and PETE). After the training period children in the treatment group were found to have superior ability to articulate the target sound in comparison to the control children. Previous studies of auditory perception had not found such positive benefits for children's speech (e.g. Williams and McReynolds, 1975) but this may have been because the segments contrasted were not specific to the child's input speech difficulties. Locke (1980a) noted that much speech perception training is too general to be of specific value, and that treatment should involve stimuli representing the error sounds and the child's substitution for this sound. Hodson and Paden (1991) use auditory bombardment as one component of their programme. This procedure is designed to provide children with intensive exposure to specific phonological targets and contrasts; children listen to amplified speech, delivered through headphones, at the beginning and end of every session.

Another auditory input approach is that of Tallal and colleagues (Tallal, Miller and Fitch, 1993; Merzenich, Jenkins, Johnson *et al.*, 1996; Tallal, Miller, Bedi *et al.*, 1996) who evaluated the effect of intensive auditory training on children, using acoustically modified speech. They found that children's language scores improved significantly, mainly in terms of speech discrimination and language comprehension. This was taken as support for their theory that temporal processing deficits underlie children's language difficulties. However, the results revealed that although auditory training has the potential to improve speech input, the effect on speech output remains limited.

Effectiveness Studies

Effectiveness studies are concerned with treatment outcomes in routine clinical settings. A large (n = 159) RCT aimed to determine the effectiveness of community-based speech and language therapy for pre-school children was carried out by Glogowska *et al.* (2000). This study found no evidence for the effectiveness of speech and language therapy when compared to 'watchful waiting' for this group. However, in evaluating such studies the dosage and nature of therapy given needs to be considered; the children participating in this RCT received limited amounts of therapy. The lack of progress is therefore the result of limitations of a particular service delivery model, rather than any particular approach to speech and language intervention (see Law and Conti-Ramsden, 2000, for discussion of this issue, as well as Chapter 13). The level of input that children need in order to make progress is an important issue when trying to justify resources and one that requires further investigation. Broomfield and Dodd (2005) describe the RCT conducted on a population of 320 children with speech disorders referred to a paediatric speech and language therapy service in the north of England. Children were grouped according to Dodd's (1995) diagnostic categories, and the outcomes of each sub-group evaluated. The authors concluded that there are a range of different factors that influence outcome, e.g. age, gender, socio-economic status; nature and severity of difficulties. These factors need to be untangled further through additional research. While RCTs are a powerful means for testing experimental hypotheses using methods designed to reduce bias, they leave many specific questions unanswered.

Effectiveness studies often evaluate specific treatment programmes with small numbers of children using single-case studies and multiple-baseline techniques. Law (1995) notes that while initially there was a slow shift to the use of single-case designs, it was in the area of phonological therapy in which convincing evidence for change by use of this design was shown successfully. Single-case studies have become increasingly well established in the intervention literature (e.g. Weiner, 1981; Chiat and Hirson, 1987; McGregor and Leonard, 1989; Bryan and Howard, 1992; Stackhouse and Wells, 1993; Dodd and McCormack, 1995; Broom and Doctor, 1995a,b; Constable, Stackhouse and Wells, 1997; Easton, Sheach and Easton, 1997; Holm and Dodd, 1999; Crosbie and Dodd, 2001; Ebbels, 2000; Spooner, 2002; Pascoe *et al.*, 2005) and are an important method for providing insights into the nature of individual patterns of change. These case studies cover a range of areas including speech processing and production, receptive and expressive language, reading and spelling.

Case studies vary widely in their theoretical starting point, design and nature of assessment and intervention. In terms of theoretical starting point, the single subject design is well suited for evaluating the effectiveness of model-based interventions. For example, psycholinguistic and cognitive neuropsychological models of speech, language and/or literacy provide a detailed framework for assessment and investigation of children's underlying difficulties. Such detailed, theoretically-motivated assessment allows one to generate hypotheses about the locus of difficulty and to evaluate intervention outcomes within this framework by returning to original hypotheses. Examples of such model-based interventions include the single-case studies reported by Bryan and Howard (1992), Broom and Doctor (1995a, b), Vance (1997), Waters *et al.* (1998), Norbury and Chiat (2000), Crosbie and Dodd (2001), Stiegler and Hoffman (2001) Spooner (2002), and Pascoe *et al.* (2005).

While many single-case studies have been published, not all of these involve intervention. Many of the model-based approaches require extremely detailed investigation of children's difficulties, and as such provide interesting insights about the nature of the difficulties in their own right (e.g. Chiat and Hirson, 1987; Stackhouse and Wells, 1993; Constable *et al.*, 1997; Ebbels, 2000; Crosbie, Dodd and Howard, 2002). Many of these studies offer suggestions for treatment and discuss the clinical implications of difficulties without systematically evaluating intervention. While single-case studies focus on individual children, in some cases comparisons with groups of normally-developing controls are necessitated due to a lack of normative data for particular tasks (e.g. Stackhouse and Snowling, 1992; Constable *et al.*, 1997; Crosbie and Dodd, 2001).

Not all single-case studies use psycholinguistic models as their theoretical springboard. Many single-case studies have relied mainly on linguistic theory (e.g. Weiner, 1981; Monahan, 1986; Saben and Ingham, 1991; Bernhardt, 1992; Stiegler and Hoffman, 2001) or are less theoretically explicit in their approach (e.g. Johnson and Hood, 1988). Pratt, Heintzelman and Deming (1993) evaluated the efficacy of the IBM *Speech-Viewer's* Vowel Accuracy Module for the treatment of vowel productions. Six pre-school children received the treatment within a single-subject research design, allowing for each child's progress to be evaluated as well as comparisons and contrasts to be made between children. Four children improved their performance on the vowels addressed, and these same children demonstrated some generalization to other vowels. While much of this single-case research has focused on younger, pre-school children, there are some examples of single-case interventions with older children. For example, Gibbon *et al.* (2003) carried out intervention using EPG (electropalatography) with a 10-year-old girl with PSDs, and Shuster, Ruscello and Haines (1992) worked with an adolescent who exhibited longstanding multiple articulation errors. Both of these interventions were shown to bring about significant changes in the children's speech. (See Chapter 7 by Hilary Dent in Book 2, Stackhouse and Wells, 2001, for further reading on EPG.)

Efficiency Studies

Efficiency studies are concerned with finding the best intervention for particular difficulties. The starting point for such studies is the assumption that intervention works. Thus, many of these studies use tried and tested techniques that have already been validated in effectiveness research. One of the main questions that this type of study aims to answer is: Does intervention A work better than intervention B? In these inter-intervention studies two different approaches to therapy are compared (e.g. minimal pair treatment vs. metaphonological approach), or alternatively providers of therapy (e.g. therapist vs. parent) or service delivery models (e.g. group vs. individual). In these types of study 'better' may be measured by means of the effect size achieved, or the speed with which a given criterion level for improvement is reached. Effect size is a statistical term that refers to the size of a relationship between two variables, e.g. speech intervention and PCC. Another approach to efficiency is that of intra-intervention studies, which look within a given therapy approach for specific ways of maximizing treatment success. For example, many of the studies in the realm of phonological therapy have focused on target selection, asking which targets result in more widespread change and greater improvements. These different approaches to efficiency evaluation are discussed in the following sections as they relate to phonological intervention.

Inter-intervention Studies: Does Intervention A Work Better than Intervention B?

Metaphonological approaches

Efforts to improve the effectiveness of intervention for children with phonological difficulties have focused on approaches to treatment. Phonological awareness is an area that has received increased attention over the past few years. It is the ability to reflect on the sounds of one's language rather than the meaning, and to manipulate these in various ways, e.g. rhyme, segmentation, blending. Phonological awareness is considered to be an integral aspect of both oral and written language (Stackhouse *et al.*, 2002). Researchers have begun to consider 'meta' approaches to phonological intervention. For example, Hesketh, Adams and Hall (2000) carried out a study comparing the effect of metaphonological therapy vs. traditional articulation therapy with a group of pre-school children with speech difficulties. They found little difference between the two groups in terms of both phonological awareness and speech production. They concluded that:

> the study in effect raises more questions than it can answer in that what actually happens in therapy still remains poorly understood, and there is a need for controlled longitudinal research to address the complex set of factors involved in a diverse set of individual children.
>
> (Hesketh *et al.*, p. 349).

Stackhouse *et al.* (2002) suggest that researchers need to be clear about what underlying aspects of the speech processing system are being tapped in intervention. There may have been no difference between the two groups in Hesketh *et al.*'s study because traditional articulation therapy implicitly requires metaphonological knowledge, and is not as different from the metaphonological approach as one might suppose.

Gillon (2000, 2002) used a phonological awareness intervention approach with children (ages 5;6–7;6) with spoken language impairments and control children. The study found that children who received phonological awareness training obtained age-appropriate levels of literacy performance, and in addition their speech articulation improved (see Chapter 10 for further details of this study). This is an efficient approach to intervention since both speech and phonological awareness skills underpinning literacy were addressed.

Another efficiency study involving phonological awareness is that of Major and Bernhardt (1998). These authors investigated the relationships between the phonological and metaphonological skills of 19 children aged 3–5 years with moderate to severe phonological disorders. Their phonological intervention programme relied on non-linear phonological analyses for goal setting (see Baker and Bernhardt, 2004, for a detailed example of this process). Non-linear phonological theory focuses on the hierarchical nature of phonological forms. A distinction is made between higher level phrase and word structures, and lower level segments (i.e. speech sounds) and features. Non-linear treatment programmes typically include systematic alternations of higher level and lower level targets. For example, targets for a specific child might include the following.

- Higher level (word and phrasal structure) targets: production of weak syllables in phrases and three-syllable words.
- Lower level (segmental and feature) targets: velars, e.g. [k, g].

Non-linear intervention studies emphasize the importance of addressing many levels of the phonological hierarchy, and linking the levels wherever possible, e.g. in words like CATERPILLAR based on the goals given above. The metaphonological intervention programme included rhyming and alliteration tasks. Intervention outcomes indicated that both phonological and metaphonological intervention may result in a significant increase in children's metaphonological task performance. It was further observed that children with more moderate phonological disorders and good morphosyntactic production skills tended to improve on the metaphonological tasks after phonological intervention alone. Children with more severe phonological and morphosyntactic disorders improved their task performance only after phonological plus metaphonological intervention. Bernhardt and Major (2005) followed up the children's speech, language and literacy development three years later, since their history of early speech and language difficulties puts them at risk for literacy difficulties and persisting speech difficulties (See Chapters 1 and 10). Results of this study revealed that five of the 19 children had PSDs. The strongest predictor for literacy development was performance on metaphonology tasks at the end of the early intervention study. The strongest predictor for ongoing speech impairment was phonological skill at the end of the early study.

Broad-based language approaches

Hoffman, Norris and Monjure (1990) compared phonological intervention targeting specific processes with broad-based, whole-language treatments for phonologically delayed pre-schoolers. They used a narrative-based discourse task, aiming to tap into a variety of levels of language, i.e. semantics, syntax, and phonology. The outcome of the whole-language intervention was positive with gains being made in each of these areas after six weeks of intervention. The results were accounted for in terms of a synergistic relationship between the different components of language. This approach of working on higher-level language functions without specifically addressing phonology, seemed promising as an efficient means of remediation. However, subsequent studies (e.g. Tyler and Watterson, 1991; Fey *et al.*, 1994) using similar whole-language treatments did not find the same results. These later studies found that whole-language treatments affected syntax, but that phonological difficulties needed to be addressed directly if gains were to be made in this area. Although the treatments may have been similar in these studies, the children were very different. Younger children with phonological delays may respond positively to whole-language treatments while children with speech disorders or older children with PSDs may require interventions more specifically focused on speech.

Parents and therapists

Traditionally speech and language therapists were solely responsible for providing intervention. However, there has been increasing acceptance of the important role parents and teachers can play in helping children with speech and language difficulties, and this accords well with the typically limited time and resources that constrain therapists from giving intensive individual therapy themselves to all children who require it. Furthermore, it is logical to include parents and teachers where possible since they spend a great deal of time with children. Ruscello, Cartwright, Haines and Shuster (1993) investigated service delivery approaches for pre-school children with speech difficulties. The children were randomly assigned to one of two treatment groups that differed in relation to service delivery. Group I received a treatment that was administered exclusively by a speech–language pathologist (SLP). Group II received a combination that included SLP administered treatment and parent administered instruction. Both groups improved significantly, but they did not differ significantly from each other in the degree of change, suggesting that at least for this younger client group, parents have an important contribution to make.

Law and Garret (2003) carried out a systematic review to examine the effectiveness of speech and language interventions for children with primary speech and language delay/disorder. A systematic review (also sometimes referred to as a meta-analysis) is a review of studies in which evidence has been systematically searched for, studied, assessed, and summarized according to predetermined criteria. Law and Garret found intervention studies by searching databases such as The Cochrane Controlled Trials Register, ERIC, MEDLINE and PsychINFO. They also used references taken from reviews of the literature and reference lists from articles. Data from these studies were categorized according to the control group used in the study; type of treatment, e.g. no treatment, general stimulation, or traditional therapy; and the effects of intervention on expressive and receptive phonology, syntax and vocabulary. The effects of therapy were investigated at the level of the target of therapy, measures of overall linguistic development and broader measures of linguistic functioning taken from parent report or language samples. Results of the review suggested that parent-based intervention is effective in treating children with expressive language delays, but that for children with phonological difficulties practitioner administered therapy is more effective.

In evaluating results from these studies, it is important to consider the age of the children involved; the type of speech difficulties referred to, and the resources and support offered to the parents. Young children with phonological delays seem to be more receptive to parental intervention than older children with PSDs. Research suggests that structured, direct work is required for children with specific difficulties developing linguistic skills (Lahey, 1988; Tannock and Girolametto, 1992; Fey, Cleave, Long and Hughes, 1993). This finding is not new, but is important given the increasing number of parent programmes being developed, and the decreasing opportunities for direct 1 : 1 work in schools. This issue is discussed in greater detail in Chapter 13.

Using computers

There are conflicting findings regarding the effectiveness of using computers in speech and language therapy for children. One of the most widely known computer interventions is that of *Fast ForWord®* (Scientific Learning, http://www.scilearn.com/), software aimed at addressing children's auditory processing deficits and promoting language and literacy skills. *Fast ForWord®* is a CD-ROM and Internet-based training programme based on the research of Merzenich *et al.* (1996) and Tallal *et al.* (1996). Numerous studies have been carried out to evaluate the effectiveness of the software in bringing about changes in children's auditory processing, speech, language and literacy. Loeb, Stoke and Fey (2001) investigated the language changes of four children (CA 5;6–8;1) who received *Fast ForWord* language intervention in their homes. Language change was assessed immediately post-intervention and 3 months later using standardized language measures, spontaneous measures of syntactic complexity, reading measures, pragmatic measures, and parental and teacher reports. Three of the four children successfully completed the programme, and all made gains on some of the same standardized measures, although the improvements the authors observed were generally smaller than those previously reported by Tallal *et al.* (1996). All children also made gains on measures of pragmatic performance. However, very few changes were observed in the children's Developmental Sentence Scores. Sixty-one per cent of the gains observed at post-testing were maintained 3 months following intervention.

Computers have also been used effectively in reading interventions. For example, Davidson, Elock and Noyes (1996) evaluated a computer system which gives pre-recorded speech prompts on request to aid with reading. Sixty children aged 5–7 years were tested on three measures of sight vocabulary (*British Ability Scales* (BAS) Word Recognition, Frequently Occurring Words, words from the books read) before and after the intervention period of one month during which 30 of the participants in the intervention group had access to the system. These children made significantly higher gains on the tests than the remaining 30 children who comprised the control group. The amount of practice undertaken by participants in the intervention group was highly positively correlated with their gains.

There are some studies that have found no difference in the outcomes of children who received computer therapy when compared with traditional table-top approaches (O'Connor and Schery, 1986; Ruscello *et al.*, 1993). Other studies examined the effect of combining computer therapy with general classroom work (Schery and O'Connor, 1997) or with more traditional approaches to phonology therapy (Rvachew, Rafaat and Martin, 1999). In all these cases, greater improvement was noted in children who received both computer therapy and standard therapy, rather than standard therapy alone. It seems clear that computers offer the potential for increasing children's motivation and enjoyment of intervention, as well as the means of maximizing intervention dosage, and as such are likely to become an increasingly important tool in the delivery of intervention.

Groups and individuals

Another way of coping with limited resources is by offering group therapy, as opposed to one-to-one approaches. Group interventions also offer individual children opportunities for interacting and working together with their peers. They can also decrease the pressure to perform that some children feel in a 1 : 1 situation. Sommers *et al.* (1961) investigated the outcomes of group therapy for children with speech problems as opposed to individual treatments. They found that over eight months there was no significant difference between the outcomes obtained for each of the two groups. Similarly, results of the meta-analysis carried out by Law and

Garret (2003) showed group therapy to be as effective as individual therapy. These studies may tell only part of the story since it seems likely that the children would not have been homogeneous, and differences in response to the intervention may have been obscured by the group means.

Intra-intervention Studies: How Can We Make Intervention Better?

Target selection is an important decision facing practitioners as they plan intervention. Which targets (e.g. segments, words or other linguistic units) will be addressed and in what order? These issues are important since the ultimate aim of intervention is to encourage generalization across speech production, and careful selection of targets may maximize the generalization achieved, and thus ultimately the efficiency of intervention. An efficient approach to intervention is one that results in widespread change throughout a child's system. (See Chapter 9 for further information about generalization.)

ACTIVITY 12.4

Read the following abstract from Gibbon and Wood (2003) published in *Clinical Linguistics and Phonetics*, and answer the questions that follow.

Using electropalatography (EPG) to diagnose and treat articulation disorders associated with mild cerebral palsy: a case study.

> Some children with mild cerebral palsy have articulation disorders that are resistant to conventional speech therapy techniques. This preliminary study investigated the use of electropalatography (EPG) to diagnose and treat a longstanding articulation disorder that had not responded to conventional speech therapy techniques in an 8-year-old boy (D) with a congenital left hemiplegia. The targets for EPG therapy were speech errors affecting velar targets /k, g, n/, which were consistently fronted to alveolar placement [t, d, n]. After 15 sessions of EPG therapy over a 4-month period, D's ability to produce velars improved significantly. The EPG data revealed two features of diagnostic importance. The first was an unusually asymmetrical pattern of tongue-palate contact and the second was unusually long stop closure durations. These features are interpreted as a subtle form of impaired speech motor control that could be related to a mild residual neurological deficit. The results suggest that EPG is of potential benefit for diagnosing and treating articulation disorders in individuals with mild cerebral palsy.
>
> (Gibbon and Wood, 2003 p. 365)

Questions

(a) What research question was posed by these authors?
(b) What outcomes measures were used in this study?
(c) Does this study evaluate efficacy, effectiveness or efficiency?
(d) What were the main findings of the study?

Now turn to the Key to Activity 12.4 at the end of this chapter and then read the following.

Case-study Evaluations

Detailed cases presented in this book have described the intervention that took place with children with PSDs, i.e. Oliver (Chapter 4), Joshua (Chapter 6), Katy (Chapter 8), Rachel (Chapter 9) and Ben (Chapter 10). Outcomes measures, which range comprehensively from the very specific (i.e. the micro measures such as evaluating Katy's use of final consonants in specific words) to the more general (i.e. the macro measures used for each of the children such as changes in their speech profiles or performance on standardized speech tests), seem most likely to yield a complete picture of the type of change occurring for each child as a result of intervention. While it has been argued that outcomes measures need to be socially and functionally relevant to children's lives (Lees and Urwin, 1997), they should also be sufficiently sensitive to measure small changes in the underlying processing system.

Improving intelligibility (see Chapter 11) is an important aim for many interventions so that children are able to make themselves better understood to unfamiliar listeners (Flipsen, 1995; Dodd and Bradford, 2000). Clearly, this is an ambitious aim for children with severe and persisting problems that may take many years of intervention to achieve. Gains in literacy and underlying processing skills are also important for these children. If we rely only on macro measures such as standardized tests, we might erroneously conclude that no progress had been made. Using micro measures allows us to provide a more complete picture of the cumulative changes that have occurred. From this point of view, intervention is considered successful if any significant change has been brought about on appropriately selected and measured stimuli. These micro and macro levels are similar to the outcomes measures presented by Frattali (1998) and Bunning (2004) to describe a range of intervention settings. These authors refer to intermediate, instrumental and ultimate outcomes.

- *Intermediate outcomes* are analogous to the micro measures employed in many of the intervention cases we have described.

They use specific stimuli to evaluate change relative to the child's own performance.

- *Instrumental outcomes* are outcomes that indicate whether to continue or close an episode of intervention. It is noted that once an individual has achieved an instrumental outcome 'it is assumed that progress will continue beyond the intervention episode' (Bunning, 2004, p. 105). For example, in Katy's case an instrumental outcome may have been achieving 95% accuracy in her final consonant production.
- *Ultimate outcomes* are analogous to the macro measures employed in the case studies: they relate to functional communication (e.g. intelligibility) and the child's performance in relation to their peers (e.g. on standardized tests).

Each of the psycholinguistically-oriented intervention programmes described in this book with the five children was successful at the intermediate outcome level in that the children's production of specific stimuli items addressed in the therapy improved. However, the extent of the generalization varied widely. Figure 12.3 provides an overview of the levels of change that occurred for each of the children participating in the study.

Significant changes in:	Oliver (Chap 4)	Joshua (Chap 6)	Katy (Chap 8)	Rachel (Chap 9)	Ben (Chap 10)	
standardized tests				√		MACRO
speech processing profile		√	√	√		
intelligibility			√*	√	√	
generalization to untreated stimuli	√	√	√	√	√	---
treated stimuli	√	√	√	√	√	MICRO

* Significant change in severity indices (PCC, PPC) not intelligibility.

Figure 12.3: Indices of change for each of the child participants (√ = positive and significant change; Chap = chapter of the book in which each child's case is presented).

ACTIVITY 12.5

Consider the data presented in Figure 12.3. Then answer the following questions:

(a) Did the children make changes at the micro level and how was this change measured?
(b) Comment on the pattern of changes observed at the macro level?
(c) Contrast the outcomes for Oliver and Rachel.
(d) Comment on the pattern of outcomes observed for Joshua and why it does not appear to follow the outcomes hierarchy presented in Figure 12.3.

Now turn to the Key to Activity 12.5 at the end of the chapter, then read the following for further discussion of the children's outcomes.

All five children made gains at the micro level, although the extent of the generalization occurring to untreated items varied widely. Rachel was the child with most wide-ranging positive change and this resulted in changes at the macro level in improved intelligibility and standardized test performance. Oliver, on the other hand, did not show significant change at the macro level with all his change occurring at the micro level. Oliver's speech difficulties were severe and pervasive - possibly associated with a diagnosis of apraxia, e.g. compare Oliver's pre-intervention PCC of 23% with Rachel's of 96%. There is a very small body of research regarding treatment outcomes for children with apraxia (e.g. Helfrich-Miller, 1994; Rosenthal, 1994; Velleman, 1994; Bornman, Alant and Meiring, 2001). The limited (or very slow) success arising from intervention with these children, as well as confusion over giving the diagnosis, has limited the publishing of such intervention cases. Oliver's case contributes to the evidence base for treatment of children with apraxia of speech. Significant change was demonstrated in Oliver's speech production at a micro level, i.e. for the targeted stimuli words as well as matched control lists of words. These findings suggest that while children with apraxia may make slow progress, intervention can be effective in bringing about change to a wide range of speech processing skills. Joffe and Reilly (2004) review the evidence base for treatment of motor speech disorders such as childhood apraxia of speech and dysarthria. Based on the extremely limited body of evidence available, they conclude that 'the evidence for improving speech intelligibility outcomes in children with motor speech disorders is weak' (p. 247). Long-term intervention studies of children like Oliver may yield a more complete picture of the outcomes of intervention over time: is there a point at which macro changes are noted, and what is the intervention dosage required to reach this level? Like Oliver, Joshua showed mainly micro gains with macro changes limited to a few changes on his speech processing profile and not extending to intelligibility or standardized tests.

Ben's pattern of change was slightly different to that of the other children. He made changes at the micro level, but revealed no difference in his speech processing profile or at the level of standardized tests. However, his intelligibility had improved significantly. The intelligibility evaluation, as described in Chapter 11, involved comparison of each child's intelligibility before and after intervention. The children acted as their own control and comparisons were not made with normative data for other children, since this was not readily available or helpful at this stage. In contrast, the standardized tests (and tests used to compile the speech processing profile) involved comparison of each child's performance with that of normally-developing age-matched peers. As such, the intelligibility evaluation is placed adjacent to the micro-level changes in the hierarchy in Figure 12.3. Katy's pattern of changes was similar to Ben's; her intelligibility did not change significantly, but her speech severity reduced. Although intelligibility and severity are closely related concepts, they are different. Intelligibility is defined as word or utterance recognition in natural communication situations and assessment of intelligibility should thus involve listeners attempting to discern meaning from an individual's speech in a way that approximates a real-life environment. Severity indices give an indication of the degree of difficulty individuals experience with their speech and this is usually estimated by carrying out counts such as percentage consonants correct (PCC) based on recordings or transcriptions or single words or connected speech.

The intervention cases presented in this book took place with children with PSDs in mainstream schools. It has been shown that the outcomes varied widely from child to child, but all children made some significant, positive changes. Having an explicit theoretical rationale for the intervention carried out in each case, and the outcomes we aimed to achieve enabled us to learn from each case and contribute to the evidence base in this area. The principles employed in each of these cases are ones that can be applied by anyone working with children with PSDs. The following section provides suggestions for turning routine therapy sessions into intervention case studies.

Thinking Therapy: Turning Routine Therapy Sessions into Case Evaluations

It has been noted that intervention research with children poses greater challenges to researchers than any other client group (Enderby and Emerson, 1995). Evaluations of intervention are less well developed in the paediatric domain than for work with adults probably because of the problems in evaluating therapy with this group: children change as they mature and one cannot depend on a stable baseline. Children with speech difficulties constitute a heterogeneous group that is resistant to grouping by medical diagnoses or even by surface speech disorders (Stackhouse and Snowling, 1992; Crosbie *et al.*, 2002). In this book, and Volumes 1 and 2 of the series, we have described how a psycholinguistic approach moves beyond diagnostic categorization and can directly inform intervention. We have also attempted to suggest ways in which some of the challenges associated with intervention studies can be addressed. Indeed, we should not be put off by the challenges associated with carrying evaluations of intervention with children, since for the most part practitioners are ideally placed to carry out therapy that can not only meet an individual child's needs but also inform our clinical and theoretical knowledge more generally.

The single-case methodology has been widely advocated (e.g. by authors such as Barlow and Hersen, 1984; Hegde, 1985; Howard, 1986; Attanasio, 1994; Enderby and Emerson, 1995; Seron, 1997; Millard, 1998; Adams, 2001) who suggest it is the method of choice for clinical sciences involving intensive interaction, such as speech and language therapy. This approach solves the problem of subject homogeneity in that subjects serve as their own control and treatment can be tailor-made to their specific needs. By varying aspects such as the time treatment commenced, or the type of treatment given, it may be possible to identify change on particular tasks as being due to specific techniques of therapy rather than the effects of treatment in general, or of external factors and maturation. The strength of single-case and small-group studies is in the detail of particular approaches to treatment. The following sections provide some suggestions for ways in which we can turn routine therapy sessions into case study evaluations.

What Questions Should be Asked?

Thinking practitioners will generate questions about their intervention all the time: Does it work? How can I make it work faster? When should I stop treating? These are all key questions that can be the starting point of an intervention project. It is, however, important to focus questions so that they are clear, unambiguous and answerable! For example, in our intervention with Katy (Pascoe *et al.*, 2005) we were driven by the overriding question: Will the intervention work? But in order to answer this question we needed to set about defining what the intervention was, and what our criteria for success would be. This led to the formation of several more specific questions regarding pre- and post-intervention comparisons such as:

- Will Katy use significantly more final consonants in the treated single words from List A?
- Will Katy use significantly more final consonants in the control matched single words from List B?

Many of the case studies in this book give examples of this process of intervention planning and question formation.

The theoretical frameworks from Frattali (1998, see Figure 12.2) and Robey and Schultz (1998) also give a useful starting point for devising and conceptualizing research evaluation. Using Frattali's model it seems logical that we should start out by gathering information about a particular intervention and whether it works with a particular child. If it does work, we may want to ask questions about specificity: looking at the clients who benefit, how much treatment they receive and under what conditions. Once more data have been gathered at this level we may want to reflect about the mechanics of the intervention: what is actually happening (e.g. in terms of client–practitioner interactions; interactions between speech, language and neurophysiology) to bring about the change? Going into each of these levels will provide us with a solid body of evidence about a particular intervention. The specific level of enquiry and question that one poses will dictate the design of the intervention. Robey and Schultz's model allows us to think about where a particular intervention falls in terms of its evidence-building process. In the interventions described with Oliver, Joshua, Katy, Rachel and Ben we argued that since there is minimal information about speech therapy for school-age children with PSDs, our starting point would be at the early levels of Robey and Schultz's phase model using single-case studies to establish efficacy/effectiveness as well as some details about specificity.

How Will Progress be Evaluated?

There are many different micro and macro ways of evaluating and measuring intervention outcomes, e.g. see Figure 12.3. The use of standardized tests allows us to compare the child's performance over time as well as how their performance relates to normally-developing peers of the same chronological age. However, such tests can be too gross to tap into the effect of specific interventions. Using tailor-made stimuli specific to a child can give one more useful answers to specific questions. Such stimuli need to be carefully designed, as discussed in Chapters 3 and 4. If we have only one set of stimuli used in intervention, it could be argued that any improvement noted from pre- to post-measurement may be due to maturation: the child was getting older and would have progressed without the intervention. Control stimuli can help overcome this argument, but the untreated stimuli need to be closely matched to the treated stimuli so that the only difference between the items is the fact that one set was treated and the other was not. In many of our intervention cases, this is the approach we used, e.g. Joshua's intervention described in Chapter 6, and Katy's intervention described in Chapter 8. When drawing up such lists, factors to take into account are numerous, and include:

- lexical factors such as age of average acquisition; frequency in spoken or written language, and imageability;
- phonological factors such as phonotactic structure, word length, intonation and stress.

Obtaining lists of matched words or phrases can be a real challenge, and perfectly balanced lists need time to prepare if not readily available. Being aware of the weaknesses in any lists we prepare is key; we need to try our utmost to create matched lists although this may never be perfect. In Katy's intervention study we strived to create lists of CVC words that met a range of criteria. This was not always feasible and thus some words with initial consonant clusters were used. Where this was the case we made sure that they were balanced across the lists.

Another way of measuring outcomes is by setting a criterion level at which intervention should stop. Thus, instead of asking: 'Will intervention bring about significant changes following 10 hours of therapy?' we ask how much therapy is required to achieve 90% (or some other criterion) success with a particular target. The *Metaphon* studies described in Chapter 9 (Dean *et al.*, 1995b) used this type of approach and the authors were able to conclude that *Metaphon* is an economical treatment procedure for pre-school children since five hours of therapy was able to bring about significant change for most children in the study. For children with PSDs it may be more practical for practitioners to evaluate changes occurring after a predetermined number of sessions, since there may be insufficient resources for a practitioner to continue working with a child until 90% accuracy is achieved.

How Should Intervention be Described?

Speech and language therapy is a complex activity, typically not one unified treatment. The exact content of therapy sessions is highly variable depending on the children involved, the professionals or carers involved, the intervention setting and the type of therapy taking place. One of the challenges faced in attempting and understanding intervention research is in detailing the components of intervention. Gallagher (1998) notes that procedural description is vital in understanding intervention work: intervention procedures should be clearly and fully specified including programme characteristics such as information about participants, frequency of intervention, length of programme, number of trials per procedure, materials used and feedback given. The components of intervention can be summarized in the following formula:

Intervention = Therapy approach + Materials (inc. stimuli) + People + Setting + Frequency/Dosage + Outcomes measures

Descriptions of tasks can be taken a level further. Authors such as Stackhouse and Wells (1997), Rees (2001a,b) and Stackhouse *et al.* (2002) place great emphasis on analysis of tasks from a psycholinguistic perspective: What do tasks really tap? (see Chapter 2, Activity 2.2). The pro-forma provided in Appendix 7 may be a useful tool for this purpose. Many studies provide broad descriptions of the intervention that takes place, e.g. traditional articulation therapy or minimal pair work. Depending on the exact nature of stimuli used, the modality in which the tasks are presented and the nature of the feedback given, these tasks could be seen to be tapping into entirely different parts of a child's speech processing system. Apparently simple tasks can tap into many different processes and component levels in a functional architecture (Seron, 1997). In order to evaluate and compare different types of intervention, one first needs to be aware of what exactly is taking place in intervention. Single-case studies contextualized within a psycholinguistic approach are well suited to providing this level of detail.

How Should Results be Interpreted?

McReynolds and Kearns (1983) raise interesting methodological issues about research designs in speech and language therapy. These authors suggest that the most important questions when evaluating results of intervention are: 'Can change be attributed to therapy?' and 'Is the change real and is the change important?' It is important to consider these questions if we are to avoid a shift from having too little outcomes data, to having too many weak data (Frattali, 1998). Intervention needs to be carried out in a carefully controlled way. Speech and language therapy is delivered alongside the educational curriculum, which in itself should bring about positive change. We need to make every attempt to separate out the effects of our interventions from other effects. Ways of doing this were discussed in Chapter 9, and included, for example, establishing a stable pre-intervention baseline and selecting control tasks unrelated to the focus of intervention, which would thus not be expected to improve significantly over the course of intervention. There are examples of these control procedures in the literature, e.g. Dodd and Bradford (2000) monitored their participants for at least one month prior to intervention.

Therapists may find this information relatively easy to obtain via case notes. Another way of demonstrating specific effects of intervention is to focus on more general areas that are thought to be separate and not directly addressed in therapy. For example, Bryan and Howard (1992) aimed to improve their participant's phonology. They measured progress on an unrelated control task, sentence comprehension, which was thought not to be tapped by the intervention. Similarly, Crosbie and Dodd (2001) measured reading age before and after therapy as an unrelated skill so that any change in auditory perception as a result of their auditory training programme could be attributed to treatment. Again, therapists may find such information easy to obtain via class teachers and national assessment results, e.g. national *Statutory Assessment Tests* (SATs) in the UK.

The other question remains, 'Is the change real and is it important?' Long-term follow-up through routine review appointments is one way of showing that change brought about is permanent and not transitory. Again, routine assessment data can be used for this purpose. The reality and importance of change to people's lives is best addressed by considering the opinions of the children involved as well as the significant people in their environment. For this a range of outcomes measures that include both impairment- and disability-focused measures are needed. We have carried out interviews with children with PSDs before and after intervention, aiming to understand their knowledge of speech difficulties and attitude to intervention. For example, Katy was interviewed in a semi-structured way with the aim of discovering more about the following areas:

- her experience of speech and language therapy;
- her perception and awareness of her own speech;
- her perceptions of communication more generally;
- her attitudes to literacy.

A summary of the findings from her interview is presented in Table 12.1.

Appendix 8 provides a sample of questions and prompts that might be used when collecting evaluative data from children. Questionnaires for parents and teachers are also useful ways of collecting evaluative data. In the longitudinal study by Nathan *et al.* (2004a) a set of questionnaires were used (see Stackhouse *et al.*, forthcoming).

Interventions that do not have positive outcomes are valuable, but are seldom discussed or published. Nevertheless these are valuable opportunities for learning and developing the evidence base, and should be shared with colleagues. Replications of intervention studies are also much needed in order to build a strong and substantial evidence base.

Table 12.1: Summary of findings from Katy's semi-structured interview following Phase I of intervention

Area of questioning	Main findings	Examples of Katy's responses
Katy's experience of SLT		
Present (comments on Phase I)	Enjoyed therapy despite initial reservations	'when I met you I said to myself I don't really want to go to her. And now I really want to go to you'
	Particularly enjoys games, stickers, toys, and being video/audio-taped	'I don't want to go . . . back to class'
	Does not enjoy hard work, e.g. writing things and practising words	'hard work . . . I don't really like hard work'
	Therapy helps children to improve their speech through hard work	(do you know how their speech gets better?) Because it all hard work
Past	Remembers previous therapy and therapists	'drawing, doing painting'
Katy's perception and awareness of own speech	Speech has improved a lot as she has grown older	'at first . . . no. And then, got better because I'm a big girl'
	Talking is fun and easy when she talks to certain people (e.g. her mother, her teacher) but is hard and makes her frustrated when people don't understand her	'If my mommy were here I can talk to her then' (You like talking to her) 'yeah' (And who don't you like talking to?) 'other people, horrid people . . . sometimes I go away. I say I don't want to talk to you' 'it happens to me over and over again'

Table 12.1: *Continued*

Area of questioning	Main findings	Examples of Katy's responses
	A lot of the time people don't understand her and she feels frustrated	'(I feel) a bit grumpy . . . because I might go away, and other people say come back. And I won't come back because they won't listen to me'
	Wishes that she had more control of volume of voice so that she could whisper to her friends in class	(And would you like to do more talking in your classroom?) 'yeah but I talk quietly . . . more quiet . . . don't let anybody else hear'
Katy's perceptions of communication more generally	Talking and listening are generally positive. She likes listening to her teacher, therapists and mother	'talking is nice; listening is nice'
	When communication breaks down you should just walk away	'I just walk away'
	Most people in England talk the same language but people in other countries talk different languages	'Some people in different countries talk a different language'
Katy's attitudes to literacy	Reading and writing can be fun if she is doing something easy at home but is harder and less enjoyable at school	'I don't like reading books. I like reading my own books but not the school's books because it's hard work'
	Did not know why reading and writing are important for children to learn	'(I like writing) a bit but don't like writing lots of words'

Summary

This chapter has aimed to bring together what is known about outcomes for children with PSDs, as well as how we can set about adding to the evidence base. The key points are as follows.

- Evaluating intervention is an important part of the intervention process needed for developing the evidence base and our theoretical knowledge.
- An outcome is defined as the result of intervention.
- Outcomes measurements should be as numerous as possible; tailor-made for specific individuals and the intervention they receive, as well as being socially meaningful.
- Efficacy is defined as the outcome of an intervention in an ideal situation.
- Effectiveness is the outcome of an intervention in a non-ideal, real-life situation.
- Efficiency is the outcome of an intervention as evaluated in terms of cost effectiveness and time effectiveness.
- Two theoretical models were presented: Frattali's (1998) hierarchy of outcomes evaluation; and the phase model from Robey and Schultz (1998).
- Both these models emphasize that intervention research is a process and as speech and language therapy is a young profession with a minimal evidence base we should start at the early stages of the process.
- Research suggests that phonological intervention for children generally has positive outcomes, although a greater number of detailed studies are needed to pinpoint why intervention is more successful for some children than others.
- The outcomes of our study of children with PSDs varied widely from child to child, and without a range of outcomes measures we would not have been able to capture this.
- Practitioners can turn routine therapy sessions into intervention case studies with very little extra work, and a few carefully constructed research questions.
- Research questions should be specific and answerable. A broad question such as 'Is intervention successful?' needs to be broken down further, for example by defining the nature of intervention, the clients who will receive it; how success will be defined and outcomes measured.
- Outcomes measures should be carefully selected based on the research questions posed.
- Intervention should be carefully and precisely described by asking: What do tasks really tap?

- Intervention case studies and replications of these are much needed.

KEY TO ACTIVITY 12.1

(a) Define the outcomes by which you will evaluate the success of your intervention.

The main or primary outcome measures would be Daisy's ability to (a) produce /s/ clusters accurately in single words or connected speech, and (b) produce /t/ in word-initial position with a decreased frequency of backing.

(b) How would you measure these outcomes?

Pre-intervention baseline assessment would need to take place and comparisons made with Daisy's post-intervention production of these stimuli. Stimuli would be at a single word or phrase level depending on the psycholinguistic focus of the intervention. The stimuli words would need to be selected to include /s/ clusters and /t/ in word-initial position. Control wordlists would be designed with these words not included in intervention but used to evaluate the extent of Daisy's generalization to untreated items.

(c) What other information would you gather post-intervention to evaluate outcomes?

It would be interesting to know if Daisy's ability to spell words with /s/ clusters and /t/ in word-initial position had improved as a result of intervention. This could be done if spelling was included as a pre-intervention baseline measure. However, comments from Daisy herself, her teachers and parents about the effects of the intervention on her speech and spelling would be important in contributing to an overall impression of outcomes.

KEY TO ACTIVITY 12.2

This activity emphasizes the importance of selecting appropriate outcomes. The children considered in the activity might have been placed in very different quadrants if different, specific outcomes had been selected and described in that activity.

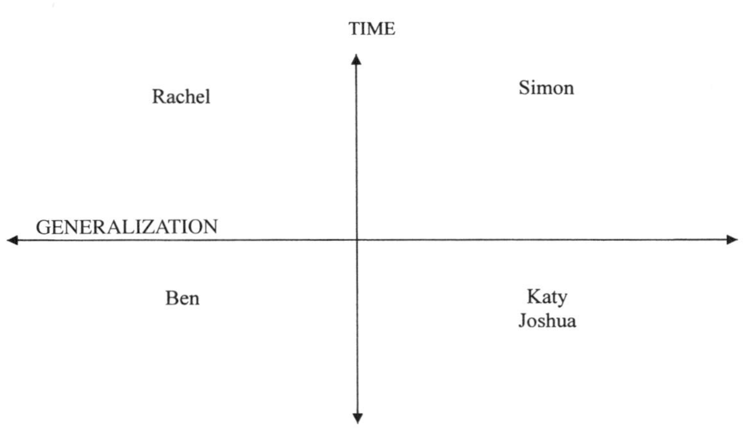

KEY TO ACTIVITY 12.3

(a) What were the intervention outcomes? How do you know?

The primary outcome measure was evaluation of Oliver's speech production of single words containing specific segments. He made significant gains on three of the four wordlists of targeted stimuli. The secondary outcome measures were evaluation of Oliver's spelling of these words, and his ability to make auditory discriminations between closely related words. He also improved significantly in these areas. We know about these outcomes because they were clearly defined prior to the intervention. Comparisons between pre-intervention and post-intervention performance were made using statistical analyses (t-tests, ANOVA's) which informed us about whether the changes were significant.

(b) Can you comment on the intervention's effectiveness? What steps might have been taken to enable further comments to be made about this?

Effectiveness is the outcome of an intervention in a non-ideal, real-life situation. Oliver's intervention was carried out at his school and in this sense was representative of how therapy is typically carried out. However, the intervention was more intensive than is typical in many parts of the UK and was carried out by an experienced therapist on a 1 : 1 basis. Working through classroom assistants and on a less intensive basis would inform us more about the effectiveness of the psycholinguistic intervention in the real world.

(c) Can you comment on the intervention's efficiency? How do you think it might compare to a different intervention (e.g. different procedures, aims, duration, intensity)?

Efficiency is the outcome of an intervention as evaluated in terms of cost effectiveness and time effectiveness. It typically involves a comparison with other interventions, e.g. asking if X intervention brings about changes more rapidly or cost effectively than Y intervention? Oliver's intervention was not specifically contrasted with other interventions, although we can use case-notes to inform us about previous interventions and outcome. Oliver had received less intensive therapy in the past, which had resulted in less significant gains in his speech.

KEY TO ACTIVITY 12.4

(a) What research question was posed by these authors?

Can the speech production of a child with PSDs be improved by means of carefully targeted EPG intervention?

(b) What outcomes measures were used in this study?

The primary outcome measure was the child's production of velars, although from the abstract we do not know if these were in isolation, single words or sentences.

(c) Does this study evaluate efficacy, effectiveness or efficiency?

Efficacy. The study evaluates the outcomes of EPG intervention in a fairly ideal clinical situation.

(d) What were the main findings of the study?

The boy's production of velars improved significantly from pre- to post-intervention, suggesting that the intervention was successful. It also allowed for qualitative comments to be made about the nature of his articulation difficulties.

KEY TO ACTIVITY 12.5

(a) Did the children make changes at the 'micro' level and how was this change measured?

Yes, all the children made significant improvements at the micro level. This was evaluated by designing specific stimuli for each child based on the intervention targets. Change was evaluated using the treated stimuli that were addressed in intervention as well as untreated stimuli not directly addressed in intervention.

(b) Comment on the pattern of changes observed at the macro level?

At this broader level, the results varied widely from child to child.

(c) Contrast the outcomes for Oliver and Rachel.

Oliver's changes did not extend beyond the specific stimuli, but Rachel's intervention was effective in bringing about changes at all levels evaluated.

(d) Comment on the pattern of outcomes observed for Joshua and why it does not appear to follow the outcomes hierarchy presented in the table.

Joshua showed specific changes on the micro measures and in his speech processing profile. However, significant changes in intelligibility were not shown. Some may consider that intelligibility should appear at a higher level of the hierarchy, although this is open to debate, e.g. compare with Ben's patterns of changes.

Note

1. Between 2001 and 2005, an additional 11 studies were carried out with a developmental focus and involving intervention.

Chapter 13
Service Delivery Issues

> Gary seems like a sharp enough kid, but he doesn't talk much and Mum has him referred for SLT. In contrast Dad is really impressed by his new company car, which is going a treat. Now which will get more attention in the coming year? Sadly the car will spend more time being serviced than Gary will spend receiving SLT . . . I hope there are no SLTs who think that language impairments can be sorted in 6 hours per year.
>
> (Pring, 2005 p. 217)

Children with PSDs have complex difficulties which can affect academic progress and social development. These children require intervention that is tailor-made to their individual needs, managed by trained professionals and intensive. Broomfield and Dodd (2004) suggest that the severity and complexity of children's speech problems shows the need for expanded and enhanced speech and language therapy services. As a profession we need to provide evidence of this to influence policy makers: one way we can do this is through carefully designed intervention studies.

It may be argued that such rigorous, tailor-made and intensive intervention is not practical for many therapists working in constrained service delivery settings. However, we argue that the psycholinguistic approach is an approach 'carried in the head of the user' (Stackhouse and Wells, 1997) – not in a bag of therapy materials! The approach does not require specific, expensive materials. Before discarding out of date therapy materials, we should ask ourselves 'what do these tasks really tap?' (Rees, 2001a,b), since it is likely that even the most unfashionable therapy equipment has some important psycholinguistic properties when used appropriately with the right child. Intervention that is specifically targeted at a child's difficulties and tailor-made to their needs will be more cost effective in the long term than a general programme of intervention that does not work! The psycholinguistic approach can also be delivered by trained and supported assistants or parents, either to individual children or to groups. In this chapter we focus on these issues of service delivery – the practical constraints that may make application of some of the ideas in this book a challenge. Let us start first by considering terminology and what is meant by service delivery as opposed to intervention.

How Does Service Delivery Differ from Intervention?

It is important to clarify the difference between service delivery and intervention - especially when talking about the evaluation of outcomes, as the two can be very different. Evaluations of interventions look at a specific approach to treating a specific child in a specific set of circumstances. The intervention needs to be clearly described in a way that would allow it to be replicated. For example, Crosbie and Dodd (2001) describe in detail the rationale and procedures they used to address auditory discrimination in a 7-year-old girl with severe language difficulties. The study is described in such a way that a practitioner faced with a similar child and agreeing with Crosbie and Dodd's rationale could carry out the same or similar intervention. Pring (2005, Chapter 15) provides a comprehensive discussion of single cases and specific therapies.

Evaluations of service delivery look more generally at how a service, i.e. speech and language therapy, which might include any number of specific or more eclectic approaches to intervention, brings about changes in clients. The randomized control trial carried out by Glogowska *et al.* (2000) aimed to compare routine speech and language therapy in 159 pre-school children with delayed speech and language against 12 months of 'watchful waiting'. The routine treatment provided by the practitioners participating in the study varied widely, but tended to focus on several areas simultaneously. Therapy techniques included activities from the *Derbyshire Language Scheme* (Masidlover and Knowles, 1982), as well as everyday play and games used as contexts for modelling language for the child. Goals covered a wide range of language stages - for example, understanding and building single words, using narratives, and identifying consonants in words. The study aimed to evaluate NHS speech and language services routinely offered in the UK to pre-school children (see Chapter 12 for further details of the study). If the study had been carried out with a group of independent practitioners, or in a different country, different outcomes may have been found. However, that is not to say that there might not have been individual therapists in the NHS, independent setting or a different country carrying out very similar interventions. The service delivery evaluation gives only a broad overview of what was done by the average professional in a particular context, not what was actually happening in individual therapy rooms across the country (see Pring, 2005, Chapter 14 for a discussion of such studies).

Evaluations of service delivery and intervention are both important and have their place in building an evidence base. Authors like Robey and Schultz (1998) and Pring (2004) argue that we need the specific intervention case studies before we can start answering questions about service delivery in an informative way. However, service delivery issues are urgent for therapy managers, who need to know how many sessions of intervention are needed and how to deliver these in a cost-effective and practical manner bearing in mind constraints of money, staff and time. Let us consider what is known about some of these issues specifically as they relate to older school-age children with persisting difficulties.

Therapy Frequency or Dosage

Intervention dosage is an important issue about which relatively little is known. We often have feelings about how much therapy a child may need, but there is little evidence to back up our intuitions. The intervention given to the children presented in this book was relatively intensive compared to what they had been receiving. It seems logical that for children who have had low dose therapy and whose problems persist, dosage intensity may need to be increased. However, therapy dosage is a relative concept! The definition of intensive varies from practitioner to practitioner and from work setting to work setting. Rosenbek (1985), when discussing therapy for adults with apraxia, defines intensive as meaning that the patient and the practitioner should have daily sessions; Haynes (1985, in Hall, Jordan and Robin, 1993) also advocates daily therapy sessions. Blakeley (1983, in Hall, Jordan and Robin, 1993, p. 27) stated, 'I do not expect to provide speech education for children with developmental apraxia of speech on a cursory basis for it may be the most important part of their entire education.' The intervention in our study was not as intensive as that given by Tallal *et al.* (1993, 1996) in their intervention studies using computerized auditory training. The intervention might have had different results if the dosage was daily and the children were seen for a shorter time period rather than twice weekly over the space of many months.

Few studies have addressed the issue of how much intervention is typically needed to bring about progress (Jacoby, Lee, Kummer *et al.*, 2002). ASHA developed the *National Outcomes Measurement System* (NOMS) for the purpose of tracking functional gains in individuals receiving therapy. NOMS data revealed that after 17 hours of treatment, 16.4% of children with a severe articulation disorder moved to a functional level for discharge. However the large majority of children (83.6%) did not evidence significant change and required additional treatment. This information shows that short-term intervention can benefit a small percentage of children, but that most children with severe speech and language disorders require more treatment time to achieve a functional communication level that enables them to participate in age-appropriate activities (Zeit and Johnson, 2002). Our children received from 10 hours (Rachel) to 36 hours (Ben) of intervention with an average dosage of 25 hours per child. Apart from Rachel whose specific difficulties were addressed after

10 hours of intervention, the other children all required further intervention.

Campbell (1999, 2002) answers the question of 'How many treatment sessions are required to improve my child's speech?' by drawing on data from his study of intervention. Interestingly, he used parental estimates of the child's intelligibility to unfamiliar listeners (see Chapter 11) as his primary outcomes measure. For the participants with phonological difficulties an average of 29 individual, 45-minute treatment sessions (range of 21 to 42 sessions) were required for parents to increase their ratings from having less than half of their child's speech understood by an unfamiliar listener to having about three-quarters of their child's speech understood. For the eight children with apraxic speech, parents considered that 75% of their child's speech could be understood following an average of 151 individual treatment sessions (ranging from 144 to 168 sessions). Campbell (1999) concludes that:

> In other words, the children with apraxia of speech required 81% more individual treatment sessions than the children with severe phonologic disorders in order to achieve a similar functional outcome. (i.e. 3/4 of speech judged to be understood by unfamiliar listeners).

What is also interesting about this study is the fairly large amount of therapy needed for the children with severe phonological difficulties – 29 sessions is a relatively large amount of individual therapy for a child to receive, but we should not be surprised at all given the complexity of the speech processing system!

Dosage and the amount of therapy a child requires is a potential minefield, especially when the evidence base is limited. Studies such as those cited in this section go some way towards helping us through this fraught area. In the UK speech and language therapists are often asked to assess children to determine whether or not they should be given a Statement of Special Education Needs. This is a legal document which describes a child's special educational needs and how these should be met by service providers. Speech and language therapists carrying out such assessments are often asked to quantify the amount of therapy a child needs. This is very difficult since we never know how a child will respond to therapy. The therapist needs to consider what is known about the child as well as what is known about the evidence base regarding dosage. The therapist's opinion may then be used by the parents at tribunal to obtain the suggested therapy dosage from local health and educational services. Conflicts can arise when an independent practitioner suggests an amount of therapy that a child might need, which cannot be provided by the local service as illustrated anecdotally below:

> In my report I suggested that the child – a child with severe speech difficulties and dyslexia – required 1 hour of speech and language

> therapy each week for the forthcoming term, in addition to recommendations about additional classroom support. I felt that this was reasonable given the nature of the child's difficulties and what I know and have read about intervention for similar children. The manager of the local service then rang me to say that I had put the local service in a difficult position since they were unable to offer this amount of therapy. She suggested that in future we decide on the recommended dosage together bearing in mind what could realistically be offered.
>
> (Independent Speech and Language Therapist)

This interesting but not uncommon scenario poses some interesting ethical issues that are discussed further in the following activity. Hall, Jordan and Robin (1993) suggest that in such cases, 'The practitioner may be thrust into the position of becoming an advocate on behalf of the child to assure that services are provided as frequently as possible.' From the other perspective of those constrained by the service delivery, Law and Conti-Ramsden (2000, pp. 909–10) note:

> Offering limited amounts of speech and language therapy is not a tenable solution to the problem. The six hours [in the Glogowska *et al.*, 2000 study] provided did not necessarily reflect the choice of the speech and language therapists in the study but rather a constraint imposed on them by the . . . model of service delivery . . .

ACTIVITY 13.1

When seeing a child for an initial assessment, what are the factors that might make you think the child is a long-term case rather than a short-term one? Make a list of these factors. Compare your list to ours in the Key to Activity 13.1 at the end of this chapter, and then read what follows.

There is a great deal of research still to be done regarding the shape of intervention and the type of dosage that is optimum for children with different types and severity of speech problems, i.e. is it better to have weekly therapy (1 hour each time) for a year's duration or to have all those 52 hours of therapy given on consecutive days, or to have blocks of intensive therapy with follow-ups? It seems likely that the answer to this question depends on the nature of the child's difficulties, circumstances and style of learning.

In a longitudinal study carried out by Nathan *et al.* (2004a) the authors investigated the outcomes for young pre-school children with speech difficulties. The results of that study are reported in Nathan *et al.* (2004a, b) as well as being discussed in Stackhouse *et al.* (forthcoming). However, of interest here is questionnaire data that were gathered for each of the children about the intervention they had (or had not) received. Although the study was not an efficacy study, the authors gave questionnaires to therapists working with the participants asking for details of any intervention the children had received. They found a relationship between the amount of therapy a child received at 4;6 years and the severity of the speech difficulties and grammatical language difficulties at 6;8 years. There was also a relationship between the amount of therapy a child received at 6;8 years and the severity of difficulty with speech output, grammar, phonological awareness and literacy at that time. The children with resolving or resolved problems at 6;8 years were likely to be receiving less therapy than those with persisting problems. Interestingly there was no relationship between the severity of a child's speech difficulties and the amount of intervention at 4;6 years and 5;8 years. Altogether these results revealed that the children with the more severe speech problems in the study were receiving therapy but, as with those pre-schoolers in the Glogowska *et al.* (2000) paper, they were receiving varying amounts and types of speech and language therapy. This study supported the view that children whose speech difficulties persist beyond the critical age of around 5;6 are likely to have persisting difficulties with both their spoken and written language development and are in need of long-term, intensive management by therapy and teaching services.

In the randomized control trial carried out by Glogowska *et al.* (2000), the pre-schoolers with language delay were seen on average for 6.2 hours of therapy, with the range for each child varying from 0 to 15 hours. The average number of contacts with the therapist was 8.1 with a range from 0 to 17 contacts. On average therapy frequency was once a month, although again variation was wide: from once a week to once every two and a half months. The average session length was found to be 47 minutes, but varied from 20 to 75 minutes. The children in Glogowska *et al.*'s study were young pre-school children with language difficulties. Nevertheless the data re dosage is illuminating generally because so few studies provide such an overview of what actually happens in a typical service. The fact that the intervention outcomes were not positive in comparison to the watchful-waiting group is not very useful given the wide range of variability in terms of dosage. In a commentary about this study by James Law and Gina Conti-Ramsden (2000) entitled: 'Six hours of therapy is not enough!', these authors emphasize the dosage issue and how it should be used to inform our practice.

> Offering limited amounts of speech and language therapy is not a tenable solution to the problem. Practitioners . . . should be able to offer a more flexible package of interventions. This is likely to require a reor-

> ganisation of . . . services, but this is the point of practising evidence-based medicine: when you fill the evidence gap you need to act.
>
> (Law and Conti-Ramsden, 2000, pp. 909–10)

Cost Effectiveness

Health service managers are under great pressure to justify the services they deliver not only in terms of positive outcomes, but also in terms of cost effectiveness. For a child with severe speech difficulties achieving basic communicative independence will typically require intensive and ongoing speech therapy (Hall, Jordan and Robin, 1993). Persisting speech difficulties are not solely a medical problem and as such will not be addressed by a cure culture. The associated social and educational issues require ongoing and integrated management. As health care costs continue to rise, it will become even more important to justify frequent speech therapy sessions over a long period of time. Cost effectiveness, cost–benefit, and cost–utility are terms used to link the expenses associated with providing intervention to the outcomes obtained as a result of that intervention. Cost effectiveness links the monetary cost of an intervention to improvement of direct health/educational outcomes, e.g. the cost of an intervention compared to the cost savings of preventing additional expenses (e.g. admission to a special school, need for counselling or psychotherapy). Cost–benefit compares the monetary cost of the intervention with the monetary benefit of the outcome measured more broadly in terms of increased income and improved leisure time. Cost–utility compares the monetary cost of the treatment most broadly with quality of life outcome. Some interventions may not be justifiable in terms of cost effectiveness, but may be argued for in terms of cost–utility (Golper, 2001). Sackett, Richardson, Rosenberg and Haynes (1997, p. 4) observe that:

> Some fear that evidence-based medicine will be highjacked by purchasers and managers to cut the cost of health care. This would not only be a misuse of evidence-based medicine but suggests a fundamental misunderstanding of its financial consequences.

Certainly, practitioners subscribing to evidence-based practice should identify and provide the most efficacious treatments to maximize their client's quality, and if applicable, quantity, of life. Ultimately, this may raise rather than lower the cost of care. Robey and Schultz's (1998) five-phase outcome research model (outlined in Chapter 12) provides a systematic method for developing a treatment; testing its efficacy; testing its effectiveness; examining its efficiency; and determining its cost effectiveness, cost–benefit, and cost–utility. While cost effectiveness may be at the forefront of managers' and purchasers' minds, it is the researcher/practitioner's role to move through the five outcomes phases, concerned with building a solid foundation of evidence for a particular intervention and considering cost effectiveness at the appropriate point once a fairly substantial amount of outcomes data has been amassed.

School-age children with PSDs may be particularly vulnerable to the effects of cost cutting and rationalization: many health authorities consider early intervention to be a greater priority than intervention for the school-age child. Increasingly consultative models are being adopted in schools, with speech and language therapists having limited opportunity for providing one-to-one intervention for children. Therapy programmes are often carried out by classroom assistants and other members of the teaching staff (Law *et al.*, 2002). The use of this consultative model with assistants is discussed in the following sections.

A Consultative Approach

A survey carried out by Lindsay, Soloff, Law *et al.* (2002b) found that speech and language therapy services in UK schools vary widely with respect to size of caseload and the number of children per therapist. Children with PSDs need to develop their communication skills and access the curriculum. These needs come together in school settings especially at Key Stage 1 of the education system in the UK (Lindsay *et al.*, 2002b). Lindsay *et al.* suggest that a consultative model can be helpful in empowering school staff. Law *et al.* (2002) define consultation as being characterized by 'an emphasis shift from direct work with children to consultation between the SLT, and other key professionals, particularly teachers, assistants . . . and parents' (p. 148). Consultative approaches may be appropriate for some children, but may not be appropriate for children with severe and persisting difficulties that have not responded to previous intervention. The interventions described in this book have shown that work with such children requires comprehensive assessment and ongoing consideration and re-evaluation of their difficulties, something which untrained personnel would not be able to do.

Despite the need for school-age children with persisting difficulties to access intensive intervention, it is difficult to justify enormous amounts of time and effort spent on just a few children (Law *et al.*, 2002). It is estimated that 14.3 speech and language therapists work with children in any given health trust in the United Kingdom and the average ratio of SLT to child population is estimated at 1 : 4257. Recent prevalence data suggest that 7.4% of school-age children have speech and language difficulties (Tomblin, Records, Buckwalter *et al.*, 1997). This equates to a typical caseload of 315 children per therapist. Law *et al.* (2002) have suggested that 40 children is a more desirable level for a notional caseload. There is obviously a considerable difference and a clear discrepancy here. A consultancy model with limited therapist–child contact, combined with opportunities for hands-on 1 : 1 work with a speech and language therapist may be best. It is suggested that it remains for researchers and practitioners who are able to carry out intervention beyond the confines of a particular service delivery model (e.g. independent practitioners) to investigate more intensive, tailor-made interventions. Collecting and providing data from this type of intervention will be a valuable addition to the evidence base, and may ultimately allow for a justification of tailor-made, intensive, one-to-one interventions for those children who need it (Zeit and Johnson, 2002). There is a growing body of evidence suggesting that in order to bring about long-term changes in speech and language, intensive input and carefully targeted intervention is needed (Law *et al.*, 1998; Glogowska, Campbell, Peters *et al.*, 2002).

Velleman (2004) comments on the role of parents, teachers, peers and siblings in a child's program of remediation, suggesting that it will vary with the circumstances. She suggests that for a child with apraxia the speech and language therapist 'may include family and/or teachers in the overall programming to provide additional response opportunities for the child to reinforce and strengthen performance on a particular speech target'. Creaghead, Newman and Secord (1989, p. 274) stated that 'nightly parental drill . . . is a necessity'. However, in today's society we need to realize that the involvement of the family in giving extra input and practice is not always a practical recommendation to pursue. As noted in Chapter 8, speech and language therapists for a long time were solely responsible for providing intervention in a 1 : 1 way. Increasingly there has been awareness of the important role parents and teachers can play in helping children with speech and language difficulties. Parents see children in different contexts and can therefore make therapy activities more meaningful. This also fits well with the limited time and resources constraining therapists from giving intensive individual therapy to all children who require it. Results of the review carried out by Law and Garret (2003) confirmed that parent-based intervention is effective in treating children with expressive language delays, but that for children with phonological difficulties practitioner-administered therapy is more effective. In evaluating results from these studies, it is important to consider the age and type of difficulties of the children in the studies, and also the resources and support offered to the parents. Young children with phonological delays may be more receptive to parental intervention than older children with persisting problems.

Working with Assistants

Law *et al.* (2002) discuss prerequisites for the successful implementation of a consultative approach. One of these is the adequate training of support workers in schools. Lindsay *et al.* (2002b) recognize the increasing numbers of learning support assistants who have received limited training in the areas of speech and language, and McCartney, Boyle, Bannatyne *et al.* (2005) reiterate the need for therapists to provide ongoing training and support of assistants, as well as the difficulties in adapting and updating therapy plans when working indirectly. While authors such as McCartney *et al.* (2005) emphasize the time required to support assistants, they also acknowledge that respondents to their survey could see the value in working through assistants. Law *et al.* (2002, p. 152) note that '. . . if there are not enough appropriately skilled learning support assistants in place, it is unlikely that SLTs will be able to function effectively in the educational context'.

Velleman (2004) notes with regard to children with apraxia that at least some of the therapy, on a regular basis (e.g. once a week) must be provided by a registered speech and language therapist. Other professionals who work with the child in other sessions must be supervised by the certified person (e.g. meet with her/him weekly to discuss progress and strategies). For school-age children with persisting speech difficulties, working with classroom assistants and speech and language therapy assistants can be a helpful way of increasing dosage, integrating therapy into school, and making intervention more cost effective in the long term. For this to happen, time needs to be invested in the appropriate training of the assistants.

Wood, Wright and Stackhouse (2000) devised a training package for use with multi-disciplinary professionals involved with children in the early years. The package contains all the materials required to run a course, along with a training video and instruction manual for tutors. The course, entitled *Language and Literacy: Joining Together* is based on research literature and on a training needs analyses (see Wright and Wood, 2006). The course, which benefits practitioners from all agencies, including those with and without professional qualifications, aims to 'enable early years practitioners to work effectively with each other and with parents, in order to identify and support children with speech, language and literacy difficulties'. Although this training package has been specifically designed with younger children in mind, many of the principles in the training are applicable to those working with school-age children with PSDs, e.g. the use of a simplified psycholinguistic model to provide a clear conceptualization of the links between speech, phonological awareness and literacy (see Figure 10.1 in Chapter 10).

Hilary Gardner has devised a training programme for speech and language therapists to use to train assistants - classroom assistants, speech and language therapy assistants, student practitioners or parents - in working with children with speech problems (Gardner, 2006). This programme makes explicit some of the interactions that therapists take for granted, and is based on her research into therapy interactions (Gardner, 1989, 1998). Two important aspects of therapy interaction which form an important part of the programme are:

(a) giving the child precise information about the target behaviour;
(b) moving the child towards self-correction.

Findings from Gardner's work suggest that this type of intensive interactional training for key workers can make the implementation of speech programmes more effective.

An interactional approach is not incompatible with the psycholinguistic and phonological approaches outlined in this book. Rather, it fits with the eclectic approach to intervention outlined in Chapter 1 of this book. An eclectic approach is likely to maximize our chances of success with a challenging client group. The psycholinguistic approach informs our knowledge of what we are targeting in the speech processing system and how we aim to bring about change. The phonological approach gives us more detail: exactly what stimuli will we use in intervention? An interactional approach tells us how we 'do therapy' itself and how the child is responding to the inputs we give him or her, making repairs and learning in therapy. We conceptualize this three-way eclectic view of therapy in Figure 13.1.

In Activity 13.2 we focus on the overlap between psycholinguistic, phonological and interactional approaches to intervention, and how one might support an assistant delivering sessions based around this triad.

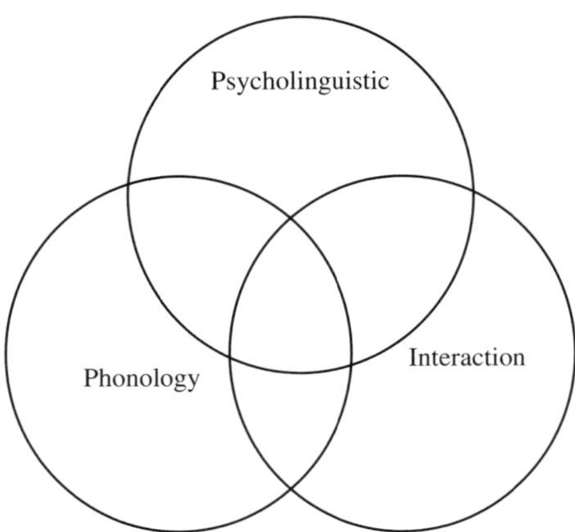

Figure 13.1: Three-way conceptualization of phonological therapy.

ACTIVITY 13.2

Read through the following transcript from a therapy session. The child was a boy called Matthew aged 6;3 with PSDs. The activity is an auditory lexical decision task in which the therapist names pictures and the child is required to make judgments about the therapist's productions and whether these are right ('sensible') or wrong ('silly'). Answer the questions that follow.

Therapist: T
Child: C

T: OK – so I'll go first, you listen carefully
Are you ready?
C: Yip
T: (puts picture of a SPOON on the table)
'boon' – is that a boon?
C: um . . . No
T: great, very clever
Your turn now
Remember, you can say something silly or sensible
C: (puts picture of SKIN on the table)
. . . (thinks)
/kɪnə/
T: /kɪnə/. . . . Mmm (pauses)
I didn't hear that /sk/ sound, the one with two parts that we practised
So I'm thinking it was silly
I'll say no
(puts picture of a SPINNING TOP on the table)
Pinning top
Is that it?
C: Uh
T: Listen carefully, I'll say it again
Pinning top
C: Yes
T: Are you sure? I said 'pinning top', and that's different to 'spinning top'
Can you hear the snakey sound when I say sssspinning top?
C: Yeah . . . sssss . . . pinning top
T: Great! You said it there!
That was brilliant
You need a prize for that . . . and a turn
C: (puts picture of someone SKI-ING on the table)
Ssssss . . . ki-ing

T: Oh that was sensible! I'll say yes
It sounded so good
C: I did it on purpose

Now consider the following questions:

1. Focus on the psycholinguistic: What do you think the psycholinguistic demands of the task were for the child?
2. Focus on the phonological: What do you think the phonological demands were for the child?
3. Focus on the interactional: Can you give examples of places where the therapist
   (a) makes the target explicit to the child?
   (b) encourages the child towards self-repair?

Now turn to the Key to Activity 13.2 at the end of the chapter before reading the following.

In the task above, the three interconnected elements – psycholinguistic, phonological and interactional – are all at play. Although they are all taking place at the same time, it is helpful to our understanding of the complex therapy process if we consider each lens separately before bringing them back into overlap.

In psycholinguistic terms, the game has two aspects. It is tapping both input and output. In terms of input the child is required to process auditory information from the therapist, and make a decision as to whether this auditory information matches the child's stored representation for the pictured item. The therapist is checking whether the child's phonological representation is accurate. This is done by drawing on the child's strengths of auditory perception, i.e. that he can hear the sounds themselves accurately, and through his good visual recognition/semantic knowledge, i.e. that he knows what the item is. The child also names some of the pictures on occasion and copies the therapist's modelled production giving him an opportunity to map from his phonological representations onto motor programmes.

Phonologically, the therapist is working on /sk/ and /st/ in word-initial position. We have no further information about the child's speech but it seems from the transcript that his speech is largely intelligible. From an interactional point of view, the following are all examples of drawing the child's attention to the target in a very explicit way:

> 'I didn't hear that /sk/ sound, the one with two parts that we practised'

> 'Can you hear the snakey sound when I say sssspinning top?'

Gardner (1998) notes that experienced speech and language therapists tend to do this automatically, but we need to remember that it may not come naturally to parents and assistants. Moving the child towards self-repair takes place at several points in the transcript. After the child says /kɪnə/ for skin, the therapist repeats what he has said, ponders his utterance in an exaggerated way ('mmm') and then pauses, giving him opportunity to change or clarify what he has said, if he wants to. She also asks him, 'Are you sure?' at one point, encouraging him to reflect on what he has said. At the end of the episode when he has produced the target word correctly, he reflects that that was precisely what he intended to do, showing knowledge of the fact that he understands the task is about actively making a decision to produce the word correctly or incorrectly.

From our experience, there are many challenges associated with the consultative model. When it works well, the assistant feels in control, stimulated and empowered to help a child and ask for support as needed. The therapist feels that his or her time has been well utilized and a child is getting the intervention needed in the most cost effective manner. The child progresses. When it works badly, the assistant feels ill-equipped to help the child, and his or her self-esteem and job satisfaction may be low; the child makes slow or minimal progress, and the therapist feels disheartened and frustrated. Given that hands-on work with clients is one of the main reasons why people enter the profession, we need to be careful about replacing this with a majority of consultative work. Both approaches have their strengths; ideally a mixture of the two is the best way of achieving optimum outcomes.

Group vs. Individual

One way of coping with limited resources is by offering group therapy, as opposed to one-to-one approaches. Sommers *et al.* (1961) investigated the outcomes of group therapy for children with speech problems as opposed to individual treatments. They found that over eight months there was no significant difference between the outcomes obtained for group vs. individual therapy. Similarly, results of the meta-analysis carried out by Law and Garret (2003) showed group therapy to be as effective as individual therapy. These studies may tell only part of the story since it seems likely that the children would not have been homogeneous, and differences in response to the intervention may have been obscured by the group means.

There are some therapists who do not favour group therapy, especially in the case of children with severe speech difficulties. Velleman (2004) suggests that for children with apraxia most therapy should be individual. She cautions that if group therapy is provided, 'It will not help unless the other children in the group have the *same diagnosis and are at the same level phonologically*.' Therapists working with older children and adults who stammer typically advocate a combination of group and individual therapy (e.g. Ramig and Bennett, 1997). There are many aspects associated with group therapy in addition to addressing the issue of resource shortages. The advantages of group approaches to intervention include:

- opportunities to share a common problem and solutions;
- a supportive environment to decrease feelings of isolation;
- communication opportunities that take place in a real social setting;
- opportunities for individuals to take responsibility for own speech difficulties.

These reasons are applicable to children who stammer, but have wider applicability to children with any sort of communication difficulty, including those falling under the umbrella of 'persisting speech problem'. Although such children are also likely to benefit from therapy that is delivered 1 : 1, the group setting also provides valuable opportunities for growth, the generalization of specific skills to a wider social setting and the management of some of the self-esteem issues that can be a problem for some children with intractable speech problems.

Nash *et al.* (2001) have devised a programme for the management of persistent communication difficulties in children. The programme aims to fill the need for psychosocial intervention using intensive, residential group work. Although originally piloted with children with cleft palate (or velopharyngeal incompetence), the programme focuses on total communication and would be appropriate for any child meeting a broad definition of having PSDs. Children are encouraged to discuss their specific difficulties with others, learn to develop strategies for forging friendships and focus on specific positive aspects of their communication in a daily activity called 'prouding'. Results from a pilot study suggested four key areas in which children benefited:

- self-confidence
- improved speech
- friendship development
- use of effective coping strategies.

Again, we suggest that socially-oriented programmes are a valuable part of the eclectic armoury of the speech and language therapist working with children with PSDs. Such an approach complements a psycholinguistic approach and the two work well together with the psycholinguistic focusing directly on speech performance and the psychosocial focusing at a more functional, social level (Nash, 2006). If one has clear knowledge of the strengths and weaknesses of all group participants, then there is no reason why some psycholinguistically oriented activities cannot be carried out in a group setting. An example of this is provided from a session working with Katy (the child who formed the focus of Chapter 8) and Rachel (Chapter 9) together.

A Small Group Session with Rachel (CA 7;1) and Katy (CA 6;5)

Katy's intervention aimed to improve her ability to produce final consonants in simple CVC words (see Pascoe, Stackhouse and Wells, 2005; and Chapter 8 for further details of her intervention). In the second phase of her intervention we aimed to work on a larger set of words to promote generalization. Each session was structured around a theme such as household items, holidays or animals. Katy greatly enjoyed being in control in the therapy situation, and she particularly liked to pretend that she was a teacher. In this session, she was told that she was the teacher, and the therapist and Rachel were children in the classroom. Katy was to give us a spelling test, and was given pictures of words that fitted in with our theme. As Katy said the word that the 'children' needed to write, there was great confusion on Rachel's (and the therapist's) part as to what the words were. Katy was often irritated when asked to repeat words since she knew that the therapist must actually know the words having thought of them herself and put the pictures on cards for her! The therapist kept quiet and Rachel on several occasions then spontaneously asked for clarification from Katy, e.g. saying:

> 'Katy, is it CAR or CARD or CART we must write?'

Katy refused to relinquish her teacherly control and let Rachel see the card she held. She was thus obliged to repeat what she had said and make clear the target item to which she referred, i.e. CART. This helped Katy to realize the importance of final consonants. She was able to repeat the words and make them clearer. The session was effective in highlighting communicative importance of the final consonants in a naturalistic way. This final session in Katy's Phase II seemed more useful than many sessions earlier in the intervention when Katy was not motivated to make repairs to her productions because she knew the therapist really knew what she was saying. However, a group must have advantages for all participants. What about the benefits for Rachel for sharing her therapy time with Katy? Rachel's therapy aims were to improve her ability to produce word-final consonant clusters such as /sp/ and /sk/ in words like WASP and MASK. Rachel was also given an opportunity to be the teacher, and her role involved telling us about these words: what they mean as well as how to write and say them. Here she was given the opportunity to think very explicitly about the final consonants as she instructed a younger and less adept talker and writer in producing these sounds.

Service Delivery and the Psycholinguistic Approach: Ideas for Best Practice

This section draws together some suggestions for best practice for delivering intervention for school-aged children with PSDs. Some of the ideas have been evaluated systematically through research, and where this is the case a reference is supplied. Some of the suggestions have yet to be tested, and these ideas might be turned into research questions for practitioners to try out in their routine practice or for student projects.

- School-age children with PSDs require intensive intervention that is carefully targeted at the appropriate parts of the child's speech processing system (Pascoe *et al.*, 2005), and supervised by trained professionals following detailed assessment (Ebbels, 2000).
- The psycholinguistic approach is a flexible approach that should be overlapped with phonological approaches (Ebbels, 2000; Pascoe *et al.*, 2005) and can be adapted to service delivery constraints, e.g. it can also be delivered in groups or by key workers.
- Working in groups has additional advantages and benefits for older children in managing their confidence and talking in real-life social situations (Nash *et al.*, 2001; Nash, 2006).
- We suggest that a combination of group and individual therapy may be most appropriate for this client group.
- Key workers (e.g. assistants and parents) are a valuable resource that can help make intervention more cost effective in the long term. However, assistants must be well supported and appropriately trained to do this. In the short to medium term this can mean a greater time and financial commitment than if the therapist was working only with children (Gardner, 2006).
- Experienced therapists tend to automatically manage sessions through facilitation of interaction, but when training key workers this is a vital aspect that needs to be explicitly addressed.
- We need studies of both service delivery and intervention (Pring, 2005).
- Individual therapists are well placed to make studies of their own intervention, but most therapists will also have access to data about dosage and intervention shape that they can use to inform their clinical decision making.

Summary

The key points are as follows.

- Children with persisting speech problems typically require intervention that is tailor-made to their individual needs, delivered by trained professionals and intensive.
- As a profession we need to provide evidence of this to influence policy makers; we can do this through carefully designed intervention studies.
- We need to acquire an understanding of what takes place in intervention and its outcomes, before service delivery studies will be fully understood.
- In general children with persisting speech difficulties require intensive intervention, but there is a need for more work focusing on the optimal 'shape' of intervention for children with different profiles.
- A psycholinguistic approach is an approach carried in the head of the user - not in a bag of therapy materials. The approach does not require specific, expensive materials.
- Intervention that is specifically targeted at a child's difficulties and tailor-made to their needs will be more cost effective in the long term than a general programme of intervention that does not work.
- Group work is not simply a way of overcoming resource issues; rather it offers positive experiences for children with PSDs to share with peers and develop friendships.
- The consultative approach has both advantages and challenges associated with it.
- Psycholinguistic/phonological approaches to intervention can be delivered by properly supervised and supported assistants or parents.

KEY TO ACTIVITY 13.1

Child might be a longer-term case if:

- older;
- had previous intervention but problems persisted;
- disordered speech rather than delayed;
- severe and pervasive difficulties, e.g. speech and language affected;
- associated difficulties with reading and spelling and phonological awareness;
- environmental factors, e.g. limited support at home or school;

- low self-esteem;
- poor attention.

Child might be a short-term case if:

- young;
- never had therapy before;
- delayed rather than disordered speech pattern;
- mild difficulties rather than severe/pervasive;
- no associated problems, e.g. self-esteem, literacy.

KEY TO ACTIVITY 13.2

1. Psycholinguistically, the child is required to: (a) process auditory information from the therapist; (b) make a decision as to whether this auditory information matches the child's stored representation for the pictured item; (c) programme and produce accurate target words.
2. Phonologically, the therapist is working on /sk/ and /st/ in word-initial position.
3. (a) From an interactional point of view, the following are all examples of drawing the child's attention to the target in a very explicit way:

   'I didn't hear that /sk/ sound, the one with two parts that we practised'

   'Can you hear the snakey sound when I say sssspinning top?'

   (b) The child produces SKIN → /kɪnə/. The therapist repeats what he has said and reflects on his production in an exaggerated way. She then pauses and gives him the opportunity to change or clarify what he has said. She asks him: 'Are you sure?' at one point, encouraging him to reflect on his own productions.

Chapter 14
Putting the Speech Back into Speech Therapy

In this book we have stressed the importance of contextualizing a child's intervention in real life. We firmly believe that intervention for children with PSDs should combine knowledge and expertise from a number of perspectives, e.g. educational, medical, linguistic, psycholinguistic, psychosocial. However, in this book we have unashamedly focused on the speech aspects of intervention because there are few books that do this specifically (exceptions being Dodd, 2005; and Hodson and Edwards, 1997 which are recommended for further reading).

Developments of inclusive education policies mean that there are more children in the classrooms with speech problems than ever before. The subsequent well-intentioned but perhaps misdirected move by some to advocate for all speech and language therapy (SLT) to be carried out within the classroom has diluted the intervention delivered to children with PSDs. Policies banning on principle any child with PSDs from having one-to-one sessions with an SLT or from being seen in a small group outside the classroom should be viewed with suspicion - as should any intervention carried out for a prescribed number of sessions regardless of individual needs and in isolation from the school or family. In short, there is no one size to fit all; flexible policies of service delivery need to reflect this. It is up to the professionals and carers involved, and depending on the age of the children themselves, to work out what an individual with PSDs needs and what aspects of the intervention can be carried out in the classroom and what cannot. The children presented in this book were seen within a mainstream school setting where there was contact with teaching staff, but all received individual and/or small group direct speech work with a speech and language therapist or assistant. This model is not dissimilar from the one adopted by teachers of, e.g. children with specific literacy difficulties (dyslexia). Studying individual needs like this will enable more realistic service delivery policies to emerge for the group of children with PSDs.

One thing is clear, children in this group cannot be ignored. By definition they are over the critical age (over 5 years of age) when spontaneous and complete recovery will happen. If left without support, educational and psychosocial consequences will be costly not only to the children and their families but also to the services involved in the long term. This is a point reiterated in *Communicating Quality 3*, the document outlining professional standards for UK SLTs, and guidance for service provision (RCSLT, CQ3, forthcoming). 'Children with Specific Speech Impairment' are included as one of the key client groups in CQ3 (see Chapter 8), where it is noted that such children typically require direct input from SLTs in order to progress, and avoid negative educational and social consequences.

The rise of the consultancy model in speech and language therapy practice (see Chapter 13) has been positive in strengthening the SLT's role in training others to understand and manage clients with communication difficulties. However, a downside has been the time taken away from direct work with children with PSDs. Ironical, given that research evidence suggests that children with PSDs, possibly more than any other group, require direct, intensive and specialist help and what is more can benefit from this. Most of the children presented in this book had not received specific intervention for their speech difficulties for some time but had been managed via a consultancy model of advice being given to the teachers and assistants involved. At a recent Special Interest Group in Developmental Cognitive Neuropsychology where we presented one of our intervention case studies of a child with PSDs, the convenor of the meeting, announced that 'This just goes to show that children with speech difficulties need speech therapy!'

How true and stated by an SLT manager who carries out direct hands-on work within a school setting. However, this slogan needs to be promoted strongly in these days of competing demands on SLTs' time and resources. This is not just important for the children with PSDs and their families, but also for the survival of our own profession. Arguably, the study of speech difficulties, and in particular the study and practice of phonetics and phonology, is the only truly unique characteristic of a speech and language therapist's training and job. If SLT students do not get hands-on experience with children with communication difficulties our future consultants will never have practised with children with PSDs and the profession will become deskilled in one area where they could make a real impact. Worrying signs that this is already happening are emerging; hence, the title of this chapter.

The cases presented in this book are not to show how intervention should be carried out with all children with PSDs, but rather to present how therapy *might* be done with individual children and to consider other approaches. The approach we put forward does not have to be carried out in such detail in everyday settings; nor does it need to be documented in such detail. It is presented here to disseminate research findings and to share therapy ideas. Through doing this we are attempting to add to a developing theory of intervention and address questions such as 'Why do we do what we do? How often should we do it? Who else can do it and when? How can we do it better?'

A psycholinguistic approach is one way of understanding the complex interaction of strengths and weaknesses that are likely to underlie longstanding speech difficulties, and it can help to address the questions above. However, we stress that this type of approach is not sufficient on its own. Each of the case studies presented demonstrates how phonological and psycholinguistic information and hypotheses can be brought together. This last chapter highlights some of the key strands of the book, e.g. links with literacy, importance of stimuli and research design; practitioners' contributions to a growing evidence base; focus on connected speech and intelligibility; questions about intervention dosage and delivery; the individual nature of children with PSDs; and the importance of moving away from diagnostic labels when planning intervention.

Links with Literacy

A theme running through the books in this series is that literacy is written language and that this arises from a foundation of spoken language. It is not surprising then that children with spoken language difficulties often have associated literacy problems. Where a child with PSDs also has language difficulties, all aspects of literacy may be affected. Some children with PSDs, however, may have age-appropriate verbal comprehension, for example, and in theory be able to abstract meaning from print. However, their difficulties with decoding print - cracking the alphabetic code - are a barrier to them doing this. Problems with phonological awareness can be compounded by speech difficulties that prevent a child from carrying out the rehearsal (or repetition) of targets out loud or subvocally. This rehearsal is necessary to hold on to the item and reflect on what a word sounds like which in turn is essential for new word learning (storage and retrieval) and allocating letters to sounds segmented for accurate spelling.

As we stated in Chapter 10, it is not the role of the SLT to teach literacy - an enormous job well placed in the hands of trained teachers. Rather, the SLT's role is to ensure the foundations for literacy are in place before a child receives formal literacy instruction at school (around the age of 5 years in the UK). Early years' programmes to promote language and literacy skills need to include training of the professionals and carers involved (Wood, Wright and Stackhouse, 2000; Wright and Wood, 2006). Through the school years and beyond the SLT's role is to support literacy development as an integral aspect of their intervention programmes (see CQ3, Section 8.21, RCSLT). We have tried to demonstrate this in our cases and in particular in Ben's programme presented in Chapter 10 (see also Stackhouse and Wells, 2001; Gillon, 2004; Snowling and Stackhouse, 2006, for further reading).

Stimuli Design

The stimuli chosen for intervention are a vital ingredient of the intervention process. The psycholinguistic approach suggests which aspects of a child's speech processing system might be targeted in intervention (e.g. auditory discrimination) but it is the phonetic/phonological analyses that determine the type of stimuli that should be used to address this area, e.g. auditory discrimination of words starting with /s/ and contrasted with words starting with /ʃ/, as in /sɪp/ vs. /ʃɪp/. Ben's case study presented in Chapter 10 reminds us that different stimuli may be needed to work on different speech processing levels.

Chapters 3 and 4 focused on the selection of individual segments in single words. However, stimuli design is not just about single segments in isolated words. The case studies presented in this book also give examples of intervention with consonant clusters (see Chapters 5 and 6) and with connected speech (see Chapters 7 and 8). Further, stimuli may be selected not only for active targets in intervention but also for control items. These matched sets of untreated words allow the effects of intervention and the extent of generalization to be monitored. The following needs to be done for this to happen:

- criteria for stimuli selection need to be listed;
- as many items as possible which meet these criteria need to be generated;
- the total number of items need to be divided randomly into two lists, one which serves as the treatment item list and the other as the untreated controls.

There are databases to help with this process, e.g. the MRC psycholinguistic database, an online resource freely available for all to use (http://www.psy.uwa.edu.au/mrcdatabase) and see Appendices 5 and 6 of this book for some of our own wordlists. Non-words can also provide a useful means of monitoring intervention if based on explicit criteria (see Appendix 5 at the end of this book, or again use web-based programmes that create novel words based on specific criteria). In some of our case studies we have used a number of treatment and control stimuli (e.g. see Rachel's intervention in Chapter 9) to help us to understand patterns of generalization. However, it is not necessary to have such a large number of stimuli in order to do this, e.g. see Oliver's case study in Chapter 4, where the treated wordlists consisted of just 10 CVC items each.

There are many challenges associated with the design and selection of stimuli for intervention. It is also often a time-consuming and frustrating task: just as a word has been added to the list, one realizes that it is not semantically appropriate, is phonotactically unsuitable, or contains some of the child's favoured segments that are likely to hinder rather than support! However, we suggest that the careful selection of stimuli that draw on our specialist phonetic and linguistic knowledge is key to successful intervention outcomes. The compilation of such stimuli lists is likely to be a skill unique to speech and language therapists and which no other profession working in education, health or the private sector possesses (given that clinical linguists/phoneticians are not normally employed in these settings).

Research Design

This is not a book on research design per se; there are already many excellent books which deal comprehensively and accessibly with the subject, e.g. see Pring (2005), and Middleton and Pannbacker (1994). Nevertheless, principles of research design underpin much of the text. We have emphasized that thinking therapists can be working like researchers without making big changes in their routine clinical practice, and can contribute to the evidence base. Single-case studies are an important and accessible way of making this contribution if one considers how this method fits into the bigger picture of outcomes research, e.g. as outlined by Robey and Schultz (1998) in their model of clinical-outcome research (see Chapter 12, and also Robey, 2005). Most of the single-case studies presented involved use of a simple ABA design (or modified version thereof) where assessment (A) is followed by intervention (B) and then followed by re-assessment (A). Such a design is typical of routinely evaluated practice and not specific to the research domain.

A key question for both researchers and practitioners is 'How do you know that the child improved because of what you did . . . and that they would not have improved anyhow?' Some suggestions for ways of answering this challenging and pertinent question were given in Chapter 12. These included fairly simple measures such as demonstrating stable pre-intervention baselines, measuring outcomes in areas not directly addressed in the intervention, and following up children to demonstrate the lasting effects of intervention. Again, many of these are measures incorporated into a routine clinical setting without too much difficulty. Other ways of evaluating intervention outcomes might involve group studies (e.g. comparing two treatments); different methods are appropriate for different research questions at different times.

Generalization

How to evaluate changes in speech performance after intervention needs careful consideration. If only standardized tests are used (e.g. of expressive language or naming a random selection of pictures), it might be concluded that minimal progress has been made. Indeed relative to their peers, this may well be the case for many children with severe PSDs. However, if we can demonstrate that in comparison to their own previous performance they are making significant gains, then this suggests that progress is rather more positive (see Chapter 8). Thus, the selection of outcomes measures is critical. A comprehensive range of outcomes measures is desirable when wanting to demonstrate the effects of intervention as this ensures that a complete picture of generalization effects is obtained. It may not, however, always be practical to choose a number of outcomes measures but a clear rationale for the measures that have been chosen is necessary. Outcomes measures should be fine-grained enough to allow change to be demonstrated if it has occurred, and should also be functionally relevant to a child's life. Generalization remains a key issue in intervention studies and is important for both theory and practice to develop (see Chapter 9 for further discussion).

Scoring

Scoring is not always given sufficient attention when evaluating outcomes for children with PSDs. Adopting a right/wrong level of scoring can miss how a child has changed qualitatively during even a short course of therapy where he or she may not have reached a performance level to be scored as 'correct'. In the case studies presented we often used graded scoring systems in which children were given partial credit for a change in their speech that suggested a move towards the target response. For example, Katy who had serious PSDs (see Chapter 8) omitted codas; following intervention we awarded 1 point for responses containing any coda segment, and 2 points for responses containing the correct coda segment. Thus, we could mark that Katy had made progress with adding codas to her speech after intervention even if these were not yet the right ones. A right/wrong scoring system would not have captured this and would have suggested that our intervention was not working. Similarly, in the intelligibility evaluation carried out in Chapter 11 we compared the listeners' written responses to the adult target responses by giving credit for any match of place, manner or voicing features.

A child's right to SLT may hinge on such issues. If an inappropriate scoring method is used then it may be argued that SLT is ineffective since no gains are being demonstrated; the next step could be to withdraw SLT from that child. Studies suggesting that SLT does not work may be misleading if, for example, an inappropriate design was adopted or too gross a scoring system used (see Pring, 2004, 2005, for further discussion of appropriacy of research designs for intervention studies). Critical reading of research papers is essential for practice to develop (see Chapter 2, and the template for doing this in Appendix 4) and for an appropriate service to be delivered. It is essential that research design skills are an integral part of any SLT's training and job. This does not mean that all SLTs are researchers - they are not typically given the time and resources to do this - but rather that all *think* like researchers. It is hoped that the research-related themes in this text might stimulate development of research methods in practice and service management further.

Building the Evidence

An important thread running through this book is evidence-based practice. There is a constant need for all practitioners to be evaluating and adding to the evidence already accrued. The evidence base for children with PSDs is not large but it is growing. There is increasing evidence from the case studies presented here and elsewhere that long-held traditions in SLT may not be well supported by the evidence base. For example, work on consonant clusters has often been added later in a therapy programme. This may not necessarily be the most effective way to approach intervention. Barbara Hodson has demonstrated successful outcomes by working on clusters through her cycles approach with young children and at an early stage in therapy (Hodson, 1997; Gierut, 1999). Similarly, work on connected speech has been traditionally placed at a later stage in therapy but could be worked on much earlier (Pascoe, Stackhouse and Wells, 2005, and see Chapter 7). Another myth may be that non-speech oral-motor work or oral-motor exercises are a necessary prerequisite for speech work; certainly this is not the case for all children (see Forrest, 2002, for a review). Adopting a psycholinguistic approach and completing a speech processing profile on a child allows appropriate therapy to be planned.

Children with PSDs are all different, making our understanding and treatment of their difficulties a real challenge. However, we suggest that it is vital to build the body of case studies so that we can not only show the wide variation between children, but also the commonalities in their responses to intervention. Such a database would allow one to identify generalization trends that could be analysed in terms of variables such as age, profile of difficulties and amount of intervention given. A problem with some intervention research has been that it was not made clear what precisely was done in the intervention. Labels sometimes applied to intervention, e.g. 'traditional', 'phonological awareness' can be confusing and need to be defined. Comparing approaches can be difficult as they often overlap, e.g. one cannot easily block speech input when carrying out speech output work; speech-related interventions with children involve at least a tacit level of phonological awareness (Stackhouse, Wells, Pascoe and Rees, 2002). A psycholinguistic approach enables one to evaluate not only 'What do tests really test' but also answer the question 'What do tasks really tap?' in intervention in a systematic and thorough way (Rees, 2001a, b). Some of our interventions may not be as different as we think they are! (see Chapter 10 for further discussion of this issue and Plante, 2005, for further discussion of evidence-based practice).

Connected Speech

Traditionally, assessment and intervention for children with PSDs has focused on single words and a literature search for journal papers focusing specifically on children's connected speech and intervention revealed few articles (see Chapter 7). Further, connected speech has often appeared late in intervention programmes and there has been little published about the practice of using, e.g. junction between words to facilitate speech production skills (for an example of how this might be done, see Wells, 1994). Certainly from our case study of Katy (Chapter 8) we suspect that we could have taken a short cut by working on the connected speech level earlier in therapy than we did, i.e. working at the 'assembly phase' of speech development (see Chapter 2 for a summary of the developmental phase model). In normal development, children do not build up speech sound by sound. Rather, they start by processing large chunks of speech and only later develop understanding of the smaller segments that then allows them to reflect on speech production (the metaphonological phase). Therapy based on developmental lines should therefore follow this pattern. A skill in devising therapy is to make such a decision: should the child's therapy be planned along typical or atypical developmental lines? Neither is right nor wrong; it depends on what the child needs.

Intelligibility

The concept of intelligibility is closely tied to connected speech given that children and adults rarely speak in single isolated words in everyday situations. Although the word 'intelligibility' is used a lot in the literature and when discussing children's speech difficulties, there is surprisingly little objective reporting and measuring of what appears to be one of the most crucial outcome measures for speech and language therapists working with children with PSDs (see Chapter 11). Refining and developing ways of reliably and practically evaluating the intelligibility of spontaneous speech before and after intervention is important. A longitudinal perspective is needed to show how changes in speech output and communication skills generally might impact on intelligibility.

Dosage and Delivery

The trend away from seeing children with PSDs for 1 : 1 tailor-made intervention increases as they move into secondary education (from around the age of 11 years in the UK). Two main reasons for this are: (a) an assumption that children grow out of their speech difficulties and will not need speech and language therapy as they get older; (b) therapy services may well prioritize younger children for their resources in the belief that this will pre-empt the need to have ongoing therapy with older children. Both are valid reasons but not true of all children. The majority of children do improve their speech difficulties but others do not and require ongoing support through adolescence and adulthood. Intervention in the early years can shift borderline children from delayed to typical groups. However, even the best designed and intensively delivered intervention may not cure speech difficulties that are pervasive and severe; though undoubtedly such therapy does improve the chances of progress and diminishes associated difficulties. In short, some children will just not grow out of their difficulties and we now have a better idea of who these might be (Nathan *et al.*, 2004a, b; Muter, 2006; Stackhouse, 2006).

In Chapter 13 we suggested some alternative ways of dealing with the resource issues for children who need ongoing and long-term support, e.g. the training of assistants using the consultative model (see McCartney *et al.*, 2005, for a critique of this). Technology may also have a role to play in addressing this issue. One potential way of addressing this problem and coping with cost-effectiveness issues may be through using intensive computer-based interventions. Comparisons of, for example, computer-based interventions versus learning support assistants for reliable delivery of speech and language programmes in schools would be helpful. This would require:

- development of a flexible, user-friendly software application to support assessment and intervention for children with speech disorders;
- creation of computerized tasks and games to be used for children's speech and language assessments;
- creation of computerized forms for the storage of information arising from such assessments;
- creation of computerized tasks and games to be used in intervention for children.

Stackhouse and Wells's psycholinguistic framework has already been used as a theoretical basis for a software application addressing input aspects of the model (Wren and Roulstone, 2001), but there is further scope for development of other aspects of the framework (e.g. games for speech output work). Discovering optimal intervention dosage remains a pressing need, as does an evaluation of consultative approaches as they are currently implemented, the use of assistants and the hands-on therapy carried out by SLTs.

Moving Beyond Diagnostic Labels

Medical information and diagnoses will always be important for: (a) understanding speech difficulties which arise from a medical condition and which may require medical intervention; (b) helping parents and others involved to accept and understand a child's difficulties; (c) assisting communication between professionals who share the same terminology; (d) indicating prognosis in children who have medical conditions; and (e) for securing specialist educational and therapy provision in some cases. However, diagnostic labels from the medical perspective do not lead to a prescription of what to do in therapy (see Chapter 1 in Book 1, Stackhouse and Wells, 1997, for further discussion of this issue). The psycholinguistic approach advocated in this text examines a child's strengths and weaknesses, regardless of any diagnostic label, in order to determine the best intervention programme for that child. Children such as Katy in Chapter 8 (diagnosed with ataxic cerebral palsy) and Oliver in Chapter 4 (diagnosed with childhood apraxia of speech) presented with speech processing profiles that these labels would not have predicted. For example, our therapy for Katy did not include any oral-motor work as she performed adequately on tasks tapping Level K (bottom right) on the speech processing profile. Other cases in the literature also illustrate this point, e.g. the case study by Ebbels (2000, and discussed in some detail in Chapter 3) of a child whose speech difficulties could not all be explained by what seemed an obvious cause of diagnosed hearing impairment.

What can be helpful in planning therapy though are diagnoses from a linguistic perspective, for example describing a child's speech development as delayed or deviant based on the pattern of their speech difficulties that have been analysed through a phonetic and phonological analysis. Barbara Dodd's notion of subgroups of speech difficulties is an example of how this might work (see Chapters 1 and 3, and Dodd, 2005). With each subgroup is a prescription of what approach might be helpful in therapy, e.g. children with 'inconsistent speech disorder' might benefit best from core vocabulary therapy while children with 'consistent speech disorder' may improve more through phonological therapy (Crosbie, Holm and Dodd, 2005). This finding accords well with a developmental perspective of speech development and difficulties. Children with inconsistent speech output are operating within the whole-word phase of speech development and require their speech system to be stabilized before they can enter the systematic simplification stage in which they can benefit from therapy targeting phonological contrasts (Stackhouse and Wells, 1997; and see the description of intervention carried out with Ruth in Chapter 3). It is still the case, however, that a group prescription based on a diagnostic label from whatever perspective may not take into account individual differences in underlying speech processing skills, associated strengths and weaknesses (e.g. literacy skills), or the broader environmental influences (e.g. within the family, home and school contexts, teaching opportunities, psychosocial factors). Further, the nature of children's speech difficulties will change as their speech matures or responds to intervention. This needs to be monitored so that ongoing therapy targets both their spoken and written language appropriately.

Children's difficulties with speech, language and literacy are likely to be the consequence of a combination of factors, and characterized by wide-ranging behavioural manifestations and underlying processing strengths and weaknesses. Detailed investigations of children with specific speech difficulties suggest that they often have pervasive speech processing problems (e.g. Stackhouse and Snowling, 1992; Chiat and Hunt, 1993) or more specifically problems with auditory discrimination (Crosbie and Dodd, 2001), imprecise storage of words (Bryan and Howard, 1992) or with all areas of output production (Waters *et al.*, 1998) – or various combinations of these areas (Stackhouse and Snowling, 1992). Ebbels (2000) cautions that while some reported cases (e.g. Bryan and Howard, 1992; Bryan and North, 1994) show a deficit limited to one module of the processing model, typically there are multiple levels of breakdown in children with PSDs. Profiling approaches such as Stackhouse and Wells's (1997, 2001) allow one to consider each child as an individual with their own collection of strengths and weakness, as well as causal and maintaining factors. This psycholinguistic framework with its model, profile and developmental phase model (see Chapter 2) provides a basis from which to work. However, it is not inflexible. Rather, it should be modified and developed as our knowledge and evidence of children's speech processing grows.

Conclusion

By definition children with PSDs are complex and considered hard to treat (see Foreword to this book by Professor Pam Enderby). Certainly, their difficulties would not have persisted if they were straightforward and could be remediated easily. At the same time they allow us to develop theoretical knowledge of the speech processing system and offer us glimpses into the 'complex, multilayered and dizzying' reality of children's speech and language processing (Chapman, 2000 p. 45). Children with PSDs present with a constellation of speech, language, literacy and possibly other social or behavioural difficulties. This should be acknowledged in our assessment and intervention with these children: there are no quick fixes or easy answers! We need to work closely with children, families, teachers and support workers. We need to spend time on assessments, evaluating the existing evidence- base, designing appropriate stimuli and monitoring outcomes. We need to be 'thinking therapists' - active in the process of designing and evaluating intervention programmes. Intervention with children with PSDs will always pose exciting challenges for practitioners and researchers, yet at the same time afford us the opportunity to contribute to a meaningful evidence base, bring about changes to the lives of individual children and their families and to strengthen the unique aspects of speech and language therapy/pathology more generally.

ACTIVITY 14.1

Try answering these questions and use them as a focus for discussion with your colleagues.

1. What service do you offer to:
   (a) children with PSDs
   (b) adolescents with PSDs
   (c) adults with (developmental) PSDs
   (d) parents of children with PSDs?
2. Is the service you offer to clients with PSDs research evidence-based or resource-based?
3. What specific training do you offer to professionals and carers who are working with clients with PSDs?
4. How do you link with literacy and the curriculum in your intervention programmes?
5. How are psychosocial factors taken into account in your intervention?
6. How do you train your clients with unintelligible speech to manage the listener in their conversations?
7. What outcome measures do you routinely use to evaluate the success of your intervention?
8. At what point do you introduce work on (a) clusters and (b) connected speech into your therapy programmes?
9. What criteria do you use to select a child's speech targets?
10. How do you score their responses on these targets?

There is no key for this activity here. Collectively, answering these questions will ensure appropriate intervention and service for children with PSDs and their families. We hope that this book has provided some ideas, information and tools to do this.

Appendix 1: Speech Processing Profile (for Photocopying)

SPEECH PROCESSING PROFILE

Name: Comments:

Age: d.o.b:

Date:

Profiler:

INPUT

F Is the child aware of the internal structure of phonological representations?

E Are the child's phonological representations accurate?

D Can the child discriminate between real words?

C Does the child have language-specific representations of word structures?

B Can the child discriminate speech sounds without reference to lexical representations?

A Does the child have adequate auditory perception?

OUTPUT

G Can the child access accurate motor programmes?

H Can the child manipulate phonological units?

I Can the child articulate real words accurately?

J Can the child articulate speech without reference to lexical representations?

K Does the child have adequate sound production skills?

L Does the child reject his/her own erroneous forms?

Appendix 2: Updated List of Examples of Tests for Each Question in the Psycholinguistic Assessment Framework

(Space has been left at the end of each question to enable you to add your own test examples.)

INPUT

F. Is the child aware of the internal structure of phonological representations?

Picture onset detection: identification of pictures that begin with the same 'sound', e.g. KEY, KITE, SHOE. The tester does not name the pictures (e.g. *PHAB* subtest: Alliteration Part 2, Frederikson *et al.*, 1997).

Picture rhyme detection: identification of pictures that rhyme, e.g. RING, SWING, DUCK. The tester does not name the pictures (e.g. Vance, Stackhouse and Wells, 1994).

Picture rhyme judgment: two pictures presented, tester asks 'Do these pictures rhyme?', e.g. key~tree, shoe~bike. The tester does not name the pictures (e.g. Vance, Stackhouse and Wells, 1994).

E. Are the child's phonological representations accurate?

Silent blending: identification of a picture that corresponds with the tester's spoken presentation of segments, e.g. onset + nucleus + coda:

/pr/ + /æ/ + /m/; onset + rime: /pr/ + /æm/ (Counsel, 1993). Sound Recognition subtest (Goldman, Fristoe and Woodcock, 1978).

Auditory detection of speech 'errors', e.g. child looks at picture of a FISH. Tester asks 'Is this a "pish"?'; 'Is this a FISH?'; 'Is this a "fis"?' (Locke, 1980a, b).

Minimal pair picture discrimination: identification of the picture that corresponds with the tester's spoken presentation of stimuli, e.g. in connected speech: I LIKE THE COAT WITH THE LONG FUR ~ I LIKE THE GOAT WITH THE LONG FUR (Cassidy, 1994; and see Stackhouse *et al.*, forthcoming); and in single words: CLOWN vs. CROWN (MorganBarry, 1988).

Tests designed for individual children, e.g.

(a) sorting tasks in which children are given pictures and asked to silently sort them into piles based on onset phonemes or rhyme;
(b) picture discrimination tasks in which children carry out auditory detection of speech errors (see Locke, 1980a, b above) but the stimuli used are derived from the child's own errors.

Auditory Lexical Discrimination Test: With and without pictures (from Constable, Stackhouse and Wells, 1997; and see Stackhouse *et al.*, forthcoming).

D. Can the child discriminate between real words?

Minimal pair auditory discrimination: clusters. Same/different discrimination, e.g. LOST vs. LOTS (Bridgeman and Snowling, 1988).

Auditory rhyme detection, e.g. three finger puppets presented; the tester speaks a word for each one (JAM, FISH, PRAM). Child points to the two puppets which said the rhyming words (Vance, Stackhouse and Wells, 1994).

Auditory rhyme judgment, e.g. tester asks, 'Do boat and coat rhyme?' (Vance, Stackhouse and Wells, 1994).

Minimal pair auditory discrimination: CVC. Same/different discrimination, e.g. PIN ~ BIN (e.g. Wepman, 1958; Wepman and Reynolds, 1987).

Own error discrimination. Same/different discrimination based on child's own error productions and adult targets.

C. Does the child have language-specific representations of word structures?

Auditory discrimination of legal from illegal non-words, e.g. BLICK vs. BNICK (Waterson, 1981; Stackhouse, 1989).

Auditory discrimination of legal from exotic non-words, e.g. [sɒf] vs. [ɬɒf].

B. Can the child discriminate speech sounds without reference to lexical representations?

Auditory discrimination of complex non-words, e.g. IBIKUS~IKIBUS (Stackhouse, 1989).

Auditory discrimination of clusters in non-words, e.g. VOST vs. VOTS (Bridgeman and Snowling, 1988).

ABX auditory non-word discrimination, e.g. two puppets presented. Tester says 'This puppet says BRISH. This puppet says BRIS. Which puppet said BRIS?' (Locke, 1980a, b; Vance, 1996, and see Stackhouse *et al.*, forthcoming).

Rhyme judgment of non-words, e.g. 'Do POAT and HOAT rhyme?' (Vance, Stackhouse and Wells, 1994).

A. Does the child have adequate auditory perception?

Auditory fusion: judge when two non-speech sounds (e.g. 'beeps') are heard as one (McCroskey, 1984).

Pitch change detection: judge if two non-speech sounds are the same or different in terms of their pitch (Tallal and Piercy, 1980).

Hearing tests, e.g. audiometry.

SCAN-C (Keith, 1999): physiological processing of speech and non-speech sounds.

OUTPUT

G. Can the child access accurate motor programs?

Production of segments from a picture: e.g. coda supply: child looks at picture (FISH), tester produces 'fi-' [fɪ], child supplies 'sh' [ʃ]. (Muter, Snowling and Taylor, 1994).

Spontaneous speech data.

Picture description data (e.g. Goldman and Fristoe, 1969; Stackhouse and Snowling, 1992).

Naming tests:

(a) Lexical (e.g. German, 1989; Renfrew, 1995; Constable *et al.*, 1997).
(b) Accuracy (e.g. *Edinburgh Articulation Test,* Goldman and Fristoe, 1969; Anthony, Bogle, Ingram *et al.*, 1971; Armstrong and Ainley, 1988; *South Tyneside Assessment of Phonology (STAP)*, Dodd *et al.*, 2002; *DEAP*, Hodson, 2004; *Happ-3*, Grunwell and Harding, 1995; Vance, Stackhouse and Wells, 2005).
(c) Lexical and accuracy (e.g. Snowling, van Wagtendonk and Stafford, 1988).

H. Can the child manipulate phonological units?

Spoonerism test, e.g. Bob Dylan → 'Dob Bylan' (Perin, 1983; *PhaB*, Frederikson *et al.*, 1997).

Onset string production, e.g. 'Tell me as many words as you can that begin with /k/.' (e.g. Alliteration Fluency subtest on the *PhAB*, Frederikson *et al.*, 1997).

Rhyme string production, e.g. 'Tell me as many words as you can that rhyme with CAT' (e.g. Vance, Stackhouse and Wells, 1994; Rhyme Fluency subtest on the *PhAB*, Frederikson *et al.*, 1997; *PAT* rhyme fluency subtest (Muter *et al.*, 1997).

I. Can the child articulate real words accurately?

Sound blending of real words from verbally presented segments, e.g. /pr/ + /æ/ + /m/ → 'pram' (Hatcher, 1994; real word items on the blending subtest from the *Aston Index*, Newton and Thomson, 1982).

Repetition tasks:

(a) Connected speech, e.g. repetition of sentence: HIS UMBRELLA IS YELLOW (Vance, Stackhouse and Wells, 1995, and see Stackhouse *et al.*, forthcoming).
(b) Real words on more than one occasion, e.g. 'Say CATERPILLAR three times' (e.g. Nuffield Centre Dyspraxia Programme, Williams and Stephens, 2004; Williams and Stackhouse, 2000).
(c) Real words of increasing syllable length, with and without clusters, e.g. with clusters: GLOVE, TRACTOR, UMBRELLA (Vance, Stackhouse and Wells, 1995, 2005; Constable *et al.*, 1997; *DEAP*, Dodd *et al.*, 2002; Roy and Chiat, 2004; Nathan *et al.*, 2004a; and see Stackhouse *et al.*, forthcoming).

J. Can the child articulate speech without reference to lexical representations?

Non-word blending from verbally presented segments, e.g. D-U-P; T-I-S-E-K (non-word items in blending subtest on the *Aston Index*, Newton and Thomson, 1982).

Repetition of non-words on more than one occasion, e.g. 'Say KUDIGAN /ˈkudɪgən/ three times.' (Coffield Consistency Test, 1994; Williams, 1996; Williams and Stackhouse, 2000; and see Stackhouse *et al.*, forthcoming).

Repetition of non-words with increasing syllable length, with and without clusters, e.g. with clusters GLEV /glev/; TRECTEE /ˈtrekti/; ambrahli /æmˈbrɑli/ (Snowling, Stackhouse and Rack, 1986; Ryder, 1991; Vance, Stackhouse and Wells, 1995, 2005; Gathercole and Baddeley, 1996; Roy and Chiat, 2004; Nathan *et al.*, 2004a; and see Stackhouse *et al.*, forthcoming).

K. Does the child have adequate sound production skills?

Diadochokinetic rates: Repeated imitation of sounds in isolation, e.g. [p] and in sequences, e.g. [pə pə pə]; [pə tə kə] (Fletcher, 1978; Henry, 1990; Williams and Stackhouse, 2000).

Oral examination of structure and function (Huskie, 1989; *POSP*, Brindley *et al.*, 1996; *DEAP*, Dodd *et al.*, 2002; Nuffield Centre Dyspraxia Programme, Williams and Stephens, 2004).

Speech Accuracy, Rate and Consistency Test (Williams and Stackhouse, 2000, and see Stackhouse *et al.*, forthcoming).

L. Does the child reject his or her own erroneous forms?

Tester observes if child attempts to correct his or her own speech output spontaneously.

Appendix 3: Speech Processing Model (for Photocopying)

SPEECH PROCESSING MODEL

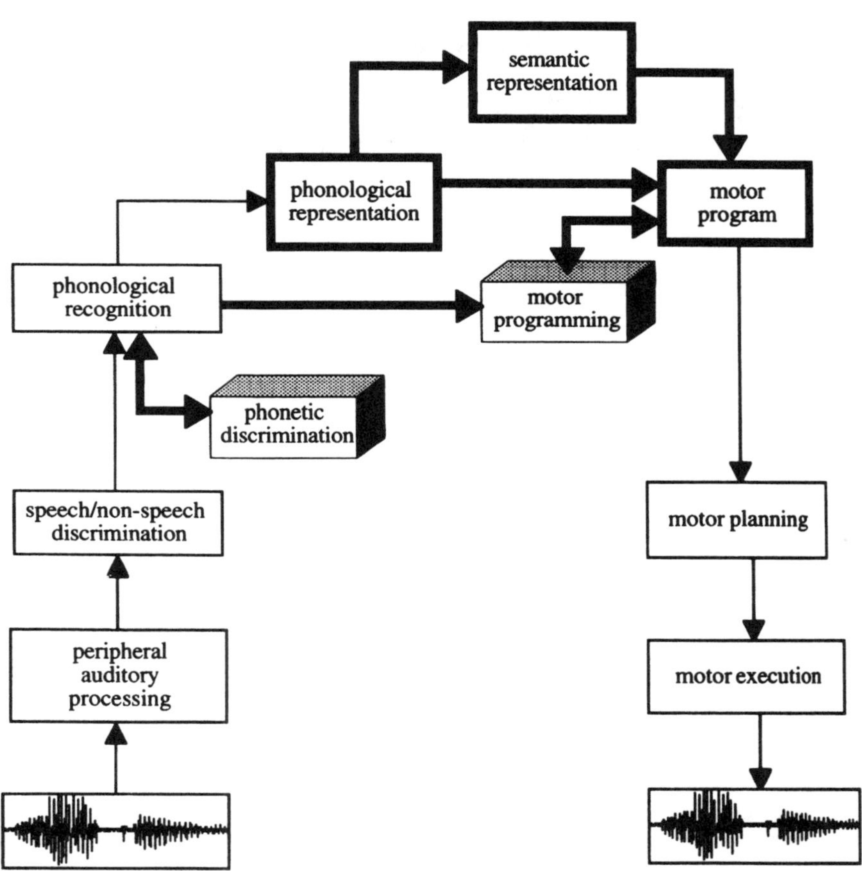

Reproduced by kind permission of © Whurr Publishers. From Stackhouse and Wells (1997) *Children's Speech and Literacy Difficulties 1: A Psycholinguistic Framework*.

Appendix 4: Template for Journal Review (for Photocopying)

Template for journal review

Title: Authors: Journal: Publication Date:	
Participant(s) details	
Theoretical framework used	
Research questions	
Intervention, e.g. tasks, dosage, stimuli	
Design	
Outcome measures used	
Changes noted in outcome measures	
Generalization observed	
Controls employed, e.g. stable baseline, inter-rater reliability; long-term follow-up	
Other Comments: Main messages	

Appendix 5: Examples of Core Vocabulary used with a Child with PSDs. Ruth (CA 6;11): Stimuli from Teal (2005)

	Core Vocabulary Word	Matched Real Word	Matched Non-Word	No. of Syllables
1	Chip	John	ʧʊp	1
2	Juice	Coke	ʤis	1
3	Bath	Sink	bʌθ	1
4	Milk	Bread	mʊlk	1
5	Tea	Ta	teɪ	1
6	Pink	Green	pæŋk	1
7	Car	Bus	kɜ	1
8	Cat	Dog	kaʊt	1
9	Colour	Number	ˈkælə	2
10	Charlie	Rachel	ˈʧɔlʌ	2
11	Pizza	Pasta	ˈputsə	2
12	Ballet	Running	ˈbɒlaʊ	2

Appendix 6: Sample Minimal Pair Lists

FINAL CONSONANT DELETION

boat/bow
goat/go
seed/see
bean/bee
meat/me
pipe/pie
rope/row
soap/sew
light/lie
cart/car

INITIAL CONSONANT DELETION

towel/owl
race/ace
my/eye
chair/air
rice/ice

VOICING

p/b

WI	**WF**
pie/bye	mop/mob
pea/bea	nip/nib
pin/bin	rope/robe

k/g

WI	**WF**
Kate/gate	back/bag
coat/goat	lock/log
cap/gap	peck/peg

t/d

WI	**WF**
tie/die	cot/cod
tea/D	pot/pod
torn/dawn	seat/seed

CLUSTER REDUCTION

sp/p
spot/pot
sport/port
spin/pin

st/t
stork/talk
stop/top
stool/tool

sk/k
school/cool
scarf/calf
scare/care

sm/m
smile/mile
smug/mug
small/mall

sn/n
snail/nail
snow/no
snap/nap

sl/l
slow/low
slap/lap
slice/lice

Appendix 7: Pro-forma for Describing Therapy Tasks (for Photocopying)

Describing therapy tasks

TASK DESCRIPTION Write a general description of the task	
MATERIALS Note the materials used	
PROCEDURES Outline what took place	
FEEDBACK What feedback was given to the child?	
(TECHNIQUES) Were any supporting techniques used?	

Appendix 8: Child Interview Questions

1. You've been coming for speech and language therapy for a while now - what do you think about it?

   Probes/prompts: What do you think about the things we do together?
   What do you like best?
   What don't you like?
   What do you think about the tape/video/being recorded?

2. You've had speech therapy with other people before - what did you think about that?

   Probes/prompts: What can you remember doing?
   What did you like?
   What didn't you like?
   Was it the same as what we do or was it different?

3. Why do you come for speech and language therapy?

   Probes/prompts: Do you think it has helped your speech?
   How do you think it helps children talk better?
   Would you like to be a speech therapist one day?
   Do you like talking - what is nice about it?
   What is hard about talking?
   What would happen if we couldn't talk?
   Do you like listening to other people talk?
   What happens when someone doesn't understand you?
   What happens when you don't understand someone?
   Why do you think talking is important?
   Why do you think listening is important?
   Do we all speak the same language?
   Even if we speak English, do we all sound the same?

4. Let's talk about reading and writing - do you like to read and write?

   Probes/prompts: Why? (What do you like and what don't you like?)
   What do you think about the reading/writing things we have done together?

Why do you think reading and writing are important for children?
Do you think reading and writing have anything to do with speech?
Which is easier for you - reading or writing?

5. Let's talk about school now - what do you think about school?

Probes/prompts: What is the best thing about school?
What don't you like about school?
Would you like to come for more/less speech therapy?
Would you like to talk more/less in the classroom?
Would you like to do more/less reading and writing?

Glossary

Across-item generalization: Generalization of performance from treated items (e.g. words directly targeted in therapy) to untreated items within the same task; the degree to which the untreated control items resemble the treated items is an important variable, i.e. these may range from very closely matched single words, to words with a different phonotactic structure, or sentences. See also **generalization**.

Across-task generalization: Generalization of performance from a treated task (e.g. naming of CVC words) to a different task (e.g. spelling of the same CVC words to dictation, or auditory discrimination of the same and closely related CVC words).

Adjunct: Term used to refer to the /s/ in word-initial /s/ clusters because these consonants are thought to be more loosely adjoined to a word than a true cluster, i.e. in SPRITE, /s/ is an adjunct (or appendix) to the remainder of the syllable.

Affricate: Consonant sound that consists of a plosive before a fricative, e.g. /dʒ/.

Approximants: Sounds that are produced by a narrowing of the vocal tract while still allowing air to flow without causing much audible turbulence, also called glides, e.g. /w/ and /l/.

Apraxia (of speech): An impaired ability to perform the coordinated movements that are required for speech (Vargha-Kadem *et al.*, 2005); One of the diagnostic categories for children with speech difficulties proposed by Shriberg, Aram and Kwiatkowski (1997a). See also **childhood apraxia of speech**; **developmental verbal dyspraxia**.

Articulation: The production of speech sounds; movements made by the speech mechanism (i.e. tongue, lips, jaw, larynx) which result in speech; one of the diagnostic sub-groups of children with speech difficulties outlined by Barbara Dodd (1995).

Aspiration: The burst of air that accompanies the release of some stop consonants, e.g. The /p/ in POT has a lot of aspiration but the /p/ in SPOT does not and sounds more like a /b/.

Assimilation: Influence that a particular sound exerts on neighbouring sounds, making them more alike, e.g. GREAT BEAR; GREAT CAT (see page 181); an important connected speech process; an example of 'close junctures'. See also **junction/juncture**.

Attention deficit hyperactivity disorder (ADHD): A behavioural difficulty in which children (or adults) show impulsivity; have difficulty in sitting still and focusing on a given task.

Auditory discrimination: The ability to distinguish between two or more different sounds or words; auditory discrimination difficulty refers to a problem in distinguishing between different sounds in isolation or words.

Auditory (picture) lexical decision: A task in which children's internal representations are tapped by asking them to make explicit decisions about how a word should be produced. For example, a child is presented with a picture of a SPOON, and asked to say whether the tester is right or wrong in how they name the picture, e.g. 'Is this a "poon"? Is this a "boon"? Is this a "SPOON"? Is this a "moon"?' If the child accepts only SPOON as correct you will have a good idea that she or he has an accurate representation of the word. If the answer is yes, for the incorrect items, it is likely that she or he has a fuzzy representation of the word.

Auditory perception: The ability to process and make sense of sounds.

Benchmarking: A process in which procedures or interventions are analysed in relation to best practice within a given field or industry; benchmarking is carried out to inform our knowledge of service delivery and has been used in the evaluation of intervention outcomes, although to date to a fairly limited extent in the field of speech and language therapy (however, see John, Enderby and Hughes, 2005a, b).

Carryover: See **generalization**.

Childhood apraxia of speech (CAS): An impaired ability to perform the coordinated movements that are required for speech (Vargha-Kadem *et al.*, 2005); one of the diagnostic categories for children with speech difficulties proposed by Shriberg, Aram and Kwiatkowski (1997a). See also **developmental verbal dyspraxia**, **apraxia**.

Co-articulation: The way in which speech segments overlap in time and in space to such an extent that it is often difficult to determine where one segment begins and another segment ends (Hardcastle and Hewlett, 1999).

Coda: The final part of a syllable; all segments following the vowel, e.g. /t/ in CAT; or /st/ in LOST.

Complexity accounts of treatment efficacy (CATE): The belief that working on more complex stimuli in intervention results in 'downward' generalization to less complex targets and thus that ultimately the approach can maximize the efficiency of intervention.

Confusion matrix: A table or grid in which target sounds (on one axis) are compared to a listener's perceptions (on the other axis); may be used in intelligibility studies to determine which consonants and vowels are not accurately perceived and exactly how these sounds are being perceived. See also **error matrix**.

Connected speech: Typical speech in conversation is in utterances of varying lengths, characterized by a flow of words connected together by specific phonetic and phonological features arising from the particular sequences of sounds that occur at word junctions.

Consistent deviant phonology: One of the diagnostic sub-groups outlined by Barbara Dodd (1995); Children who show non-developmental errors and unusual processes, and are consistent in their application of these rules. See also **inconsistent deviant phonology**.

Consonant cluster: Adjacent consonant segments in the same syllable, e.g. BLINK. Also referred to as blends or consonant sequences.

Controls: Stimuli, tasks or participants that are not the specific focus of an intervention and are not treated, but monitored to enable comparison with treated stimuli, tasks or participants.

Conversation analysis (CA): A research methodology that examines naturally occurring conversations or talk in interaction.

Core-vocabulary approach: An intervention approach for children with speech difficulties based on the work of Dodd (1995, 2005) and often used with children with inconsistent speech; a set of words, the core vocabulary, is selected and these are addressed using a drill-type approach in therapy and at home. The aim is for children to develop stable productions of these items, the first step in developing their phonological system.

Cost effectiveness: The cost of achieving a desired outcome of treatment; the final phase of the outcome research model proposed by Robey and Schultz (1998). See also **effectiveness**.

Craniofacial: Pertaining to the skull or face; craniofacial abnormalities may include cleft-lip and palate.

Critical age hypothesis: The premise that children are at increased risk of literacy problems if speech difficulties have not resolved by the time they start formal literacy instruction at school.

Cycles approach: A phonological intervention approach that involves selection of a small set of 'error sounds' to be targeted in therapy. Target sounds (or processes) are individually addressed in both input and output in a successive way with each of the targets addressed for a limited time before moving on to another target. When all targets have been addressed, the cycle begins again and continues for as many rotations as needed until a given sound has been acquired (see Hodson and Paden, 1991).

DAMP (Deficits of attention, motor control and perception): Diagnosis sometimes given by psychiatrists and paediatricians which combines elements of Asperger's syndrome and attention deficit hyperactivity disorder (ADHD) (See Gillberg, 2003).

Dependent variable: The data that are observed and measured in response to the independent variable; this variable is not under the experimenter's control but depends on the independent variable which is being manipulated, e.g. dependent variable may be accuracy of consonant production in response to an independent variable such as providing intervention/no intervention.

Developmental verbal dyspraxia: An impaired ability to perform the coordinated movements that are required for speech (Vargha-Kadem *et al.*, 2005); One of the diagnostic categories for children with speech difficulties proposed by Shriberg, Aram and Kwiatkowski (1997a).

Digraphs: Two letters representing one speech sound, e.g. <sh>.

Dysarthria: A speech difficulty due to abnormal muscle tone.

Dysfluency: Disruptions to the smooth flow of speech.

Dyspraxia: See **childhood apraxia of speech**.

Effectiveness: The outcome of an intervention in a non-ideal, real-life situation. Does the intervention work in the real world? Evaluated in the third phase of the outcome research model proposed by Robey and Schultz (1998). See also **cost effectiveness**.

Effect size: A statistical term that refers to the size of a relationship between two variables, e.g. speech and spelling; sometimes known as a treatment effect because it is often used when dealing with therapeutic interventions.

Efficacy: The outcome of an intervention in an ideal situation. Does the intervention work in optimal circumstances? Evaluated in the second phase of the outcome research model proposed by Robey and Schultz (1998).

Efficiency: The outcome of an intervention as evaluated in terms of cost effectiveness and time effectiveness. Does intervention X bring about changes more rapidly or cost effectively than intervention Y? Evaluated in the fourth phase of the outcome research model proposed by Robey and Schultz (1998).

Electropalatography (EPG): An instrumental technique used to show on a screen tongue contact with the palate when producing speech sounds.

Elision: The connected speech process in which sounds that would be pronounced in slow, careful speech disappear in everyday speech, e.g. the contracted use of 'gonna' for GOING TO.

Error matrix: A table or grid in which target sounds (on one axis) are compared to a listener's perceptions (on the other axis); may be used in intelligibility studies to determine which consonants and vowels are not accurately perceived and exactly how these sounds are being perceived. See also **confusion matrix**.

Evidence-based practice (EBP): The explicit use of current best evidence in decision making; it involves application and consideration of the various forms of evidence (e.g. published group and single-case studies of intervention and their outcomes) as they relate to the practitioner's specific problem or situation under investigation.

Fricative: Consonant sound produced with audible friction due to closure at some point in the vocal tract, e.g. /s/, /f/.

Gemination: Consonant lengthening; when a spoken consonant is 'doubled' so that it is pronounced for twice as long as is usual (from Gemini, the astrological sign for the Twins).

Generalization: Transfer of knowledge or learning from one environment or skill-set to another; also referred to as carryover. See also **across-item generalization**; **across-task generalization**; **within-class generalization**.

Grammatical representation: Information that is stored about the morphological and grammatical characteristics of a word, e.g. past tense of KICK is KICKED; THE is followed by nouns in sentences.

Grapheme: Written or printed letter.

Homonymy: The production of the same phonetic form for two or more adult words that are normally pronounced differently, e.g. where a child says 'boo' for both MOO and SHOE.

Hyperlexia: An unusually well-developed ability to read in children with cognitive deficits; children with comprehension or semantic–pragmatic difficulties are often described as hyperlexic. This term indicates that a child can read print mechanically better than they can understand it.

Inconsistent deviant phonology: One of the diagnostic sub-groups outlined by Barbara Dodd (1995). Children show delayed and non-developmental errors, but in addition they show significant variability in their speech production that does not reflect a maturing system. See also **consistent deviant phonology**.

Independent variable: Variable which is manipulated by the researcher or practitioner, e.g. giving therapy or no therapy. See also **dependent variable**.

Intelligibility: Understandability; how well an individual's speech is understood by other individuals.

Inter-rater reliability: Some studies use more than one rater to transcribe and score speech data. Where this is done, inter-rater reliability – the agreement between the two raters - can be calculated using statistical procedures. See also **intra-rater reliability**.

Intra-rater reliability: Some studies repeat a certain number of stimuli (e.g. 10%) so that an individual rater's consistency can be checked; this is termed intra-rater or intra-judge reliability and can be measured using a statistical procedure such as Pearson's product moment correlation. See also **inter-rater reliability**.

Intervention: An action that results in an outcome.

Intonation: A prosodic aspect of speech made up of changes in stress and pitch in the voice; serves to group words into cohesive utterances and contribute to the meanings of spoken phrases and sentences. See also **prosody**.

Junction/juncture: The way in which words are joined with each other across syllable boundaries. Open juncture occurs in formal, emphatic speech where all individual phonemes are precisely realized, e.g. LOST BOOK → /lɒst bʊk/; Close juncture includes assimilation which refers to the way in which sounds are influenced by the neighbouring sounds, e.g. LOST BOOK → /lɒs bʊk/.

Lexeme: Component of a lexicon; refers to a word or other small unit of meaning.

Lexical representation: Knowledge stored about a word including its meaning; what it sounds like; how it is produced; how it is written and how it can be used in sentences.

Lexicon: A dictionary or mental store of information about words; contains lexical representations.

Liaison: The phonological adjustments made when a glide is inserted between adjacent vowels across a word boundary, e.g. GO OVER → [gəʊwəʊvə].

Literacy: Ability to read (decode and comprehend what has been read) and write/spell.

Maintenance: The preservation of any changes brought about through intervention once intervention has ceased.

Markedness: The way segments or words are changed or added to, to give a special meaning. An unmarked phoneme or word (e.g. CAT) may be considered basic, but if something is added to it (e.g. plural 's'), it becomes special or marked (e.g. CATS).

Maximal oppositions: Where two very different segments are opposed or contrasted with each other, e.g. /s/ and /b/ in SEW and BOW differ in terms of place, manner and voicing; this makes the difference between segments more noticeable for a child with speech difficulties.

Mean: Average.

Mean length of utterance (MLU): An expressive language measure obtained by counting the number of morphemes (i.e. grammatical meaning units) in a series of utterances, and obtaining an average number of morphemes per utterance. See also **morpheme**.

Meaningful minimal contrast therapy (MMCT): Approach to phonological intervention in which children's attention is drawn to the difference between their own errors and adult targets through focusing on semantics and the different meanings of the words (Weiner, 1981), e.g. contrasting TEA / KEY.

Metaphonology; Metaphonological skills: The ability to reflect on the sound structure of words or utterances as distinct from the meaning. See also **phonological awareness**.

Minimal pairs: Stimuli which differ by only one feature, e.g. TEA, KEY differ only in the voicing of the initial consonant.

Morpheme: The smallest grammatical and lexical unit, e.g. DOG, FROG. A word like KICKED consists of two morphemes KICK + ED. The morpheme ED denotes past tense and is called a bound morpheme because it cannot stand alone and have meaning, whereas KICK is a free morpheme which can stand as a word in its own right.

Motor planning: The actual realization of a motor program (or output template) in connected speech; output level of the speech processing model.

Motor program: Templates or blueprints of how to produce a word; consists of a series of gestural targets for the articulators, i.e. tongue, lips, soft palate, vocal folds.

Motor programming: Level of output processing responsible for the creation of new motor programs; called upon when speakers have to produce new words for the first time. See also **motor program**.

Multiple baseline design: A research design in which two or more baselines are staggered; in a single baseline design, often called an ABA design, pre-intervention assessment is carried out (A); this is followed by the intervention phase (B); and then post-intervention assessment (A). In a multiple baseline design, baseline measures are established and then treatment is introduced at different times. There are three variations of a multiple baseline design: multiple baseline across behaviours (different behaviours are observed), across participants (different participants are observed), or across settings (different settings are used).

Multiple oppositions: Approach to phonological therapy in which a set of contrasting words are focused on all at one time; the concept of homonymy is important in designing stimuli for multiple oppositions therapy, e.g. for a child who uses a particular word such as [dɒ] to mean DOG, DAD, GOT and SOCK, all these words (DOG, DAD, GOT and SOCK) might be used in therapy with the child being encouraged to differentiate between his or her productions in order to realize the distinct meanings.

Non-linear phonology: Theoretical approach to phonology which focuses on the hierarchical nature of phonological forms; a distinction is made between higher level phrase and word structures, and lower level segments (i.e. speech sounds) and features. Non-linear treatment programmes typically include systematic alternations of structural and segmental (feature) targets.

Nucleus: The peak or central part of a syllable usually the vowel, e.g. /æ/ in CAT.

Obstruent: Consonant sound formed by obstructing the airway; subdivided into plosives, fricatives and affricates.

Onset: Part of a syllable that precedes a vowel, e.g. /d/ in DOG, or /pl/ in PLATE.

Orthographic representation: What a word looks like; necessary for automatic word recognition and spelling.

Otitis media with effusion: Middle-ear infection characterized by fluid discharge that can impact widely on speech and language development in children; one of the aetiological categories of speech disorders proposed by Shriberg, Aram and Kwiatkowki. (1997a) often abbreviated to SD-OME.

Outcome, outcomes: The result/s of intervention; see also **outcome measures**; **effectiveness**; **efficacy; efficiency**.

Outcome measures: The assessments, indices or evaluations used to determine whether intervention has brought about changes. See also **primary outcome measure**, **secondary outcome measure**.

PCC/Percentage of consonants correct: Severity index used to estimate degree of a child's speech difficulties; involves counting the number of consonants accurately produced in a representative speech sample and expressing these as a percentage. See also **PPC** and **PVC**.

PPC/Percentage of phonemes correct: Severity index used to estimate degree of a child's speech difficulties; involves counting the number of phonemes (vowels and consonants) accurately produced in a representative speech sample and expressing these as a percentage. See also **PCC** and **PVC**.

PVC/Percentage of vowels correct: Severity index used to estimate degree of a child's speech difficulties; involves counting the number of vowels accurately produced in a representative speech sample and expressing these as a percentage. See also **PCC** and **PPC**.

Persisting speech difficulties (PSDs): Difficulties with any aspect of speech processing or production that have not resolved by the time a child starts formal schooling; may be linked to literacy difficulties and social/emotional problems.

Phonetics: The study of speech sounds in any/all languages.

Phonetic discrimination: A processing level in the speech processing model; drawn on as needed when circumstances demand, e.g. when processing unfamiliar accents a child will need to draw on phonetic discrimination abilities much broader than those required by his or her own accent.

Phonetic inventory: All the speech sounds that a child can produce in a given language, irrespective of whether they are used appropriately or not; a list of a child's speech sound capabilities at a segmental level and without taking context into account.

Phonological awareness: Ability to reflect on the sound structure of an utterance rather than its meaning (Stackhouse and Wells, 1997); typical tasks may include blending, segmenting and manipulating sounds and syllables.

Phonological delay: Children whose phonology resembles that of a younger child, i.e. they show normal speech processes exhibited by younger children; one of the diagnostic sub-groups outlined by Barbara Dodd (1995).

Phonological lexicon: A store of phonological representations.

Phonological recognition: A processing level in the speech processing model at which a child's own language or languages are distinguished from other languages. If English-speaking children receive input in English then through this level of processing, they will recognize that further processing needs to occur. If the language is unknown to the children, then no further processing will take place, unless of course they are trying to learn a new language. This level of speech processing can be thought of as similar to tuning a radio and selecting only, for example, English-speaking channels.

Phonological representation: The knowledge that individuals have stored about the sound structure of words in their language.

Phonology: The study of sounds in a specific language, e.g. English, and how these sounds are used contrastively for meaning; the representation, processing and actual pronunciation of speech sounds, syllables and words in phrases (Bernhardt, 2004 p. 195).

Phonotactics: Relates to the permissible sequence of sounds in a language, e.g. which combination of vowels, consonant clusters are permitted.

Plosive: Consonant sounds produced by complete closure of the vocal tract, e.g. /p/, /b/: also referred to as stops.

Primary outcome measure: The main assessment or area used to evaluate outcome of an intervention.

Productive phonological knowledge (PPK): Attempts to classify children's knowledge about specific sounds of their language into categories; use of surface speech errors to infer children's knowledge about individual phonemes; the degree to which children have internalized a particular phoneme into their phonological system; see also **complexity accounts of treatment efficacy**.

Prosody: Term applied to patterns of intonation and rhythm in human speech; can be categorized as either lexical (word stress) or supra-lexical, moving beyond single words. See also **intonation**.

Psycholinguistics: Study of the psychological factors involved in processing and producing language; the study of the relationship between language in its different forms (e.g. spoken, written or signed) and the mind.

Randomized control trial (RCT): A study involving relatively large numbers of participants who are randomly assigned into two groups: one group receives a particular treatment or therapy, and the other group receives no treatment. Assigning participants at random reduces the risk of bias (i.e. where individuals are aware that they are being treated and change in anticipation of the treatment) and increases the probability that differences between the groups can be attributed to the treatment.

Realization rules: Linguistic rules or statements used to make links between a child's inaccurate production of a specific adult target, e.g. a realization rule used to account for a child's consistent reduction of consonant clusters might be expressed $C_1C_2VC \rightarrow C_2VC$.

Recency effect: A transitory change due to the recent work done but not of any lasting benefit to the child. See also **maintenance**.

Reliability: Evaluation of the stability or consistency of results over repeated observations or measurements under the same conditions each time. See also **inter-rater** and **intra-rater reliability**.

Replication: The duplication of a study, experiment or program to determine if the same findings as in the original study can be found.

Representation: The abstract knowledge stored about words; see also **lexical representation**, **phonological representation**.

Rime: The part of a word that rhymes with another word, e.g. CAT/HAT where the rime for both is AT.

Secondary outcome measures: Outcome measures following an intervention that are of secondary importance to the main or primary outcome measure. See also **primary outcome measure**.

Semantic representation: A level in the speech processing model at which knowledge of the meaning of words is stored.

Severity indices: Measures of the degree of difficulty a child experiences with his/her speech based on accuracy counts of vowels and consonants in a representative speech sample. See also **PCC**, **PPC**, **PVC**.

Single-case study design: Studies in which intervention given to one participant, or a small number of participants, is considered in great detail in terms of the individual response to that intervention. Single-case reports can be descriptive, simply outlining what took place with a specific child. Experimental single-case designs have specific research questions and are set up in such a way as to provide answers to them.

Social stories: Short stories written according to a formula, and used to describe social situations that a child, typically on the autistic spectrum, finds difficult (see Gray, 1994; Rowe, 1999). They are tailor made for an individual child based on specific scenarios with which the child has difficulty, and can also be used for children with PSDs.

Sonority: Refers to the openness of the vocal tract when a sound is spoken: vowels are most sonorous, stop consonants least sonorous, e.g. /p, b, t, d, k, g/.

Sonority sequencing principle: A linguistic rule that governs the way in which consonants are combined within syllables; the components of the syllable are placed on a continuum ranging from most sonorous to least sonorous; the principle suggests that a syllable should have a sonorous peak, i.e. a vowel, and sonority must decrease towards the edges.

Specific language impairment (SLI): A developmental language disorder in the absence of neurological, sensori-motor, non-verbal cognitive or social emotional deficits; children with SLI have difficulties with language production and language comprehension which impacts on educational performance.

Specificity: Knowledge of intervention outcomes as they relate to specific circumstances, e.g. which children benefit? How much treatment have they received and under what conditions?

Speech processing: The complex psycholinguistic skills encompassing input speech processing, storage of representations in the lexicon, and output speech production that enable us to make sense and produce speech, and develop phonological awareness skills for literacy.

Speech processing model: Visual representation, typically using 'boxes and arrows' to show what is thought to happen when speech is processed and produced.

Speech processing profile: A practical tool that can be used to organize assessment data from a child into appropriate processing levels, in order to evaluate their speech processing strengths and weaknesses.

Standard deviation: A measure of the variation of measurements around the average score for a group; the higher the standard deviation, the greater the spread of data, i.e. the variation of performance within the group.

Stimulability: The degree to which a misarticulated sound can be articulated correctly (Hodson, 1997). If children can physically produce a particular sound not normally used in their speech, e.g. they can produce it when given specific instructions and modelling, it is described as stimulable.

Stimulus, stimuli: All items presented in assessment or intervention tasks; including distractors and untreated control items.

Stridency: Forceful airflow striking the back of the teeth as in /s, f, v/.

Systematic review: A review of studies in which evidence has been searched for, studied, evaluated and summarized according to predetermined criteria.

Target: What is being worked on in therapy; what a child is aiming for.

Task: An intervention activity; made up of materials, procedures, feedback and optionally the use of specific techniques. This can be written as an equation as follows (from Rees, 2001b):

TASK = Materials + Procedure + Feedback (+ Technique)

Therapy Outcome Measures (TOM) (Enderby and John, 1999): An approach to evaluating outcomes of speech and language therapy that involves rating the dimensions of impairment, disability, handicap and well-being based on the World Health Organization's (WHO, 2001) *International Classification of Functioning, Disability and Health.*

Validity: The extent to which a measure accurately reflects what it is intended to measure.

Variable: A factor that can be measured and is likely to change, e.g. age, speech production skills; see also **independent** and **dependent variable**.

Velar consonant: Consonant produced with the back of the tongue touching or near the soft palate, e.g. /k/.

Within-class generalization: Patterns of change which take place within a family of sounds, e.g. consonant clusters. See also **generalization**.

References

Adams, C. (2001) Clinical diagnostic and intervention studies of children with semantic-pragmatic language disorder. *International Journal of Language and Communication Disorders*, **36**(3), 289-305.

Allen, C., Nikolopoulos, T., Dyar, D. and O'Donoghue, G. (2001) Reliability of a rating scale for measuring speech intelligibility after pediatric cochlear implantation. *Otology and Neurotology*, **22**(5), 631-3.

Allerton, D. (1976) Early phonotactic development: some observations on a child's acquisition of initial consonant clusters. *Journal of Child Language*, **3**, 429-33.

Almost, D. and Rosenbaum, P. (1998) Effectiveness of speech intervention for phonological disorders: a randomized controlled trial. *Developmental Medicine and Child Neurology*, **40**, 319-52.

Andrews, N. and Fey, M. (1986) Analysis of the speech of phonologically impaired children in two sampling conditions. *Language, Speech and Hearing Services in Schools*, **17**, 187-98.

Anthony, A., Bogle, D., Ingram, T. and McIsaac, M. (1971) *Edinburgh Articulation Test*. Edinburgh: Churchill Livingstone.

Armstrong, S. and Ainley, M. (1988) *South Tyneside Assessment of Phonology (STAP)*. Ponteland: STASS Publications.

ASHA Special Emphasis Panel in Treatment Efficacy (2002) Meeting held at City University, Department of Language and Communication Science, London.

Attanasio, J. (1994) Inferential statistics and treatment efficacy studies in communication disorders. *Journal of Speech and Hearing Research*, **37**, 755-9.

Baker, E. and Bernhardt, B. (2004) From hindsight to foresight: Working around barriers to success in phonological intervention. *Child Language Teaching and Therapy*, **20**(3), 287-319.

Baker, E. and McLeod, S. (2004) Evidence-based management of phonological impairment in children. *Child Language Teaching and Therapy*, **20**(3), 261-86.

Baker, E., Croot, K., McLeod, S. and Paul, R. (2001) Psycholinguistic models of speech development and their application to clinical practice. *Journal of Speech, Language and Hearing Research*, **44**, 685-702.

Barlow, J. (2001) The structure of /s/-sequences: evidence from a disordered system. *Journal of Child Language*, **28**, 291-324.

Barlow, J. and Gierut, J. (2002) Minimal pair approaches to phonological remediation. *Seminars in Speech and Language*, **23**, 57-68.

Barlow, D. and Hersen, M. (1984) *Single-case Experimental Designs: Strategies for Studying Behaviour Change*. Elmsford, NY: Pergamon.

Basso, A. and Caporali, A. (2001) Aphasia therapy or the importance of being earnest. *Aphasiology*, **15**(4), 307–32.

Bernhardt, B. (1992) The application of non-linear phonological theory to intervention with one phonologically disordered child. *Clinical Linguistics and Phonetics*, **6**, 283–316.

Bernhardt, B. (2004) Editorial: Maximizing success in phonological intervention. *Child Language Teaching and Therapy*, **20**(3), 195–8.

Bernhardt, B. and Major, E. (2005) Speech, language and literacy skills three years later: Long-term outcomes of non-linear phonological intervention. *International Journal of Language and Communication Disorders*, **40**(1), 1–27.

Best, W. (2005) Investigation of a new intervention for children with word-finding problems. *International Journal of Language and Communication Disorders*, **40**(3), 279–318.

Bishop, D. (1997a) *Uncommon Understanding*. London: Psychology Press.

Bishop, D. (1997b) Cognitive neuropsychology and developmental disorders: uncomfortable bedfellows. *Quarterly Journal of Experimental Psychology*, **50**(4), 899–923.

Bishop, D. and Adams, C. (1990) A prospective study of the relationship between specific language impairment, phonological disorders and reading retardation. *Journal of Child Psychology and Psychiatry*, **31**, 1027–50.

Bishop, D. and Clarkson, B. (2003) Written language as a window into residual language deficits: A study of children with persistent and residual speech and language impairments. *Cortex*, **39**, 215–37.

Bishop, D. and Robson, J. (1989) Accurate non-word spelling despite congenital inability to speak: phoneme-grapheme conversion does not require subvocal articulation. *British Journal of Psychology*, **80**(1), 1–13.

Blache, S., Parsons, C. and Humphreys, J. (1981) A minimal-word-pair model for teaching the linguistic significance of distinctive feature properties. *Journal of Speech and Hearing Disorders*, **46**, 291–6.

Bornman, J., Alant, E. and Meiring, E. (2001) The use of a digital voice output device to facilitate language development in a child with developmental apraxia of speech: A case study. *Disability and Rehabilitation*, **20**(14), 623–34.

Bourassa, D. and Treiman, R. (2003) Spelling in dyslexic children: Analyses from the Treiman-Bourassa Early Spelling Test. *Scientific Studies of Reading*, **7**, 309–33.

Bowen, C. and Cupples, L. (1998) A tested phonological therapy in practice. *Child Language Teaching and Therapy*, **14**(1), 29–50.

Bridgeman, E. and Snowling, M. (1988) The perception of phoneme sequence: A comparison of dyspraxic and normal children. *British Journal of Disorders of Communication*, **23**(3), 245–52.

Bridges, A. (1991) Acceptability ratings and intelligibility scores of alaryngeal speakers by three listener groups. *British Journal of Disorders of Communication*, **26**(3), 325–36.

Brindley, C., Cave, D., Lees, J., Crane, S. and Maffat, V. (1996) *Paediatric Oral Skills Package (POSP)*. Whurr Publishers: London.

Broom, Y. and Doctor, E. (1995a) Developmental phonological dyslexia: A case study of the efficacy of a remediation programme. *Cognitive Neuropsychology*, **12**(7), 725–66.

Broom, Y. and Doctor, E. (1995b) Developmental surface dyslexia: A case study of the efficacy of a remediation programme. *Cognitive Neuropsychology*, **12**(1), 69–110.

Broomfield, J. and Dodd, B. (2004) The nature of referred subtypes of primary speech disability. *Child Language Teaching and Therapy*, **20**(2), 135–51.

Broomfield, J. and Dodd, B. (2005) Clinical effectiveness, in *Differential Diagnosis and Treatment of Children with Speech Disorder* 2nd edn (ed. B. Dodd). London: Whurr Publishers.

Bruck, M. and Treiman, R. (1990) Phonological awareness and spelling in normal children and dyslexics: The case of initial consonant clusters. *Journal of Experimental Child Psychology*, **50**, 156–78.

Bryan, A. and Howard, D. (1992) Frozen phonology thawed: The analysis and remediation of a developmental disorder of real word phonology. *European Journal of Disorders of Communication*, **27**, 343–65.

Bryan, A. and North, C. (1994) Developmental cognitive neuropsychology: a comparison of two case studies. *Child Language Teaching and Therapy*, **10**, 313–27.

Bryan, K. (2004) Preliminary study of the prevalence of speech and language difficulties in young offenders. *International Journal of Language and Communication Disorders*, **39**(3), 391–400.

Bunning, K. (2004) *Speech and Language Therapy Intervention: Frameworks and Processes*. London: Whurr Publishers.

Byng, S., Van der Gaag, A. and Parr, S. (1998) International initiatives in outcomes measurement: A perspective from the United Kingdom, in *Measuring Outcomes in Speech-language Pathology* (ed. C. Frattali). New York: Thieme.

Camarata, S. (1998) Connecting speech and language: Clinical applications, in *Exploring the Speech-Language Connection*, vol 8 (ed. R. Paul). Baltimore, MD: Brookes Publishing.

Campbell, R. and Butterworth, B. (1985) Phonological dyslexia and dysgraphia in a highly literate subject: A developmental case with associated deficits of phonemic processing and awareness. *Quarterly Journal of Experimental Psychology*, **37**, 435–75.

Campbell, T. (1999) Functional treatment outcomes in young children with motor speech disorders, in *Clinical Management of Motor Speech Disorders in Children* (eds A. Caruso and E. Strand). New York: Thieme Medical Publishers Inc.

Campbell, T. (2002) Child apraxia of speech: Clinical symptoms and speech characteristics. Paper in the *Proceedings of the 2002 Childhood Apraxia of Speech Research Symposium*, California, USA.

Carlomagno, S. and Parlato, V. (1989) Writing rehabilitation in brain-damaged adult patients: A cognitive approach, in *Cognitive Approaches in Neuropsychological Rehabilitation* (eds X. Seron and S. Deloche). Hillsdale, NJ: Lawrence Erlbaum Associates.

Carroll, J. and Snowling, M. (2004) Language and phonological skills in children at high risk of reading difficulties. *Journal of Child Psychology and Psychiatry*, **45**, 631–45.

Cassidy, B. (1994) An investigation into the auditory discrimination skills of normally-developing children using single-word and sentence stimuli. Unpublished MSc thesis. National Hospital's College of Speech Sciences/ Institute of Neurology, London University.

Chapman, R. (2000) Children's language learning: An interactionist perspective. *Journal of Child Psychology and Psychiatry*, **41**(1), 33–54.

Chiat, S. (2000) *Understanding Children with Language Problems*. Cambridge: Cambridge University Press.

Chiat, S. (2001) Mapping theories of developmental language impairment: Premises, predictions and evidence. *Language and Cognitive Processes*, **16**(2/3), 113–42.

Chiat, S. and Hirson, A. (1987) From conceptual intention to utterance: a study of impaired language output in a child with developmental dysphasia. *British Journal of Disorders of Communication*, **22**, 37–64.

Chiat, S. and Hunt, J. (1993) Connections between phonology and semantics: an exploration of lexical processing in a language impaired child. *Child Language Teaching and Therapy*, **9**, 200–13.

Chin, S., Finnegan, K. and Chung, B. (2001) Relationships among types of speech intelligibility in pediatric users of cochlear implants. *Journal of Communication Disorders*, **34**, 187–205.

Chin, S., Tsai, P. and Gao, S. (2003) Connected speech intelligibility of children with cochlear implants and children with normal hearing. *American Journal of Speech Language Pathology*, **12**, 440–51.

Christensen, J. and Dwyer, P. (1990) Improving alaryngeal speech intelligibility. *Journal of Communication Disorders*, **23**(6), 445–51.

Cienkowski, K. and Speaks, C. (2000) Subjective vs. objective intelligibility of sentences in listeners with hearing loss. *Journal of Speech Language Hearing Research*, **43**(5), 1205–10.

Clarke-Klein, S. and Hodson, B. (1995) A phonologically-based analysis of misspellings by third graders with disordered-phonology histories. *Journal of Speech and Hearing Research*, **38**, 839–49.

Clements, G. (1990) The role of the sonority cycle in core syllabification, in *Papers in Laboratory Phonology I: Between the Grammar and Physics of Speech* (eds J. Kingston and M. Beckman). New York: Cambridge University Press, pp. 283–333.

Clements, G. and Hume, E. (1995) The internal organisation of speech sounds, in *The Handbook of Phonological Theory* (ed. J. Goldsmith). Oxford: Blackwell, pp. 245–306.

Coffield, C. (1994) An investigation into the speech output of four Down's syndrome adolescents. Unpublished MSc thesis, National Hospital's College of Speech Sciences/Institute of Neurology, London.

Coltheart, M. and Byng, S. (1989) A treatment for surface dyslexia, in *Cognitive Approaches in Neuropsychological Rehabilitation* (eds X. Seron and G. Deloche). Hillsdale, NJ: Lawrence Erlbaum.

Connery, V. (1992, 1994) *The Nuffield Centre Dyspraxia Programme*. London: The Nuffield Hearing and Speech Centre.

Constable, A. (1993) Investigating word-finding difficulties in children. Unpublished MSc thesis, University College London.

Constable, A., Stackhouse, J. and Wells, B. (1997) Developmental word-finding difficulties and phonological processing: The case of the missing handcuffs. *Applied Psycholinguistics*, **18**, 507–36.

Conti-Ramsden, G. and Botting, N. (2000) Social and behavioural difficulties in children with language impairment. *Child Language Teaching and Therapy*, **16**(2), 105–20.

Corrin, J. (2001a) From profile to programme: Steps 1–2, in *Children's Speech and Literacy Difficulties 2: Identification and Intervention* (eds J. Stackhouse and B. Wells). London: Whurr Publishers.

Corrin, J. (2001b) From profile to programme: Steps 3-6, in *Children's Speech and Literacy Difficulties 2: Identification and Intervention* (eds J. Stackhouse and B. Wells). London: Whurr Publishers.

Corrin, J., Tarplee, C. and Wells, B. (2001) Interactional linguistics and language development: A conversation analytic perspective on emergent syntax, in *Studies in Interactional Linguistics* (eds M. Selting and E. Couper-Kuhlen). Amsterdam: John Benjamins.

Costello, J. and Onstine, J. (1976) The modification of multiple articulation errors based on distinctive feature theory. *Journal of Speech and Hearing Disorders*, **41**, 199-215.

Counsel, J. (1993) Oral language deficits in reading-impaired children. MSc thesis, Department of Human Communication Science. University College London.

Crary, M. and Hunt, T. (1982) Sounds vs Patterns: A case comparison of approaches for articulation therapy. *Australian Journal of Human Communication Disorders*, **10**(2), 15-22.

Creaghead, N., Newman, P. and Secord, W. (1989) *Assessment and Remediation of Articulatory and Phonological Disorders*, 2nd edn. New York: Macmillan Publishing Company.

Crosbie, S. and Dodd, B. (2001) Training auditory discrimination: A single case study. *Child Language Teaching and Therapy*, **17**(3), 173-94.

Crosbie, S., Dodd, B. and Howard, D. (2002) Spoken word comprehension in children with SLI: A comparison of three case studies. *Child Language Teaching and Therapy*, **18**(3), 191-212.

Crosbie, S., Holm, A. and Dodd, B. (2005) Intervention for children with severe speech disorder: A comparison of two approaches. *International Journal of Language and Communication Disorders*, **40**(4), 467-91.

Crowe Hall, B. (1991) Attitudes of fourth and sixth graders toward peers with mild articulation disorders. *Language, Speech and Hearing Services in Schools*, **22**, 334-40.

Dagenais, P. (1995) Electropalatography in the treatment of articulation/phonological disorders. *Journal of Communication Disorders*, **28**, 302-29.

Damico, J. (1988) The lack of efficacy in language therapy: a case study. *Language, Speech and Hearing Services in Schools*, **19**, 51-66.

Dankovicová, J., Pigott, K., Wells, B. and Peppé, S. (2004) Temporal markers of prosodic boundaries in children's speech production. *Journal of the International Phonetic Association*, **34**(1), 17-36.

Davidson, J., Elock, J. and Noyes, P. (1996) A preliminary study of the effect of computer-assisted practice on reading attainment. *Journal of Research in Reading*, **19**, 102-10.

Dean, E., Howell, J., Grieve, R., Donaldson, M. and Reid, J. (1995a) Harnessing language awareness in a communicative context: a group study of the efficacy of metaphon. *Proceedings of the RCSLT Golden Jubilee Conference*, York.

Dean, E., Howell, J., Waters, D. and Reid, J. (1995b) Metaphon: A metalinguistic approach to the treatment of phonological disorders in children. *Clinical Linguistics and Phonetics*, **9**, 9-19.

De Bodt, M., Hernandez-Diaz, H. and Van De Heyning, P. (2002) Intelligibility as a linear combination of dimensions in dysarthric speech. *Journal of Communication Disorders*, **35**, 283-92.

Denne, M., Langdown, N., Pring, T. and Roy, P. (2005) Treating children with expressive phonological disorders: does phonological awareness therapy work in the clinic? *International Journal of Language and Communication Disorders*, **40**, 493–504.

Dent, H. (2001) Electropalatography: A tool for psycholinguistic therapy, in *Children's Speech and Literacy Difficulties 2: Identification and Intervention* (eds J. Stackhouse and B. Wells). London: Whurr Publishers.

Dinnsen, D., O'Connor, K. and Gierut, J. (2001) The puzzle-puddle-pickle problem and the Duke-of-York gambit in acquisition. *Journal of Linguistics*, **37**, 503–25.

Dodd, B. (ed.) (1995) Differential diagnosis and treatment of children with speech disorder. London: Whurr Publishers.

Dodd, B. (ed.) (2005) *Differential Diagnosis and Treatment of Children with Speech Disorder*, 2nd edn. London: Whurr Publishers.

Dodd, B. and Bradford, A. (2000) A comparison of three therapy methods for children with different types of developmental phonological disorder. *International Journal of Language and Communication Disorder*, **35**(2), 189–209.

Dodd, B. and Iacano, T. (1989) Phonological disorders in children: Changes in phonological process use during treatment. *British Journal of Disorders of Communication*, **24**, 333–51.

Dodd, B. and McCormack, P. (1995) A model of speech processing for differential diagnosis of phonological disorder, in *Differential Diagnosis and Treatment of Children with Speech Disorder* (ed. B. Dodd). London: Whurr Publishers.

Dodd, B., Gillon, G., Oerlemans, M., Russell, T., Syrmis, M. and Wilson, H. (1995) Phonological disorder and the acquisition of literacy, in *Differential Diagnosis and Treatment of Children with Speech Disorder* (ed. B. Dodd). London: Whurr Publishers.

Dodd, B., Hua, Z., Crosbie, S., Holm, A. and Ozanne, A. (2002) *Diagnostic Evaluation of Articulation and Phonology (DEAP)*. Psychological Corporation.

Easton, C., Sheach, S. and Easton, S. (1997) Teaching vocabulary to children with wordfinding difficulties using a combined semantic and phonological approach: an efficacy study. *Child Language Teaching and Therapy*, **13**(2), 125–42.

Ebbels, S. (2000) Psycholinguistic profiling of a hearing-impaired child. *Child Language Teaching and Therapy*, **16**(1), 3–22.

Edwards, J., Fourakis, M., Beckman, M. and Fox, R. (1999) Characterizing knowledge deficits in phonological disorders. *Journal of Speech, Language and Hearing Research*, **42**, 169–86.

Edwards, M. (1983) Selection criteria for developing therapy goals. *Journal of Childhood Communication Disorders*, **7**, 36–45.

Eksteen, E., Rieger, J., Nesbitt, M. and Seikaly, H. (2003) Comparison of voice characteristics following three different methods of treatment for laryngeal cancer. *Journal of Otolaryngology*, **32**, 250–3.

Elbert, M. (1997) From articulation to phonology: The challenge of change, in *Perspectives in Applied Phonology* (eds B. Hodson and M. Edwards), Maryland: Aspen.

Elbert, M. and McReynolds, L. (1975) Transfer of /r/ across contexts. *Journal of Speech and Hearing Research*, **40**, 380–7.

Elbert, M., Powell, T. and Swartzlander, P. (1991) Toward a technology of generalisation: How many exemplars are sufficient? *Journal of Speech and Hearing Research*, **34**, 81–7.

Elbert, M., Dinnsen, D., Swartzlander, P. and Chin, S. (1990) Generalization to conversational speech. *Journal of Speech and Hearing Disorders*, **55**, 694–9.

Ellis, A. and Young, A. (1988) *Human Cognitive Neuropsychology*. Hove, UK: Erlbaum.

Ellis, L. and Fucci, D. (1992) Effects of listeners' experience on two measures of intelligibility. *Perceptual and Motor Skills* **74**, 1099–104.

Enderby, P. (1983) *Frenchay Dysarthria Assessment*. San Diego, CA: College Hill Press.

Enderby, P. and Emerson, J. (1995) *Does Speech and Language Therapy Work?* London: Whurr Publishers.

Enderby, P. and John, A. (1999) Therapy outcome measures in speech and language therapy: Comparing performance between different providers. *International Journal of Language and Communication Disorders*, **34**(4), 417–29.

Evershed Martin, S. (1991) Input training in phonological disorder: A case discussion, in *Phonological Disorders in Children* (ed. M. Yavas). London: Routledge.

Fazio, B. (1997) Learning a new poem: Memory for connected speech and phonological awareness in low-income children with and without specific language impairment. *Journal of Speech Language and Hearing Research*, **40**, 1285–97.

Ferguson, C. (1978) Learning to pronounce: The earliest stages of phonological development in the child, in *Communicative and Cognitive Abilities – Early Behavioural Assessment* (eds F. Minifie and L. Lloyd), Baltimore, MD: University Park Press, pp. 273–97.

Ferguson, C. and Farwell, C. (1975) Words and sounds in early language acquisition. *Language*, **51**, 419–39.

Fey, M. (1988) Generalisation issues facing language interventionists: an introduction. *Language Speech and Hearing Services in Schools*, **19**, 272–81.

Fey, M., Cleave, P., Long, S. and Hughes, D. (1993) Two approaches to the facilitation of grammar in children with language impairment: an experimental evaluation. *Journal of Speech and Hearing Research*, **36**, 141–57.

Fey, M., Cleave, P., Ravida, A., Long, S., Dejmal, A. and Easton, D. (1994) Effects of grammar facilitation on the phonological performance of children with speech and language impairments. *Journal of Speech and Hearing Research*, **37**, 594–607.

Fletcher, P. (1985) *A Child's Learning of English*. Oxford: Basil Blackwell.

Fletcher, S. (1978) *The Fletcher Time-by-count Test of Diadochokinetic Syllable Rate*. Tigard, OR: C.C. Publications.

Flipsen, P. (1995) Speaker-listener familiarity: Parents as judges of delayed speech intelligibility. *Journal of Communication Disorders*, **28**, 3–19.

Flipsen, P. (2002) Chapter 9: *Phonemic Therapy*, http://web.utk.edu/~pflipsen/435.html.

Forrest, K. (2002) Are oral-motor exercises useful in the treatment of phonological/articulatory disorders. *Seminars in Speech and Language*, **23**(1), 15–26.

Forrest, K., Elbert, M. and Dinnsen, D. (2000) The effect of substitution patterns on phonological treatment outcomes. *Clinical Linguistics and Phonetics*, **14**(7), 519–31.

Fox, A., Dodd, B. and Howard, D. (2002) Risk factors for speech disorders in children. *International Journal of Language and Communication Disorders*, **37**(2), 117–33.

Frattali, C. (1998) Outcomes measurement: Definitions, dimensions and perspectives, in *Measuring Outcomes in Speech-Language Pathology* (ed. C. Frattali), New York: Thieme.

Frederikson, N., Frith, U. and Reason, R. (1997) *Phonological Assessment Battery (PhAB)*. Windsor: NFER-Nelson.

Frith, U. (1985) Beneath the surface of developmental dyslexia, in *Surface Dyslexia* (eds K. Patterson, J. Marshall and M. Coltheart). London: Routledge and Kegan Paul.

Fujimoto, P., Madison, C. and Larrigan, L. (1991) The effects of a tracheostoma valve on the intelligibility and quality of tracheoesophageal speech. *Journal of Speech, Language and Hearing Research*, **34**(1), 33–6.

Furia, C., Kowalski, L., Latorre, M., Angelis, E., Martins, N., Barros, A. *et al.* (2001) Speech intelligibility after glossectomy and speech rehabilitation. *Archives of Otolaryngology and Head Neck Surgery*, **127**(7), 877–83.

Gallagher, A. (1998) Treatment research in speech, language and swallowing: lessons from child language disorders. *Folia Phoniatrica et Logopaedica*, **50**, 165–82.

Garcia, J. and Dagenais, P. (1998) Dysarthric sentence intelligibility: Contribution of iconic gestures and message predictiveness, **41**(6), 1282–93.

Gardner, H. (1989) An investigation of maternal interaction with phonologically disordered children as compared to two groups of normally developing children. *British Journal of Disorders of Communication*, **24**(1), 41–60.

Gardner, H. (1997) Are your minimal pairs too neat? The dangers of phonemicisation in phonology therapy. *European Journal of Disorders of Communication*, **32**(2), 167–75.

Gardner, H. (1998) Children's social and metalinguistic knowledge and their respective roles in speech therapy tasks, in *Children and Social Competence* (eds I. Hutchby and S. Moran Ellis). Falmer Press.

Gardner, H. (2006) Training others in the art of therapy for speech sound disorders: an interactional approach. *Child Language Teaching and Therapy*, **22**(1), 27–46.

Gathercole, S. and Baddeley, A. (1996) *The Children's Test of Nonword Repetition*. UK Psychological Corporation.

German, D. (1989) *Test of Word Finding*. Leicester: Taskmaster.

Gibbon, F. and Wood, S. (2003) Using electropalatography (EPG) to diagnose and treat articulation disorders associated with mild cerebral palsy: a case study. *Clinical Linguistics and Phonetics*, **17**, 365–74.

Gibbon, F., McNeill, A., Wood, S. and Watson, J. (2003) Changes in linguapalatal contact patterns during therapy for velar fronting in a 10-year-old with Down syndrome. *International Journal of Language and Communication Disorders*, **38**(1), 47–64.

Gierut, J. (1989) Maximal opposition approach to phonological treatment. *Journal of Speech and Hearing Disorders*, **54**, 9–19.

Gierut, J. (1990) Differential learning of phonological oppositions. *Journal of Speech and Hearing Research*, **33**, 540–9.

Gierut, J. (1991) Homonymy in phonological change. *Clinical Linguistics and Phonetics*, **5**, 119–37.

Gierut, J. (1992) The conditions and course of clinically induced phonological change. *Journal of Speech and Hearing Research*, **35**(5), 1049–63.

Gierut, J. (1998a) Treatment efficacy: functional phonological disorders in children. *Journal of Speech and Hearing Research*, **41**, 85–100.

Gierut, J. (1998b) Production, conceptualisation and change in distinctive featural categories. *Journal of Child Language*, **25**, 321–41.

Gierut, J. (1999) Syllable onsets: clusters and adjuncts in acquisition. *Journal of Speech, Language and Hearing Research*, **42**(3), 708–26.

Gierut, J. and Champion, A. (1999) Interacting error patterns and their resistance to treatment. *Clinical Linguistics and Phonetics*, **13**(6), 421–31.

Gierut, J. and Dinnsen, D. (1987) On predicting ease of phonological learning. *Applied Linguistics*, **8**(3), 241–63.

Gierut, J. and O'Connor, K. (2002) Precursors to onset clusters in acquisition. *Journal of Child Language*, **29**, 495–517.

Gierut, J., Elbert, M. and Dinnsen, D. (1987) A functional analysis of phonological knowledge and generalisation learning in misarticulating children. *Journal of Speech and Hearing Research*, **30**, 462–79.

Gierut, J., Morrisette, M., Hughes, M. and Rowland, S. (1996) Phonological treatment efficacy and developmental norms. *Language, Speech and Hearing Services in Schools*, **27**(3), 215–30.

Gillberg, C. (2003) Deficits in attention, motor control, and perception: a brief review. *Archives of Disease in Childhood*, **88**, 904–10.

Gillon, G. (2000) The efficacy of phonological awareness intervention for children with spoken language impairment. *Language, Speech, and Hearing Services in Schools*, **31**, 126–41.

Gillon, G. (2002) Follow-up study investigating the benefits of phonological awareness intervention for children with spoken language impairment. *International Journal of Language and Communication Disorders*, **37**(4), 381–400.

Gillon, G. (2004) *Phonological Awareness: From Research to Practice*. New York: The Guilford Press.

Gillon, G. (2005) Facilitating phoneme awareness development in 3–4 year old children with speech impairment. *Language, Speech and Hearing Services in Schools*, **36**, 308–24.

Gillon, G. and Dodd, B. (2005) Understanding the relationship between speech and language impairment and literacy difficulties: the central role of phonology, in *Differential Diagnosis and Treatment of Children with Speech Disorder*, 2nd edn (ed. B. Dodd). London: Whurr Publishers.

Glogowska, M. (2001) RCTs: Myths, misconceptions and mastery. *RCSLT Bulletin, March*, 6–7.

Glogowska, M., Roulstone, S., Enderby, P. and Peters, T. (2000) Randomised controlled trial of community based speech and language therapy in preschool children. *British Medical Journal*, **321**, 923–6.

Glogowska, M., Campbell, R., Peters, T., Roulstone, S. and Enderby, P. (2002) A multi-method approach to the evaluation of community preschool speech and language therapy provision. *Child: Care, Health and Development*, **28**(6), 513–21.

Goldman, R. and Fristoe, M. (1969) *Goldman-Fristoe Test of Articulation*. Windsor: NFER-Nelson.

Goldman, R., Fristoe, M. and Woodcock, R. (1972) *Goldman-Fristoe-Woodcock Tests of Articulation*: American Guidance Service.

Goldman, R., Fristoe, M. and Woodcock, R. (1978) *Goldman-Fristoe-Woodcock Auditory Skills Test Battery, revised edition*. Windsor: NFER-Nelson.

Goldrick, M. and Rapp, B. (2002) A restricted interactions account (RIA) of spoken word production: The best of both worlds. *Aphasiology*, **16**, 20–55.

Goldstein, H. and Gierut, J. (1998) Outcomes measurement in child language and phonological disorders, in *Measuring Outcomes in Speech-Language Pathology* (ed. C. Fratteli). New York: Thieme.

Golper, L. (2001) *Evidence-Based Practice Guidelines for the Management of Communication Disorders in Neurologically Impaired Individuals: Project Introduction*. The Academy of Neurologic Communication Disorders and Sciences' ad hoc Practice Guidelines Coordinating Committee.

Gordon-Brannan, M. and Hodson, B. (2000) Intelligibility/severity measurements of prekindergarten children's speech. *American Journal of Speech-Language Pathology*, **9**, 141–50.

Gray, B. and Fygetakis, L. (1968) Mediated language acquisition for dysphasic children. *Behavioral Research and Therapy*, **6**, 263–80.

Gray, C. (1994) *The New Social Story Book*: Arlington: Future Horizons.

Griffiths, M. (2005) The relationship between speech and spelling: An analysis of the spoken and written production of consonant clusters. Unpublished MPhil thesis. University of Sheffield: Department of Human Communication Sciences.

Grigorenko, E., Klin, A., Pauls, D., Senft, R., Hooper, C. and Volkmar, F. (2002) A descriptive study of hyperlexia in a clinically referred sample of children with developmental delays. *Journal of Autism and Developmental Disorders*, **32**(1), 3–12.

Grundy, K. (1989) *Linguistics in Clinical Practice*. London: Taylor and Francis.

Grunwell, P. (1985) *PACS – Phonological Assessment of Child Speech*. Windsor: NFER-Nelson.

Grunwell, P. (1987) *Clinical Phonology*, 2nd edn. London: Croom Helm.

Grunwell, P. (1992) Principled decision making in the remediation of children with developmental phonological disorders, in *Specific Speech and Language Disorders in Children* (eds P. Fletcher and D. Hall). London: Whurr Publishers.

Grunwell, P. and Harding, A. (1995) *PACS TOYS*. Windsor: NFER-Nelson.

Grunwell, P. and Yavas, M. (1988) Phonotactic restrictions in disordered child phonology: A case study. *Clinical Linguistics and Phonetics*, **2**, 1–16.

Hadley, P. and Rice, M. (1991) Conversational responsiveness of speech and language impaired preschoolers. *Journal of Speech and Hearing Research*, **34**, 1308–17.

Hall, P., Jordan, L. and Robin, D. (1993) *Developmental Apraxia of Speech: Theory and Clinical Practice*. Austin, TX: Pro-Ed.

Harbers, H., Paden, E. and Halle, J. (1999) Phonological awareness and production: Changes during intervention. *Language, Speech, and Hearing Services in Schools*, **30**(1), 50–60.

Hardcastle, W. and Hewlett, N. (1999) *Coarticulation: Theory, Data and Techniques*. Cambridge: Cambridge University Press.

Harley, T. (2001) *The Psychology of Language*. Hove: Psychology Press.

Hatcher, P. (1994) *Sound Linkage: An Integrated Programme for Overcoming Reading Difficulties* (2nd edn, 2000). London: Whurr Publishers.

Hatcher, P. (2006) Phonological awareness and reading intervention, in *Dyslexia, Speech and Language: A Practitioner's Handbook*, 2nd edn (eds M. Snowling and J. Stackhouse). London: Whurr Publishers.

Hegde, M. (1985) *Treatment Procedures in Communicative Disorders*. London: Taylor and Francis.

Helfrich-Miller, K. (1994) A clinical perspective: melodic intonation therapy for developmental apraxia. *Clinics in Communication Disorders*, **4**(3), 175–82.

Henry, C. (1990) The development of oral diadochokinesis and non-linguistic rhymthic skills in normal and speech-disordered young children. *Clinical Linguistics and Phonetics*, **4**(2), 121–38.

Hesketh, A., Adams, C. and Hall, R. (2000) Phonological awareness therapy and articulatory training approaches for children with phonological disorders: a comparative outcome study. *International Journal of Language and Communication Disorders*, **35**(3), 337–54.

Hewlett, N. (1990) Processes of development and production, in *Developmental Speech Disorders* (ed. P. Grunwell). Edinburgh: Churchill Livingstone.

Hodson, B. (1997) Disordered phonologies: What have we learned about assessment and treatment? in *Perspectives in Applied Phonology* (eds B. Hodson and M. Edwards). Aspen: Gaithersburg.

Hodson, B. (2004) *The Hodson Assessment of Phonological Patterns-Third Edition* (HAPP-3). Texas: Pro-ed.

Hodson, B. and Edwards, M. (eds) (1997) *Perspectives in Applied Phonology*. Aspen: Gaithersburg.

Hodson, B. and Paden, E. (1991) *Targeting Intelligible Speech: A Phonological Approach to Remediation*. San Diego, CA: College-Hill Press.

Hoffman, P., Norris, J. and Monjure, J. (1990) Comparison of process targeting and whole language treatments for phonologically delayed pre-school children. *Language, Speech and Hearing Services in Schools*, **21**, 102–9.

Holm, A., Crosbie, S. and Dodd, B. (2005a) Phonological approaches to intervention, in *Differential Diagnosis and Treatment of Children with Speech Disorder*, 2nd edn (ed. B. Dodd). London: Whurr Publishers.

Holm, A., Crosbie, S. and Dodd, B. (2005b) Treating inconsistent speech disorders, in *Differential Diagnosis and Treatment of Children with Speech Disorder*, 2nd edn (ed. B. Dodd). London: Whurr Publishers.

Holm, A. and Dodd, B. (1999) An intervention case study of a bilingual child with phonological disorder. *Child Language Teaching and Therapy*, **15**(2), 139–58.

Horton, S. and Byng, S. (2000) Examining interaction in language therapy. *International Journal of Language and Communication Disorders*, **35**(3), 355–75.

Howard, D. (1986) Beyond randomised controlled trials: The case for effective case studies of the effects of treatment in aphasia. *British Journal of Disorders of Communication*, **21**, 89–102.

Howard, D. and Hatfield, F. (1987) *Aphasia Therapy: Historical and contemporary Issues*. London: Erlbaum.

Howard, S. (2004) Connected speech processes in developmental speech impairment: Observations from an electropalatographic perspective. *Clinical Linguistics and Phonetics*, **18**, 405–17.

Howell, J. and Dean, E. (1994) *Treating Phonological Disorders in Children: Metaphon – Theory to Practice*. London: Whurr Publishers.

Hulme, C. and Snowling, M. (1992) Phonological deficits in dyslexia: A 'sound' reappraisal of the verbal deficit hypothesis, in *Current Perspectives in Learning Disabilities* (eds N. Singh and I. Beale). New York: Springer-Verlag, pp. 270–301.

Hunter, L., Pring, T. and Martin, S. (1991) The use of strategies to increase speech intelligibility in cerebral palsy: An experimental evaluation. *British Journal of Disorders of Communication*, **26**(2), 163–74.

Huskie, C. (1989) Assessment of speech and language status: Subjective and objective approaches to appraisal of vocal tract structure and function, in

Cleft Palate - The Nature and Remediation of Communication Problems (ed. J. Stengelhofen). London: Whurr Publishers.

Hustad, K. and Beukelman, D. (2001) Effects of linguistic cues and stimulus cohesion on intelligibility of severely dysarthric speech. *Journal of Speech, Language and Hearing Research*, **44**(3), 497-510.

Hustad, K., Jones, T. and Dailey, S. (2003) Implementing speech supplementation strategies: Effects on intelligibility and speech rate of individuals with chronic severe dysarthria. *Journal of Speech Language and Hearing Research*, **9**, 462-74.

Ingham, R., Kilgo, M., Ingham, J., Moglia, R., Belknap, H. and Sanchez, T. (2001) Evaluation of a stuttering treatment based on reduction of short phonation intervals. *Journal of Speech Language and Hearing Research*, **44**, 1229-44.

Ingram, D. (1974) Phonological rules in young children. *Journal of Child Language*, **1**, 49-64.

Ingram, D. (1976) *Phonological Disability in Children.* New York: Elsevier.

Ingram, D. and Ingram, K. (2001) A whole-word approach to phonological analysis and intervention. *Language, Speech and Hearing Services in Schools*, **32**, 271-83.

Jacoby, G., Lee, L., Kummer, A., Levin, L. and Creaghead, N. (2002) The number of individual treatment units necessary to facilitate functional communication improvements in the speech and language of young children. *American Journal of Speech-Language Pathology*, **11**, 370-80.

Jamieson, D. and Rvachew, S. (1992) Remediation of speech production errors with sound identification training. *Journal of Speech-language Pathology and Audiology*, **16**, 519-21.

Joffe, B., Penn, C. and Doyle, J. (1996) The persisting communication difficulties of 'remediated' language-impaired children. *European Journal of Disorders of Communication*, **31**(4), 369-86.

Joffe, B. and Reilly, S. (2004) The evidence base for the treatment of motor-speech disorders in children, in *Evidence-based practice in speech pathology* (eds S. Reilly, J. Douglas and J. Oates), London: Whurr Publishers, pp. 259-87.

Joffe, B. and Serry, T. (2004). The evidence base for the treatment of articulation and phonological disorders in children, in *Evidence-based practice in speech pathology* (eds Reilly, S., Douglas, J. and Oates, J). London: Whurr Publishers, 259-87.

John, A., Enderby, P. and Hughes, A. (2005a) Benchmarking outcomes in dysphasia using the therapy outcome measure, *Aphasiology*, **19**, 165-78.

John, A., Enderby, P. and Hughes, A. (2005b) Comparing outcomes of voice therapy: A benchmarking study using the therapy outcome measure, *Journal of Voice*, **19**, 114-23.

Johnson, H. and Hood, S. (1988) Teaching chaining to unintelligible children: How to deal with open syllables. *Language, Speech and Hearing Services in Schools*, **19**, 211-20.

Jusczyk, P. (1986) Toward a model of speech perception, in *Invariance and Variability in Speech Processes* (ed. J. Perkell). Hillsdale, NJ: Lawrence Erlbaum.

Keatley, A. and Wirz, S. (1994) Is 20 years too long? Improving intelligibility in long-standing dysarthria - a single case treatment study. *European Journal of Disorders of Communication*, **29**(2), 183-201.

Keith, R. (1999) *SCAN-C: Test for Auditory Processing Disorders in Children - Revised.* San Antonio, TX: Psychological Corporation.

Kelly, J. and Local, J. (1989) *Doing Phonology*. Manchester: Manchester University Press.

Kempler, D. and Van Lancker, D. (2002) Effect of speech task on intelligibility in dysarthria: A case study of Parkinson's disease. *Brain and Language*, **80**(3), 449-64.

Kent, J., Kent, R., Rosenbek, J., Weismer, G., Martin, R., Sufit, R. *et al.* (1990) Quantitative description of the dysarthria in women with amyotrophic lateral sclerosis, *Journal of Speech and Hearing Research*, **35**, 723-33.

Kent, R. (1982) Contextual facilitation of correct sound production. *Language Speech and Hearing Services in Schools*, **13**, 66-76.

Kent, R. (ed.). (1992) *Intelligibility in Speech Disorders: Theory, Measurement and Management*. Amsterdam: John Benjamins.

Kent, R., Miolo, G. and Bloedel, S. (1994) The intelligibility of children's speech: A review of evaluation procedures. *American Journal of Speech-Language Pathology*, **3**(2), 81-95.

Kent, R., Weismer, G., Kent, J. and Rosenbek, J. (1989) Toward explanatory intelligibility testing in dysarthria. *Journal of Speech and Hearing Disorders*, **54**, 482-99.

Kirk, C. and Demuth, K. (2005) Asymmetries in the acquisition of word-initial and word-final consonant clusters. *Journal of Child Language*, **32**(4), 709-34.

Knox, E. and Conti-Ramsden, G. (2003) Bullying risks of 11-year-old children with specific language impairment (SLI): does school placement matter? *International Journal of Language and Communication Disorders*, **38**(1), 1-12.

Koegel, R., Camarata, S., Koegel, L., Ben-Tall, A. and Smith, A. (1998) Increasing speech intelligibility in children with autism. *Journal of Autism and Developmental Disorders*, **28**(3), 241-51.

Konst, E., Weersink-Braks, H., Rietveld, T. and Peters, H. (2000) An intelligibility assessment of toddlers with cleft lip and palate who received and did not receive presurgical infant orthopedic treatment. *Journal of Communication Disorders*, **33**(6), 483-99.

Kumin, L. (1994) Intelligibility of speech in children with Down syndrome in natural settings: parents' perspective. *Perception and Motor Skills*, **78**(1), 307-13.

Kvam, M. and Bredal, U. (2000) Do we understand the speech of deaf adolescents? An evaluation and comparison of intelligibility in two similar research projects from 1979 and 1995. *Logopedics Phoniatrics Vocology*, **25**(2), 87-92.

Kwiatkowski, J. and Shriberg, L. (1992) Intelligibility assessment in developmental phonological disorders: accuracy of caregiver gloss. *Journal of Speech and Hearing Research*, **35**(5), 1095-104.

Lahey, M. (1988) *Language Disorders and Language Development*. New York: Macmillan.

Lance, D., Swanson, L. and Peterson, H. (1997) A validity study of an implicit phonological awareness paradigm. *Journal of Speech, Language and Hearing Research*, **40**, 1002-10.

Law, J. (1995) Efficacy of speech and language therapy with children. *Proceedings of the RCSLT Golden Jubilee Conference*, York.

Law, J. and Conti-Ramsden, G. (2000) Treating children with speech and language impairments. *British Medical Journal*, **321**, 908-9.

Law, J. and Garret, Z. (2003) *Does Speech and Language Intervention for Children with Speech and Language Delay/Disorder Work?* (Briefing Paper). Nuffield Foundation.

Law, J., Boyle, J., Harris, F., Harkness, A. and Nye, C. (1998) Screening for speech and language delay: A systematic review of the literature. *International Journal of Language and Communication Disorders*, **33** Suppl., 21–3.

Law, J., Lindsay, G., Peacey, N., Gascoigne, M., Soloff, N., Radford, J. *et al.* (2002) Consultation as a model for providing speech and language therapy in schools: a panacea or one step too far? *Child Language Teaching and Therapy*, **18**(2), 145–63.

Lees, J. and Urwin, S. (1997) *Children with Language Disorders*, 2nd edn. London: Whurr Publishers.

Leitao, S. and Fletcher, J. (2004) Literacy outcomes for students with speech impairment: Long term follow-up. *International Journal of Language and Communication Disorders*, **39**, 245–56.

Letts, C. (1995) Speech and language therapy in a community clinic: Report of an efficacy study. *Proceedings of the RCSLT Golden Jubilee Conference*, York.

Levelt, W. (1989) *Speaking: From Intention to Articulation.* Cambridge, MA: MIT Press.

Levelt, W. (1999) Models of word production. *Trends in Cognitive Sciences*, **3**(6), 223–32.

Lewis, B., Freebairn, L. and Taylor, G. (2002) Correlates of spelling abilities in children with early speech sound disorders. *Reading and Writing*, **15**, 389–407.

Lindsay, G., Dockrell, J., Letchford, B. and Mackie, C. (2002a) Self-esteem of children with specific speech and language difficulties. *Child Language Teaching and Therapy,* **18**(2), 125–42.

Lindsay, G., Soloff, N., Law, J., Band, S., Peacey, N., Gascoigne, M. *et al.* (2002b) Speech and language therapy services to education in England and Wales. *International Journal of Language and Communication Disorders*, **37**(3), 273–88.

Liss, J., Spitzer, S., Caviness, J. and Adler, C. (2002) The effects of familiarization on intelligibility and lexical segmentation in hypokinetic and ataxic dysarthria. *Journal of the Acoustical Society of America*, **112**(6), 3022–30.

Locke, A., Ginsborg, J. and Peers, I. (2002) Development and disadvantage: Implications for the early years and beyond. *International Journal of Language and Communication Disorders*, **37**(1), 3–15.

Locke, J. L. (1980a) The inference of speech perception in the phonologically disordered child. Part I: A rationale, some criteria, the conventional tests. *Journal of Speech and Hearing Disorders*, **45**, 431–44.

Locke, J. L. (1980b) The inference of speech perception in the phonologically disordered child. Part II: Some clinically novel procedures, their use, some findings. *Journal of Speech and Hearing Disorders*, **45**, 445–68.

Loeb, D., Stoke, C. and Fey, M. (2001) Language changes associated with Fast ForWord-language: Evidence from case studies. *American Journal of Speech-Language Pathology*, **10**, 216–30.

Lof, G. (2004) Confusion about speech sound norms and their use. On-line language conference. http://www.thinkingpublications.com/LangConf04/PosterSessions/PostersessionsPDFs/Lof.pdf

Loucas, T. and Marslen-Wilson, W. (2000) An experimental and computational exploration of developmental patterns in lexical access and representation, in *New Directions in Language Development and Disorders* (eds M. Perkins and S. Howard). New York: Kluwer/Plenum.

Lynch, J. I. and Fox, D. R. (1980) *A Parent - Child Cleft Palate Curriculum: Developing Speech and Language.* Oregon: CC Publications.

MacWhinney, B. (1985) Hungarian language acquisition as an exemplification of a general model of grammatical development, in *The Crosslinguistic Study of Language Acquisition* (Vol. 2) (ed. D. Slobin). Hillsdale, NJ: Erlbaum.

Major, E. and Bernhardt, M. (1998) Metaphonological skills of children with phonological disorders before and after phonological and metaphonological intervention. *International Journal of Language and Communication Disorders*, **33**(4), 413-44.

Masidlover, M. and Knowles, W. (1982) *Derbyshire Language Scheme.* Derbyshire County Council Educational Psychology Service.

Max, L., De Bruyn, W. and Steurs, W. (1997) Intelligibility of oesophageal and tracheoesophageal speech: preliminary observations. *European Journal of Disorders of Communication*, **29**(2), 183-201.

McCartney, E., Boyle, J., Bannatyne, S., Jessiman, E., Campbell, C., Kelsey, C. *et al.* (2005) 'Thinking of two': A case study of speech and language therapists working through assistants. *International Journal of Language and Communication Disorders*, **40**(2), 221-35.

McColl, D., Fucci, D., Petrosino, L., Martin, D. and McCaffrey, P. (1998) Listener ratings of the intelligibility of tracheoesophageal speech in noise. *Journal of Communication Disorders*, **31**(4), 279-88.

McCormack, M. (1995) The relationship between the phonological processes in early speech development and later spelling strategies, in *Differential Diagnosis and Treatment of Children with Speech Disorder* (ed. B. Dodd). London: Whurr Publishers.

McCroskey, R. (1984) *Wichita Auditory Processing Test.* Oklahoma: Modern Education Corporation.

McGregor, K. and Leonard, L. (1989) Facilitating word-finding skills of language-impaired children. *Journal of Speech and Hearing Disorders*, **54**, 141-7.

McHenry, M. (2003) The effect of pacing strategies on the variability of speech movement sequences in dysarthria. *Journal of Speech, Language and Hearing Research*, **46**, 702-10.

McLeod, S. (2002) *Articulation and Phonology: Typical Development of Speech.* http://members.tripod.com/Caroline_Bowen/acquisition.html

McLeod, S. and Bleile, K. (2004) The ICF: A framework for setting goals for children with speech impairment. *Child Language Teaching and Therapy*, **20**(3), 199-219.

McLeod, S., van Doorn, J. and Reed, V. (1997) Realizations of consonant clusters by children with phonological impairment. *Clinical Linguistics and Phonetics*, **11**(2), 85-113.

McLeod, S., van Doorn, J. and Reed, V. (2001) Normal acquisition of consonant clusters. *American Journal of Speech Language Pathology*, **10**, 99-110.

McReynolds, L. and Kearns, K. (1983) *Single Subject Designs in Communicative Disorders.* Baltimore, MD: University Park Press.

Merzenich, M., Jenkins, W., Johnston, P., Schreiner, C., Miller, S. and Tallal, P. (1996) Temporal processing deficits of language-learning impaired children ameliorated by training. *Science*, **271**, 77-80.

Metsala, J.L. and Walley, A.C. (1998) Spoken vocabulary growth and the segmental restructuring of lexical representations: Precursors to phonemic awareness and early reading ability, in *Word Recognition in Beginning Literacy* (eds J. Metsala and L. Ehri). Hillsdale, NJ: Erlbaum, pp. 89–120.

Miccio, A. and Elbert, M. (1996) Enhancing stimulability: A treatment program. *Journal of Communication Disorders*, **29**, 335–51.

Middleton, G. and Pannbacker, M. (1994) *Introduction to Clinical Research in Communication Disorders*. San Diego, CA: Singular.

Millard, S. (1998) The value of single-case research. *International Journal of Language and Communication Disorders*, **33**(Supplement), 370–3.

Miralles, J. and Cervera, T. (1995) Voice intelligibility in patients who have undergone laryngectomies. *Journal of Speech and Hearing Research*, **38**(3), 564–71.

Monahan, D. (1986) Remediation of common phonological processes: Four case studies. *Language Speech and Hearing Services in Schools*, **17**, 199–206.

Monsen, R. (1983) The oral-speech intelligibility of hearing impaired talkers. *Journal of Speech and Hearing Disorders*, **48**, 286–96.

MorganBarry, R. (1988) *The Auditory Discrimination and Attention Test*. Windsor: NFER-Nelson.

Morrison, J. and Shriberg, L. (1992) Articulation testing versus conversational speech sampling. *Journal of Speech and Hearing Research*, **35**, 259–73.

Muter, V. (2006) The prediction and screening of children's reading difficulties, in *Dyslexia, Speech and Language: A Practitioner's Handbook*, 2nd edn (eds M. Snowling and J. Stackhouse). London: Whurr Publishers.

Muter, V., Hulme, C. and Snowling, M. (1997) *Phonological Abilities Test (PAT)*. London: The Psychological Corporation.

Muter, V., Snowling, M. and Taylor, S. (1994) Orthographic analogies and phonological awareness: Their role and significance in early reading development. *Journal of Child Psychology and Psychiatry*, **35**, 293–310.

Muter, V., Hulme, C., Snowling, M. and Taylor, S. (1998) Segmentation, not rhyming, predicts early progress in learning to read. *Journal of Experimental Child Psychology*, **71**, 3–27.

Nash, P. (2006) Assessment and management of psychosocial aspects of reading and language impairments, in *Dyslexia, Speech and Language: A Practitioner's Handbook*, 2nd edn (eds M. Snowling and J. Stackhouse). London: Whurr Publishers.

Nash, P., Stengelhofen, J., Toombs, L., Brown, J. and Kellow, B. (2001) An alternative management of older children with persisting communication problems. *International Journal of Language and Communication Disorders*, **36**, 179–84.

Nathan, L. and Simpson, S. (2001) Designing a literacy programme for a child with a history of speech difficulties, in *Children's Speech and Literacy Difficulties 2: Identification and Intervention* (eds J. Stackhouse and B. Wells), London: Whurr Publishers, pp. 249–98.

Nathan, L., Wells, B. and Donlan, C. (1998) Children's comprehension of unfamiliar regional accents: A preliminary investigation. *Journal of Child Language*, **25**, 343–65.

Nathan, L., Stackhouse, J., Goulandris, N. and Snowling, M. (2004a) The development of early literacy skills among children with speech difficulties: A test of the 'critical age hypothesis'. *Journal of Speech, Language and Hearing Research*, **47**, 377–91.

Nathan, L., Stackhouse, J., Goulandris, N. and Snowling, M. (2004b) Educational consequences of developmental speech disorder: Key Stage I National Curriculum assessment results in English and mathematics. *British Journal of Educational Psychology*, **74**, 173–86.

Newton, C. (1999) *Connected Speech Processes in Phonological Development: Word Glue and Other Sticky Situations*. Doctoral Dissertation, University College London.

Newton, C. and Wells, B. (2002) Between word junctures in early multiword speech. *Journal of Child Language*, **29**, 275–99.

Newton, M. and Thompson, M. (1982) *The Revised Aston Index*. Cambridge: Learning Development Aids.

Nittrouer, S. and Burton, L. (2005) The role of early language experience in the development of speech perception and phonological processing abilities: Evidence from 5-year olds with a history of otitis media with effusion and low SES. *Journal of Communication Disorders*, **38**(1), 29–63.

Norbury, C. F. and Chiat, S. (2000) Semantic intervention to support word recognition: A single-case study. *Child Language Teaching and Therapy*, **16**(2), 141–63.

Norris, J. and Hoffman, P. (1993) *Whole Language Intervention for the School-age Child*. San Diego, CA: Singular.

Nye, C., Foster, S. and Seaman, D. (1987) Effectiveness of language intervention with the language/learning disabled. *Journal of Speech and Hearing Disorders*, **52**, 348–57.

O'Connor, L. and Schery, T. (1986) A comparison of microcomputer-aided and traditional language therapy for developing communication skills in non-oral toddlers. *Journal of Speech and Hearing Disorders*, **51**, 356–61.

Ohala, D. (1999) The influence of sonority on children's cluster reductions. *Journal of Communication Disorders*, **32**, 397–422.

Onslow, M., Packman, A. and Harrison, E. (eds.) (2001) *The Lidcombe Program of Early Stuttering Interventions: A Clinician's Guide*. Austin, TX: Pro-ed.

Osberger, M. (1992) Speech intelligibility in the hearing impaired: Research and clinical implications, in *Intelligibility in Speech Disorders: Theory, Measurement and Management* (ed. R. Kent). Amsterdam: John Benjamins.

Osberger, M., Robbins, A., Todd, S. and Riley, A. (1994) Speech intelligibility of children with cochlear implants. *Volta Review*, **96**, 169–80.

Ozanne, A. (1995) The search for developmental verbal dyspraxia, in *Differential Diagnosis and Treatment of Children with Speech Disorders* (ed. B. Dodd). London: Whurr Publishers.

Ozanne, A. (2005) Childhood apraxia of speech, in *Differential Diagnosis and Treatment of Children with Speech Disorders*, 2nd edn (ed. B. Dodd). London: Whurr Publishers.

Pallant, J. (2001) *SPSS Survival Manual: A Step by Step Guide to Data Analysis Using SPSS for Windows*. UK: Open University Press.

Panagos, J. and Prelock, P. (1982) Phonological constraints on the sentence productions of language disordered children. *Journal of Speech and Hearing Research*, **25**, 171–6.

Pantelemidou, V., Herman, R. and Thomas, J. (2003) Efficacy of speech intervention using electropalatography with a cochlear implant user. *Clinical Linguistics and Phonetics*, **17**, 383–92.

Pascoe, M., Stackhouse, J. and Wells, B. (2005) Phonological therapy within a psycholinguistic framework: Promoting change in a child with persisting speech difficulties. *International Journal of Language and Communication Disorders*, **40**(2), 189–220.

Pascoe, M. and Tuomi, S. (2001) Segmental phonology and Black South African English speakers: Communicative success with standard dialect listeners. *The South African Journal of Communication Disorders*, **47**, 99–110.

Pater, J. and Barlow, J. (2003) Constraint conflict in cluster reduction. *Journal of Child Language*, **30**(3), 487–526.

Patterson, K. (1994) Reading, writing and rehabilitation: A reckoning, in *Cognitive Neuropsychology and Cognitive Rehabilitation* (eds M. Riddoch and G. Humphreys). Hove, UK: Lawrence Erlbaum.

Paul, R. and Shriberg, L. (1982) Associations between phonology and syntax in speech delayed childen. *Journal of Speech and Hearing Research*, **25**, 536–46.

Pennington, L. and McConachie, H. (2001) Interaction between children with cerebral palsy and their mothers: The effects of speech intelligibility. *International Journal of Language and Communication Disorders*, **36**(3), 371–93.

Peppé, S. and McCann, J. (2003) Assessing intonation and prosody in children with atypical language development: The PEPS-C test and the revised version. *Clinical Linguistics and Phonetics* **17**, 345–54.

Perin, D. (1983) Phonemic segmentation and spelling. *British Journal of Psychology*, **74**, 129–44.

Pilon, M., McIntosh, K. and Thaut, M. (1998) Auditory vs visual speech timing cues as external rate control to enhance verbal intelligibility in mixed spastic-ataxic dysarthric speakers: A pilot study. *Brain Injury*, **12**(9), 793–803.

Plante, E. (2005) Evidence-based practice in communication sciences and disorders. *Journal of Communication Disorders*, **37**, 389–90.

Plaut, D. (1996) Relearning after damage in connectionist networks: Toward a theory of rehabilitation. *Brain and Language*, **52**, 25–82.

Popple, J. and Wellington, W. (2001) Working together: The psycholinguistic approach within a school setting, in *Children's Speech and Literacy Difficulties 2: Identification and Intervention* (eds J. Stackhouse and B. Wells). London: Whurr Publishers.

Powell, T. (1991) Planning for phonological generalization: Approach to treatment target selection. *American Journal of Speech-Language Pathology*, **1**, 21–8.

Powell, T. and Elbert, M. (1984) Generalisation following the remediation of early- and later-developing consonant clusters. *Journal of Speech and Hearing Disorders*, **49**(2), 211–18.

Powell, T., Elbert, M. and Dinnsen, D. (1991) Stimulability as a factor in the phonological generalisation of misarticulating pre-school children. *Journal of Speech and Hearing Research*, **34**, 1318–28.

Powell, T. and Miccio, A. (1996) Stimulability: A useful clinical tool. *Journal of Communication Disorders*, **29**, 237–53.

Pratt, S., Heintzelman, A. and Deming, S. (1993) The efficacy of using the IBM Speech Viewer Vowel Accuracy Module to treat young children with hearing impairment. *Journal of Speech and Hearing Research*, **36**, 1063–74.

Pring, T. (2004) Ask a silly question: Two decades of troublesome trials. *International Journal of Language and Communication Disorders*, **39**(3), 285–302.

Pring, T. (2005) *Research Methods in Communication Disorders*. London: Whurr Publishers.

Prosek, R. and Vreeland, L. (2001) The intelligibility of time-domain edited esophageal speech. *Journal of Speech Language and Hearing Research*, **44**(3), 525–34.

Ramig, P. and Bennett, E. (1997) Considerations for conducting group intervention with adults who stutter. *Seminars in Speech and Language*, **18**(4), 343–55.

Rapp, B. C. and Caramazza, A. (1991) Lexical deficits, in *Acquired Aphasias*, 2nd edn (ed. M. Sarno). San Diego, CA: Academic Press, pp. 181–222.

RCSLT (forthcoming) *Communicating Quality 3: Information, Standards and Guidance to Support the Provision of Quality Speech and Language Services in the UK*. London: RCSLT.

Redford, M. A., MacNeilage, P. F. and Davis, B. L. (1997) Production constraints on utterance-final consonant characteristics in babbling. *Phonetica*, **54**, 172–86.

Rees, R. (2001a) Principles of psycholinguistic intervention, in *Children's Speech and Literacy Difficulties 2: Identification and Intervention* (eds J. Stackhouse and B. Wells). London: Whurr Publishers.

Rees, R. (2001b) What do tasks really tap?, in *Children's Speech and Literacy Difficulties 2: Identification and Intervention* (eds J. Stackhouse and B. Wells). London: Whurr Publishers.

Reilly, S. (2004) The move to evidence-based practice in speech pathology, in *Evidence-Based Practice in Speech Pathology* (eds S. Reilly, J. Douglas and J. Oates). London: Whurr Publishers, pp. 3–17.

Renfrew, C. (1969) *The Bus Story*. Bicester, Oxon: Winslow Press.

Renfrew, C. (1995) *Word Finding Vocabulary Test*, 4th edn. Bicester, Oxon: Winslow Press.

Riddell, J., McCauley, R., Mulligan, M. and Tandan, R. (1995) Intelligibility and phonetic contrast errors in highly intelligible speakers with amyotrophic lateral sclerosis. *Journal of Speech and Hearing Research*, **38**(2), 304–14.

Rieger, J., Wolfaardt, J., Jha, N. and Seikaly, H. (2003) Maxillary obturators: The relationship between patient satisfaction and speech outcome. *Head Neck*, **25**(11), 895–903.

Roberts, E. and Burchinal, M. (2001) The complex interplay between biology and environment. Otitis media and mediation effects on early literacy, in *Handbook of Early Literacy Research* (eds S. Neumann and D. Dickinson). NY: The Guilford Press, 232–44.

Robey, R. (2005) A five-phase model for clinical-outcome research. *Journal of Communication Disorders*, **37**, 389–465.

Robey, R. and Schultz, M. (1998) A model for conducting clinical-outcome research: An adaptation of the standard protocol for use in aphasiology. *Aphasiology*, **12**, 787–810.

Rosenbek J. (1985) Treating apraxia of speech, in *Clinical Management of Neurogenic Communicative Disorders*, 2nd edn (ed. D. Johns). Boston: Little, Brown, Co., pp. 267–312.

Rosenthal, J. (1994) Rate control therapy for developmental apraxia of speech. *Clinics in Communication Disorders*, **4**(3), 190–200.

Roulstone, S. (2001) Consensus and variation between speech and language therapists in the assessment and selection of preschool children for intervention: A body of knowledge or idiosyncratic decisions? *International Journal of Language and Communication Disorders*, **36**(3), 329–48.

Rousseau, I., Onslow, M., Packman, A. and Robinson, R. (2001) The Lidcombe program in Australia, in *The Lidcombe Program of Early Stuttering Interventions: A Clinician's Guide* (eds M. Onslow, A. Packman and E. Harrison). Austin, TX: Pro-ed.

Rowe, C. (1999) Do social stories benefit children with autism in mainstream schools? *British Journal of Special Education*, **26**(1), 12–14.

Roy, P. and Chiat, S. (2004) A prosodically controlled word and non-word repetition tast for 2–4 year olds: Evidence from typically developing children. *Journal of Speech, Language and Hearing Research*, **47**(1), 223–34.

Ruscello, D. (1995) Visual feedback in treatment of residual phonological disorders. *Journal of Communication Disorders*, **28**, 279–302.

Ruscello, D., Cartwright, L., Haines, K. and Shuster, L. (1993) The use of different service delivery models for children with phonological disorders. *Journal of Communication Disorders*, **26**, 193–203.

Rvachew, S. (1994) Speech perception training can facilitate sound production learning. *Journal of Speech and Hearing Research*, **37**, 347–57.

Rvachew, S. and Nowack, M. (2001) The effect of target-selection strategy on phonological learning. *Journal of Speech, Language and Hearing Research*, **44**, 610–23.

Rvachew, S., Rafaat, S. and Martin, M. (1999) Stimulability, speech perception skills and the treatment of phonological disorders. *American Journal of Speech-Language Pathology*, **8**, 33–43.

Ryder, R. (1991) Word and non-word repetition in normally developing children. MSc thesis. Department of Human Communication Science, University College London.

Saben, C. and Ingham, J. (1991) The effects of minimal pairs treatment on the speech-sound production of two children with phonologic disorders. *Journal of Speech and Hearing Research*, **34**, 1023–40.

Sackett, D., Richardson, W., Rosenberg, W. and Haynes, R. (1997) *Evidence-based Medicine: How to Practise and Teach EBM.* Edinburgh: Churchill Livingstone.

Samar, V. and Metz, D. (1988) Criterion validity of speech intelligibility rating scale procedures for the hearing impaired population. *Journal of Speech and Hearing Research*, **31**, 307–16.

Sapir, S., Spielman, J., Ramig, L., Hinds, S., Countryman, S., Fox, C. *et al.* (2003) Effects of intensive voice treatment (the Lee Silverman Voice Treatment [LSVT]) on ataxic dysarthria: A case study. *American Journal of Speech and Language Pathology*, **12**, 387–99.

Schery, T. and O'Connor, L. (1997) Language intervention: Computer training for young children with special needs. *British Journal of Educational Technology*, **28**(4), 271–9.

Schiavetti, N. (1992) Scaling procedures for the measurement of speech intelligibility, in *Intelligibility in Speech Disorders: Theory, Measurement and Management* (ed. R. Kent). Amsterdam: John Benjamins.

Schuell, H., Jenkins, J. and Jimenez-Pabon, E. (1964) *Aphasia in Adults: Diagnosis, prognosis and treatment.* New York: Harper and Row.

Scott, C. and Brown, S. (2001) Spelling and the speech-language pathologist: there's more than meets the eye. *Seminars in Speech and Language*, **22**(3), 197–207.

Scott, C. and Byng, S. (1989) Computer assisted remediation of a homophone comprehension disorder in surface dyslexia. *Aphasiology*, **3**, 301–20.

Searl, J., Carpenter, M. and Banta, C. (2001) Intelligibility of stops and fricatives in tracheoesophageal speech. *Journal of Communication Disorders*, **34**(4), 305–21.

Seron, X. (1997) Effectiveness and specificity in neuropsychological therapies: A cognitive point of view. *Aphasiology*, **11**, 105–23.

Shallice, T. (1987) Impairments of semantic processing: Multiple dissociations, in *The Cognitive Neuropsychology of Language* (eds M. Coltheart, R. Job and G. Sartori). London: Lawrence Erlbaum.

Shriberg, L., Aram, D. and Kwiatkowski, J. (1997a) Developmental apraxia of speech: I. Descriptive and theoretical perspectives. *Journal of Speech Language and Hearing Research*, **40**(2), 273–85.

Shriberg, L., Aram, D. and Kwiatkowski, J. (1997b) Developmental apraxia of speech: II. Toward a diagnostic marker. *Journal of Speech Language and Hearing Research*, **40**(2), 286–312.

Shriberg, L., Gruber, F. and Kwiatkowski, J. (1994) Developmental phonological disorders III: Long-term speech sound normalisation. *Journal of Speech and Hearing Research*, **37**, 1151–77.

Shriberg, L. and Kwiatkowski, J. (1982) Phonological disorders III: A procedure for assessing severity of involvement. *Journal of Speech and Hearing Disorders*, **47**, 256–70.

Shriberg, L. and Kwiatkowski, J. (1994) Developmental phonological disorders I: A clinical profile. *Journal of Speech and Hearing Research*, **37**, 1100–26.

Shriberg, L., Austin, D., Lewis, B., McSweeny, J. and Wilson, D. (1997) The speech disorders classification system: Extensions and lifespan reference data. *Journal of Speech, Language, and Hearing Research*, **40**, 723–40.

Shuster, L., Ruscello, D. and Haines, K. (1992) Acoustic patterns of an adolescent with multiple articulation errors. *Journal of Communication Disorders*, **25**, 162–74.

Sinha, U., Young, P., Survitz, K. and Crockett, D. (2004) Functional outcomes following palatal reconstruction with a folded radial forearm free flap. *Ear Nose Throat Journal* **83**(1), 45–8.

Sloane, H. and MacAulay, B. (1968) *Operant Procedures in Remedial Speech and Language Training*. Boston, MA: Houghton Mifflin.

Smit, A. (1993) Phonologic error distributions in the Iowa-Nebraska articulation norms project: Word initial consonant clusters. *Journal of Speech and Hearing Research*, **36**, 931–47.

Snowling, M. and Stackhouse, J. (1983) Spelling performance of children with developmental verbal dyspraxia. *Developmental Medicine and Child Neurology*, **25**, 430–7.

Snowling, M. and Stackhouse, J. (eds) (2006a) *Dyslexia, Speech and Language: A Practitioner's Handbook*, 2nd edn. London: Whurr Publishers.

Snowling, M. and Stackhouse, J. (2006b) Current themes and future directions, in *Dyslexia, Speech and Language: A Practitioner's Handbook*, 2nd edn. (eds M. Snowling and J. Stackhouse). London: Whurr Publishers.

Snowling, M., Stackhouse, J. and Rack, J. (1986) Phonological dyslexia and dysgraphia: A developmental analysis. *Cognitive Neuropsychology*, **3**, 309–39.

Snowling, M., van Wagtendonk, B. and Stafford, C. (1988) Object-naming deficits in developmental dyslexia. *Journal of Research in Reading*, **11**(2), 67–85.

Sommers, R., Logsdon, B. and Wright, J. (1992) A review and critical analysis of treatment research related to articulation and phonological disorders. *Journal of Communication Disorders*, **25**, 3–22.

Sommers, R., Cockerille, C., Paul, C., Bowser, D., Fichter, G., Fenton, A., *et al.* (1961) Effects of speech therapy and speech improvement on articulation and reading. *Journal of Speech and Hearing Disorders*, **26**, 27–37.

Sparks, R. (2001) Phonemic awareness and reading skill in hyperlexic children: A longitudinal study. *Reading and Writing: An Interdisciplinary Journal*, **14**, 333–60.

Spooner, L. (2002) Addressing expressive language disorder in children who also have severe receptive language disorder: A psycholinguistic approach. *Child Language Teaching and Therapy*, **18**(3), 289–313.

Stackhouse, J. (1982) An investigation of reading and spelling performance in speech disordered children. *British Journal of Disorders of Communication*, **17**(2), 53–60.

Stackhouse, J. (1989) Phonological dyslexia in children with developmental verbal dyspraxia. PhD thesis, Psychology Department, University College London.

Stackhouse, J. (1996) Speech, spelling and reading: Who is at risk and why? in *Dyslexia Speech and Language: A Practitioner's Handbook* (eds M. Snowling and J. Stackhouse). London: Whurr Publishers.

Stackhouse, J. (2001) Identifying Children at risk for literacy problems, in *Children's Speech and Literacy Difficulties 2: Identification and Intervention* (eds J. Stackhouse and B. Wells). London: Whurr Publishers.

Stackhouse, J. (2006) Speech and spelling difficulties: What to look for, in *Dyslexia, Speech and Language: A Practitioner's Handbook*, 2nd edn (eds M. Snowling and J. Stackhouse). London: Whurr Publishers.

Stackhouse, J. and Snowling, M. (1992) Developmental verbal dyspraxia II: A developmental perspective on two case studies. *European Journal of Disorders of Communication*, **27**(1), 35–54.

Stackhouse, J. and Wells, B. (1991) Dyslexia: The obvious and hidden speech and language disorder, in *Dyslexia: Integrating Theory and Practice* (eds M. Snowling and M. Thomson). London: Whurr Publishers.

Stackhouse, J. and Wells, B. (1993) Psycholinguistic assessment of developmental speech disorders. *European Journal of Disorders of Communication*, **28**, 331–48.

Stackhouse, J. and Wells, B. (1997) *Children's Speech and Literacy Difficulties 1: A Psycholinguistic Framework.* London: Whurr Publishers.

Stackhouse, J. and Wells, B. (2001) *Children's Speech and Literacy Difficulties 2: Identification and Intervention.* London: Whurr Publishers.

Stackhouse, J., Wells, B., Pascoe, M. and Rees, R. (2002) From phonological therapy to phonological awareness. *Seminars in Speech and Language*, **23**(1), 27–42.

Stackhouse, J., Wells, B., Vance, M., Nathan, L. and Pascoe, M. (forthcoming) *A Compendium of Psycholinguistic Tasks for Children – Speech and Auditory Procedures.*

Stiegler, L. and Hoffman, P. (2001) Discourse-based intervention for word-finding in children. *Journal of Communication Disorders*, **34**(4), 277–304.

Stoel-Gammon, C. (2001) Down syndrome phonology: Developmental patterns and intervention strategies. *Down Syndrome Research and Practice*, **7**, 93–100.

Stothard, S., Snowling, M. and Hulme, C. (1996) Deficits in phonology but not dyslexic? *Cognitive Neuropsychology*, **13**, 641–72.

Tallal, P., Miller, S. and Fitch, R. (1993) Neurobiological basis of speech: A case for the pre-eminence of temporal processing, in *Annals of the New York Academy of Sciences: Temporal Information Processing in the Nervous System* (eds P. Tallal, A. Galaburda, R. Llinas and C. Euler). New York: New York Academy of Sciences.

Tallal, P. and Piercy, M. (1980) Defects of auditory perception in children with developmental dysphasia, in *Developmental Dysphasia* (ed. M. Wyke). New York: Academic Press.

Tallal, P., Miller, S., Bedi, G., Byma, G., Wang, Srikantan, S. *et al.* (1996) Language comprehension in language impaired children improved with acoustically modified speech. *Science*, **271**, 81–4.

Tannock, R. and Girolametto, L. (1992) Reassessing parent-focused language intervention programmes, in *Causes and Effects in Communication and in Normal and Language Impaired Children* (eds S. Warren and J. Reichle). Baltimore, MD: Paul Brookes.

Teal, J. (2005) An investigation into classification approaches and therapy outcomes for a child with a severe persisting speech difficulty. Unpublished MMedSci. Dissertation, Department of Human Communication Sciences, University of Sheffield.

Temple, C., Jeeves, M. and Vilarroya, O. (1990) Reading in callosal agenesis. *Brain and Language*, **39**, 235–53.

Tikofsky, R. (1970) A revised list for the estimation of dysarthric single word intelligibility. *Journal of Speech and Hearing Research*, **13**, 59–71.

Tomblin, J., Records, N., Buckwalter, P., Zhang, X., Smith, E. and O'Brian, M. (1997) The prevalence of specific language impairment in kindergarten children. *Journal of Speech Language Hearing Research*, **40**, 1245–60.

Townsend, S. (2005) Therapy within the psycholinguistic framework for children with Down Syndrome. Unpublished MMedSci. Dissertation, Department of Human Communication Sciences, University of Sheffield.

Treiman, R. (1985) Onsets and rimes as units of spoken syllables: Evidence from children. *Journal of Experimental Child Psychology*, **39**, 161–81.

Treiman, R. (1993) *Beginning to Spell. A Study of First Grade Children*. New York: Oxford University Press.

Treiman, R. (1994) Use of consonant letter names in beginning spelling. *Developmental Psychology*, **30**, 567–80.

Treiman, R. and Baron, J. (1981) Segmental analysis ability: Development and relation to reading ability, in *Reading Research: Advances in Theory and Practice*, vol 3 (eds G. MacKinnon and T. Walker). New York: Academic Press, pp. 159–97.

Treiman, R. and Bourassa, D. (2000) The development of spelling skills. *Topics in Language Disorders*, **20**, 1–18.

Treiman, R. and Zukowski, A. (1991) Levels of phonological awareness, in *Phonological Processes in Literacy: A tribute to Isabelle Y. Liberman* (eds S. Brady and D. Shankweiler). Hillsdale, NJ: Erlbaum.

Tyler, A. and Watterson, K. (1991) Effects of phonological versus language intervention in pre-schoolers with both phonological and language impairment. *Child Language Teaching and Therapy*, **7**, 141–60.

Van der Gaag, A. (1993) *Outcome Research in Speech and Language Therapy. Audit: A Manual for Speech and Language Therapists*. London: RCSLT.

Van Lierde, K., De Bodt, M., Van Borsel, J., Wuyts, F. and Van Cauwenberge, P. (2002) Effect of cleft type on overall speech intelligibility and resonance. *Folia Phoniatrica et Logopaedica*, **54**(3), 158–68.

Van Riper, C. (1963) *Speech Correction: Principles and Methods*. Englewood-Cliffs, NJ: Prentice-Hall.

Vance, M. (1996) Assessing speech processing skills in children: a task analysis, in *Dyslexia, Speech and Language: A Practitioner's Handbook* (eds M. Snowling and J. Stackhouse). London: Whurr Publishers.

Vance, M. (1997) Christopher Lumpship: Developing phonological representations in a child with an auditory processing deficit, in *Language Disorders in Children and Adults - Psycholinguistic Approaches to Therapy* (eds S. Chiat, J. Law and J. Marshall). London: Whurr Publishers.

Vance, M., Stackhouse, J. and Wells, B. (1994) 'Sock the Wock the Pit-Pat-Pock' - children's responses to measures of rhyming ability. *Work in Progress, National Hospitals College of Speech Sciences*, **4**, 171-85.

Vance, M., Stackhouse, J. and Wells, B. (1995) The relationship between naming and word-repetition skills in children aged 3 to 7 years. *Work in Progress, UCL Department of Human Communication Sciences*, **5**, 127-33.

Vance, M., Stackhouse, J. and Wells, B. (2005) Speech production skills in children aged 3-7 years. *International Journal of Language and Communication Disorders*, **40**(1), 29-48.

Vargha-Khadem, F., Gadian, D., Copp, A. and Mishkin, M. (2005) FOXP2 and the neuroanatomy of speech and language. *Nature Reviews Neuroscience*, **6**, 131-8.

Velleman, S. (1994) The interaction of phonetics and phonology in developmental verbal dyspraxia: Two case studies. *Clinics in Communication Disorders*, **4**, 66-77.

Velleman, S. (2002) Phonotactic therapy. *Seminars in Speech and Language*, **23**, 1-18.

Velleman, S. (2004) Developmental verbal dyspraxia, apraxia-kids website. http://www.apraxia-kids.org/slps/velleman.html

Wagner, R. and Torgeson, J. (1987) The nature of phonological processing and its causal role in the acquisition of reading skills. *Psychological Bulletin*, **101**, 192-212.

Waters, D. (2001) Using input processing strengths to overcome speech output difficulties, in *Children's Speech and Literacy Difficulties 2: Identification and Intervention* (eds J. Stackhouse and B. Wells). London: Whurr Publishers.

Waters, D., Hawkes, C. and Burnett, E. (1998) Targeting speech processing strengths to facilitate pronunciation change. *International Journal of Language and Communication Disorders*, **33**, 469-74.

Waterson, N. (1981) A tentative developmental model of phonological representation, in *The Cognitive Representation of Speech* (eds T. Myers, J. Laver and J. Anderson). Amsterdam: North Holland. (Reprinted in Waterson, 1987.)

Waterson, N. (1987) *Prosodic Phonology: The Theory and its Application to Language Acquisition and Speech Processing*. Newcastle-upon-Tyne: Grevatt and Grevatt.

Watson, B. and Gillon, G. (1999) Responses of children with developmental verbal dyspraxia to phonological awareness training. Paper presented at the Speech Pathology Australia National Conference, Sydney.

Weiner, F. (1981) Treatment of phonological disability using the method of meaningful contrast: Two case studies. *Journal of Speech and Hearing Disorders*, **46**, 97-103.

Weismer, G. and Laures, J. (2002) Direct magnitude estimates of speech intelligibility in dysarthria: Effects of a chosen standard. *Journal of Speech, Language and Hearing Research*, **45**(3), 421-33.

Weismer, G. and Martin, R. (1992) Acoustic and perceptual approaches to the study of intelligibility, in *Intelligibility in Speech Disorders: Theory, Measurement and Management* (ed. R. Kent). Amsterdam: John Benjamins.

Weismer, G., Jeng, J., Laures, J., Kent, R. and Kent, J. (2001) Acoustic and intelligibility characteristics of sentence production in neurogenic speech disorders. *Folia Phoniatrica et Logopaedica*, **53**(1), 1-18.

Weiss, C. (1980) *Weiss Comprehensive Articulation Test*. USA: Pro-ed.
Weiss, C., Gordon, M. and Lillywhite, H. (1987) *Clinical Management of Articulatory and Phonological Disorders*. Baltimore, MD: Williams and Wilkins.
Wells, B. (1994) Junction in developmental speech disorder: A case study. *Clinical Linguistics and Phonetics*, **8**(1), 1-25.
Wells, B. and Local, J. (1993) The sense of an ending: A case of prosodic delay. *Clinical Linguistics and Phonetics*, **6**(4), 59-73.
Wells, B. and Peppé, S. (2001) Intonation within a psycholinguistic framework, in *Children's Speech and Literacy Difficulties 2: Identification and Intervention*. (eds J. Stackhouse and B. Wells). London: Whurr Publishers, pp. 366-95.
Wells, B. and Peppé, S. (2003) Intonation abilities of children with speech and language impairments. *Journal of Speech, Language and Hearing Research*, **46**, 5-20.
Wells, B., Peppé, S. and Goulandris, N. (2004) Intonation development from five to thirteen. *Journal of Child Language*, **31**, 749-78.
Wepman, J. (1958) *Auditory Discrimination Test*. Chicago, IL: Language Research Associates.
Wepman, J. and Reynolds, W. (1987) *Wepman's Auditory Discrimination Test*, 2nd edn. Los Angeles, CA: Western Psychological Services.
Werner, E. and Smith, R. (1982) *Vulnerable but Invincible: A Longitudinal Study of Resilient Children and Youth*. New York: McGraw-Hill.
Weston, A. and Shriberg, L. (1992) Contextual and linguistic correlates of intelligibility in children with developmental phonological disorders. *Journal of Speech and Hearing Research*, **35**(6), 1316-32.
Whitehill, T. (2002) Assessing intelligibility in speakers with cleft palate: A critical review of the literature. *Cleft Palate and Craniofacial Journal*, **39**(1), 50-8.
Whitehill, T. and Ciocca, V. (2000) Effects of linguistic cues and stimulus cohesion on intelligibility of severely dysarthric speech. *Journal of Speech Language and Hearing Research*, **44**(3), 497-510.
Wilcox, K. and Morris, S. (1999) *Children's Speech Intelligibility Measure (CSIM)*. USA: Psychological Corporation.
Williams, A. (1991) Generalization patterns associated with training least phonological knowledge. *Journal of Speech and Hearing Research*, **34**(4), 722-33.
Williams, A. (2000a) Multiple oppositions: Case studies of variables in phonological intervention. *American Journal of Speech-Language Pathology*, **9**, 289-99.
Williams, A. (2000b) Multiple oppositions: Theoretical foundations for an alternative contrastive intervention approach. *American Journal of Speech-Language Pathology*, **9**, 282-8.
Williams, G. and McReynolds, L. (1975) The relationship between discrimination and articulation training in children with misarticulations. *Journal of Speech and Hearing Research*, **18**, 401-12.
Williams, P. (1996) Diadochokinetic rates in children with normal and atypical speech development. MSc thesis. Department of Human Communication Science, University College London.
Williams, P. and Stackhouse, J. (2000) Rate, accuracy and consistency: diadochokinetic performance of young, normally developing children. *Clinical Linguistics and Phonetics*, **14**(4), 267-93.

Williams, P. and Stephens, H. (2004) *Nuffield Centre Dyspraxia Programme*, 3rd edn. Windsor: Miracle Factory.

Wimmer, H. (1996) The non-word reading deficit in developmental dyslexia: Evidence from children learning to read German. *Experimental Child Psychology*, **61**(1), 80–90.

Wood, J., Wright, J. and Stackhouse, J. (2000) *Language and Literacy: Joining Together*. British Dyslexia Association, Reading, UK.

Wood, S. and Scobbie, J. (2003) Evaluating the clinical effectiveness of EPG in the assessment and diagnosis of children with intractable speech disorders. *Proceedings of the Vth European CPLOL Congress. Evidence Based Practice: A Challenge for Speech and Language Therapists*.

Woodyatt, G. and Dodd, B. (1995) A treatment case study of speech disorder: A child with multiple underlying deficits, in *Differential Diagnosis and Treatment of Children with Speech Disorder* (ed. B. Dodd). London: Whurr Publishers.

World Health Organization (2001) *ICF: International Classification of Functioning, Disability and Health*. Geneva, Switzerland: WHO.

Wren, Y. and Roulstone, S. (2001) *Hear IT - Sound IT Project*. Speech and Language Therapy Research Unit, Bristol: UK.

Wright, J. and Wood, J. (2006) Supporting language and literacy in the early years: Interdisciplinary training, in *Dyslexia, Speech and Language: A Practitioner's Handbook*, 2nd edn. (eds M. Snowling and J. Stackhouse). London: Whurr Publishers.

Wright, V., Shelton, R. and Arndt, W. (1969) A task for evaluation of articulation change III: Imitative task scores compared with scores for more spontaneous tasks. *Journal of Speech and Hearing Research*, **12**, 875–84.

Wyllie-Smith, L. and McLeod, S. (2001) The use of sonority in the analysis of children's speech. *Acquiring Knowledge in Speech, Language and Hearing*, **3**(1), 37–9.

Yorkston, K. and Beukelman, D. (1981) *Assessment of Intelligibility of Dysarthric Speech*. Tigard, OR: CC Publications.

Yorkston, K., Beukelman, D. and Traynor, C. (1984) *Computerized Assessment of Intelligibility of Dysarthric Speech*. Tigard, OR: CC Publications.

Yorkston, K., Dowden, P. and Beukelman, D. (1992) Intelligibility measurement as a tool in the clinical management of dyarthric speakers, in *Intelligibility in Speech Disorders: Theory, Measurement and Management* (ed. R. Kent). Amsterdam: John Benjamins.

Yorkston, K., Hammen, V., Beukelman, D. and Traynor, C. (1990) The effect of rate control on the intelligibility and naturalness of dysarthric speech. *Journal of Speech and Hearing Disorders*, **55**(3), 550–60.

Zeit, K. and Johnson, P. (2002) Insurance advocacy: The growth of a grassroots initiative. *The ASHA Leader*, **7**(18).

Index

Other Titles in this Series

Children's Speech and Literacy Difficulties : A Psycholinguistic Framework, Book 1
Joy Stackhouse and Bill Wells
Paperback
ISBN 1-86156-030-3

Children's Speech and Literacy Difficulties: Book 2 – Identification and Intervention
Edited by Joy Stackhouse and Bill Wells
Paperback
ISBN 1-86156-131-8